Microbes and infections of the gut

T.
Book

Microbes and infections of the gut

edited by

C. S. GOODWIN
MA, MD(Cantab), DipBact(Lond.), FRCPath, FRCPA

Head, Department of Microbiology, Royal Perth Hospital,
Western Australia and Associate Professor in Clinical Microbiology,
University of Western Australia

Blackwell Scientific Publications
MELBOURNE OXFORD LONDON EDINBURGH BOSTON

© 1984 by
Blackwell Scientific Publications
Editorial offices:
99 Barry Street, Carlton
  Victoria 3053, Australia
Osney Mead, Oxford OX2 OEL
8 John Street, London WC1N 2ES
9 Forrest Road, Edinburgh EH1 2QH
52 Beacon Street, Boston
  Massachusetts 02108, USA

First published 1984

Typeset by ABB Typesetting Pty Ltd
Printed in Australia by
Globe Press Pty Ltd, Brunswick,
Victoria

DISTRIBUTORS
USA
  Blackwell Mosby Book Distributors
  11830 Westline Industrial Drive
  St Louis, Missouri 63141

Canada
  Blackwell Mosby Book Distributors
  120 Melford Drive, Scarborough
  Ontario M1B 2X4

Australia
  Blackwell Scientific Book
  Distributors
  31 Advantage Road,
  Highett, Victoria 3190

Cataloguing in Publication Data

Microbes and infections of the gut.

Bibliography.
Includes index.
ISBN 0 86793 104 3.

1. Intestines — Infections. 2. Intestines
— Bacteriology. 3. Infection. I. Goodwin,
C.S. (Charles Stewart).

616.3'4014

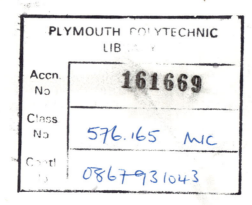

Contents

Contributors   vii

Preface   ix

1   The development of the infant gut flora; and the medical microbiology of infant botulism and necrotizing enterocolitis
S. P. BORRIELLO and S. STEPHENS   1

2   Immunological aspects of the intestinal lymphoid system
G. N. COOPER   27

3   Salmonellosis, campylobacter enteritis and shigella dysentery
B. ROWE and R. J. GROSS   47

4   *Escherichia coli* diarrhoea
R. J. GROSS and B. ROWE   79

5   Cholera and other vibrios, *Aeromonas* and *Plesiomonas*
C. S. GOODWIN   103

6   Enteric fever — due to *Salmonella typhi* and *S. paratyphi*
J. SCHNEIDER   129

7   Gastroenteritis due to *Staphylococcus aureus*, *Clostridium perfringens* and *Bacillus cereus*
J. SCHNEIDER   149

8   The virology of acute infectious diarrhoea
T. H. FLEWETT   159

9   The challenge of childhood gastroenteritis
M. GRACEY   187

10   Amoebic dysentery, intestinal protozoa and helminths
D. GROVE   209

11   *Yersinia* infections including mesenteric adenitis, and gastrointestinal tuberculosis
C. S. GOODWIN   241

12 Immunization against gut infections
    G. N. COOPER   253

13 Public health aspects of gastroenteritis
    C. S. GOODWIN   269

14 The functions and the regulation of normal gut bacteria,
    and bacterial overgrowth syndromes
    P. J. McDONALD   289

15 The antimicrobial management of gut-derived sepsis complicating
    surgery and cancer chemotherapy
    P. J. McDONALD, J. McK. WATTS and J. J. FINLAY-JONES   307

16 *Clostridium difficile* and gut disease
    S. P. BORRIELLO   327

17 Carcinoma of the colon and gut bacteria
    S. P. BORRIELLO   347

Index   365

Contributors

S. P. BORRIELLO BSc(Hons), PhD
Research Fellow, Division of Communicable Diseases, Clinical Research
Centre, Harrow, Middlesex, England

GEOFFREY N. COOPER MSc, PhD, MASM
Professor of Medical Microbiology, University of New South Wales and
Honorary Consultant Microbiologist, Prince Henry, Prince of Wales and
St George's Hospitals, Sydney, Australia

JOHN J. FINLAY-JONES BSc, PhD
Lecturer, School of Medicine, Flinders University, Bedford Park,
South Australia

T. H. FLEWETT MD, FRCP, FRCPath
Director, Regional Virus Laboratory and World Health Organization,
Collaborating Centre for Reference and Research on Rotaviruses,
East Birmingham Hospital, and Honorary Reader, University
of Birmingham, Birmingham, England

MICHAEL GRACEY MD, PhD, FRACP
Associate Professor and Head, Gastroenterology and Nutrition Unit, Princess
Margaret Children's Medical Research Foundation, Perth, Western Australia

ROGER J. GROSS MA MSc
Principal Microbiologist, Division of Enteric Pathogens, Central Public
Health Laboratory, London, England

DAVID I. GROVE MD, FRACP, DTM&H
Associate Professor of Medicine, University of Western Australia, Perth,
Western Australia

PETER J. McDONALD MB BS, FRACP, FRCPA
Associate Professor and Head, Department of Clinical Microbiology,
Flinders Medical Centre, Bedford Park, South Australia

JAMES McKINNON WATTS MB BS, FRACS
Professor, Department of Surgery, Flinders University, Bedford Park,
South Australia

B. ROWE MA, MB BChir, FRCPath, DTM&H
Director, Division of Enteric Pathogens, Central Public Health Laboratory,
Colindale Avenue, London, England

JACOB SCHNEIDER MD, DMed, FRCP, FRACP, DTM&H
Consultant Physician, Sir Charles Gairdner Hospital, Perth, Western Australia

SUSAN STEPHENS MSc, MIBiol
Research Officer, Division of Communicable Diseases, Clinical Research
Centre, Harrow, Middlesex, England

Preface

Microbes in the human gut are involved in gastrointestinal disease in a wide variety of ways. This book was originally designed to include in one volume a discussion of bacterial, viral, protozoal and helminthic gut infections, bacterial overgrowth syndromes, and the role of gut bacteria in carcinoma of the colon and abdominal wound infection. Some microbes such as hepatitis A virus and poliovirus are found in the gut but as their primary pathology is outside the gut they have not been discussed. While space has not permitted an exhaustive description of each condition, the range of references should be useful to readers who seek more information. The metabolic activities of gut bacteria have been fully delineated by Drasar and Hill,[2] and have not been included in this book. Descriptions of the management of clinical conditions, such as dehydration and shock, and of microbiological bench techniques are already available in textbooks. The practising physician will not need to be told the necessity to examine faeces for leukocytes, and the value of this in distinguishing enteroinvasive and enterotoxic diarrhoeal disease.[6] A succinct but clear title for this book was a problem, and we trust that after reading the chapter headings and their contents you will not be disappointed.

The pathogenesis of bacterial gut disease is aided by an understanding of the bacteriology of the normal gut and its development, and the immunological mechanisms in the gastrointestinal tract. Thus the bacteria in the infant gut are discussed in Chapter 1 and gut anaerobes in Chapter 14. At the present time our understanding of gut immunology is based largely on work in rodents. Simplistic theories of the immunological mechanisms of the gut do not satisfactorily explain all the observed facts. In Chapter 2 our knowledge of these mechanisms is reviewed and this provides the basis for discussion of immunization procedures against microbial gut infections in Chapter 12.

Pathogenic gut bacteria may produce toxin in food, and such bacteria are enterotoxigenic *Staphylococcus aureus* and *Bacillus cereus*; other bacteria produce toxin in the intestine, such as enterotoxigenic *Escherichia coli*, *Vibrio cholerae*, and *Aeromonas hydrophila*. The other group of gut pathogens is enteroinvasive, such as *Salmonella*, *Shigella*, *Campylobacter*, *Yersinia* and enteroinvasive *Escherichia coli*. However, these two mechanisms of pathogenesis are not mutually exclusive; for example toxin production by salmonellae has been reported and is briefly discussed in Chapter 3. Our intention in this book is to provide for the physician and surgeon, the paediatrician and the oncologist, and the microbiologist and immunologist, a synthesis of the old with recent developments in microbial gut disease, and also to bring together subjects that usually appear in different specialist textbooks, on infectious diseases, gastro-enterology, surgery, microbiology or immunology.

Furthermore an attempt has been made to take a global view. In developed countries with chlorinated water supplies and efficient sewage disposal the pathway of enteric pathogens from faeces to new hosts is usually interrupted. In such countries a patient with gastrointestinal symptoms may be suffering from pyschosomatic disease, a malabsorption syndrome, nonmicrobial inflammatory bowel disease or food intolerance; and if the major initial symptom is vomiting, heavy metal poisoning could be the cause. A patient returning from overseas may present with vomiting and diarrhoea due to malignant tertian malaria caused by *Plasmodium falciparum*. However, microbial causes of gastroenteritis are still surprisingly frequent in developed countries. In developing countries many millions of people, particularly children, suffer from microbial gastroenteritis, and each year at least 5 million children die from this cause alone; such problems deserve the attention of doctors and scientists outside developing countries even though many of us will not be faced with these problems personally. This book includes a discussion of the public health problems of gastroenteritis in developing countries with an emphasis on practical solutions. Enteric pathogens that still make life a misery for so many inhabitants of this planet must be curbed.

The example of Costa Rica as a country where high rates of diarrhoeal disease and death have been sharply reduced should be an encouragement to all who seek to produce a similar result in other developing countries. The principles enunciated in Chapter 13 have been strikingly successful in Costa Rica. In 1981 98% of the urban population, and 70% of the rural population enjoyed a piped water supply, and latrines and toilets have been widely available. In 1930 the death rate from diarrhoea in Costa Rica was 400 per 100 000 but in 1978 had fallen to 12 per 100 000. Also an intelligent programme of oral rehydration of children with diarrhoea has been implemented. Surveys revealed that in the countryside one litre containers were scarce, but 8 ounce (230 ml) bottles were in 98% of the homes. A new pack was therefore designed at the Institute of Health Research which contained the correct concentration of oral rehydration salts for the 230 ml bottles. Oral rehydration in the countryside saves money because children do not need to be brought into hospital. Breast-feeding is also encouraged.[5]

Until a few years ago a surprisingly high percentage of fluid stool specimens submitted to microbiology laboratories were returned with a report that 'No pathogens have been isolated'. However, new bacteriological culture media, different temperatures of incubation, and direct tests for enterotoxin production have indicated that gastroenteritis may be caused frequently by *Campylobacter* species, and less frequently by *Yersinia enterocolitica, Aeromonas hydrophila*, or *Clostridium difficile*. Newer techniques in virology, such as immunoelectron microscopy, have revealed that some explosive outbreaks of diarrhoea are due to Norwalk virus, that diarrhoea in infants is often due to rotavirus, and that a few patients are infected with other newly-recognized agents such as calicivirus.

Stools submitted from patients suffering from antibiotic-associated diarrhoea should be cultured for *Clostridium difficile*, and tested for the presence of *C. difficile* cytotoxin. The enterotoxin of *C. difficile* will require a different test and some details of this toxin are given in Chapter 16.

Although much is known about microbial gut disease there are still areas of ignorance such as the exact relationship of intestinal bacteria to tropical sprue, and whether spirochetes other than *Campylobacter*, can cause human disease. In 1940 a study of 13 patients with chronic gastritis and duodenal ulcer was reported. Spirochetes were found in the gastric mucosa of two patients; also 16 patients with duodenal or gastric ulcer were studied, and the authors concluded that in the absence of ulceration spirochetes were rarely found.[3] Robin Warren, histopathologist at the Royal Perth Hospital, again drew attention to these bacteria in gastric biopses,[7] and they were first obtained in culture in 1982 in my department at the Royal Perth Hospital, from biopses taken by Barry Marshall.[8] They are *Campylobacter*-like organisms which are new to human microbiology. The interplay of microbial and nonmicrobial factors in producing gut symptoms may become clearer in the years to come. The role of gut-brain peptides in gut physiology and pathology is a vast new field.[1]

This book has been a joint effort of many authors. Some were able to write their chapters promptly, at an earlier date than others, inevitably without some of the most recent information in this rapidly advancing field. Unfortunately, discussion of a few microbes including fungi, had to be omitted. *Edwardsiella tarda* was one of these omissions, even though Western Australia has a high isolation rate of this organism due to the snake-eating habits of the desert Aboriginal, and the industry of John Iveson, who has shown that strontium chloride B broth at 43°C is suitable for the isolation both of *Salmonella* and *Edwardsiella*.[4]

I am grateful for the tolerance of my fellow authors to my editorial suggestions, and I would like to record my sense of privilege to be associated with so many acknowledged experts in the area of microbial gut disease. Blackwell Scientific Publications have been consistently supportive, and I have especially appreciated the encouragement of Mr Peter Saugman. I thank my secretaries Mrs Soula Manganas and Mrs Faye Coverley who have typed uncomplainingly. My wife Jean and my children, who lived with me in India, Hong Kong and Ethiopia, and also my parents, have consistently encouraged me.

C. Stewart Goodwin   *Perth, Western Australia, 1983*

REFERENCES

1. Bloom S.R. and Polak J.M. (1982) Clinical aspects of gut hormones and neuropeptides. *Brit. Med. Bull.* **38**, 233.
2. Drasar B.S. and Hill M.J. (1974) *Human Intestinal Flora*, Academic Press, London.
3. Freedberg A.S. and Barron L.E. (1940) The presence of spirochetes in human gastric mucosa. *Am. J. Dig. Dis.* **7**, 443.
4. Iveson J.B. (1971) Strontium chloride B and E.E. enrichment broth media for the isolation of *Edwardsiella*, *Salmonella* and *Arizona* species from tiger snakes. *J. Hyg. (Camb.)* **69**, 323.
5. Mata L. (1981) Diarrhoeal diseases — How Costa Rica won. *World Health Forum* **2**(1), 141.
6. Satterwhite T.K. and Dupont H.L. (1976) The patient with acute diarrhea. An algorithm for diagnosis. *J. Am. Med. Ass.* **236**, 2662.
7. Warren J.R. (1983) Unidentified curved bacilli in gastric epithelium in active chronic gastritis. *Lancet* **i**, 1273.
8. Marshall B. (1983) Unidentified curved bacilli in gastric epithelium in active chronic gastritis. *Lancet* **i**, 1273.

1 The development of the infant gut flora; and the medical microbiology of infant botulism and necrotizing enterocolitis

S. P. Borriello and S. Stephens

Introduction	1
Development of the flora of the gut	2
Factors controlling the development of the gut flora	3
Non-immunological factors	6
Immunological factors	7
Maternal factors	8
Non-specific factors in milk	9
Specific factors in milk	11
Cells of colostrum and milk	13
Infant botulism	15
Necrotizing enterocolitis	15
References	19

INTRODUCTION

The environment in which the fetus develops is normally sterile resulting in a sterile gastrointestinal tract at birth. Within hours of birth, bacteria start to colonize the gut and a delicate balance between host and organisms develops. The establishment of the gut flora is of vital importance to the host throughout infant and adult life, not only for nutritional and digestive purposes but also for the normal development of the gut and its defences. The quantity and species of bacteria found vary enormously throughout the length of the gut, and the factors controlling the establishment of the normal flora involve not only the environment and exposure to organisms but also numerous host factors (Table 1.3). In the second part of this chapter two diseases are described — infant botulism and infant necrotizing enterocolitis — both of which are probably a result of deficient protective activity of the 'normal' gut flora.

1

DEVELOPMENT OF THE FLORA OF THE GUT

The presence of bacteria in infant stools was described as long ago as 1866 by both Escherich[53] and Breslau.[25] These observations were confirmed by Billroth in 1874[16] and Nothnagel in 1881.[113] Since these early observations many workers have looked at the development of the infant faecal flora.[29,30,51,69,141,143] Much of the recent work on infant faecal flora development has centred on investigations into the relationship between type of infant feed — breast milk or formula preparations — stool pH, stool buffering capacity, and relative concentrations of lactobacilli and *Escherichia coli*.[29,30,31,77,167]

We are of the opinion that a review of these findings would serve little purpose. Instead, a brief statement of the conclusions to be drawn from the findings will be made, followed by a detailed description of the factors controlling this development.

Many published studies have shown that infants start to become colonized very soon after birth; organisms can be recovered as early as the first day of life. Although usually the first organisms to be found are aerobes, anaerobes have also been found (Table 1.1). The flora at this time is relatively simple (Table 1.1) especially when compared with the situation in the adult. In addition the type of diet can affect the faecal flora in infants. In general, it appears that breast-fed

Table 1.1 Development of faecal flora during first week of life in (a) breast-fed infants and (b) bottle-fed infants (modified from Borriello 1981[21])

	Day (no. of samples analysed)						
	1 (1)	2 (3)	3 (2)	4 (4)	5 (4)	6 (4)	7 (4)
(a)							
Coliforms	1*(7.0)†	3 (8.0)	1 (8.8)	4 (9.4)	4 (9.2)	4 (8.6)	4 (9.4)
Bifidobacteria	1 (5.2)	1 (6.7)	1 (9.2)	3 (7.0)	3 (8.4)	3 (8.3)	4 (8.0)
Streptococci	—	1 (7.1)	1 (10.2)	2 (8.0)	3 (6.7)	2 (7.1)	1 (9.2)
Bacteroides	—	2 (4.0)	2 (8.5)	3 (9.0)	3 (7.4)	3 (8.1)	3 (5.6)
Clostridia	—	1 (2.1)	1 (2.3)	2 (3.5)	4 (3.7)	3 (1.0)	4 (4.6)
Lactobacilli	—	—	1 (4.3)	—	3 (4.4)	3 (3.9)	4 (4.8)
Micrococci	—	1 (5.8)	—	—	—	1 (7.5)	—
Veillonella	—	—	—	—	1 (4.7)	1 (4.3)	—
Proteus	—	—	—	—	—	—	—
	1 (2)	2 (3)	3 (4)	4 (3)	5 (4)	6 (3)	7 (2)
(b)							
Coliforms	1 (2.7)	2(10.0)	4 (9.1)	3 (10.5)	4 (8.6)	3 (8.9)	2 (9.3)
Bifidobacteria	—	—	1 (3.9)	—	3 (3.5)	2 (4.7)	1 (4.0)
Streptococci	—	—	—	—	—	1 (7.6)	1 (9.7)
Bacteroides	—	1 (2.9)	3 (4.9)	3 (4.1)	3 (4.6)	2 (8.1)	1 (7.1)
Clostridia	1 (2.5)	1 (+)	2 (2.3)	3 (4.3)	3 (5.8)	2 (6.0)	2 (6.4)
Lactobacilli	1 (2.7)	—	2 (2.9)	2 (3.4)	4 (4.1)	3 (4.7)	—
Micrococci	—	—	—	—	—	—	—
Veillonella	1 (2.7)	—	—	—	2 (4.6)	—	1 (5.1)
Proteus	—	1 (7.0)	1 (4.0)	—	—	—	1 (4.0)

* No. of positive samples; † Mean $\log_{10}$ no. of organisms per gram stool in carriers; (+) obtained only on enrichment.

Table 1.2 Development of clostridial flora in infants (modified from Borriello[21])

No. of samples		Mean age (weeks)	Mean clostridia/g in carriers ($\log_{10}$)	% of positive samples	No. of clostridial species
Breast-fed	(28)	<1	3.7	68	5
Bottle-fed	(23)	<1	4.8	70	3
Breast-fed	(16)	2.7	5.2	38	7
Bottle-fed	(11)	5.8	6.0	73	10
Breast-fed (weaned)	(5)	37.4	4.5	100	7
Bottle-fed (weaned)	(14)	26.6	5.8	93	12

infants have a simpler faecal flora with less putrefactive microorganisms, fewer *E. coli* and higher counts of lactobacilli than their bottle-fed counterparts. However, this association between type of feed and relative counts of lactobacilli and *E. coli* has not been demonstrated in all of these studies. The proportions of different bacteria present during the first week of life in the two feeding groups persist as the infant becomes older. The differences between the feeding groups, such as a simpler flora composed of fewer putrefactive type organisms, become accentuated. This situation persists until weaning when the faecal flora becomes much more complex and similar in both groups. This situation is highlighted by the findings presented in Table 1.2. Most of the changes towards an adult type faecal flora pattern take place between 4 and 12 months, resulting in a flora similar to that found in adults being established between 1 and 4 years of age.

FACTORS CONTROLLING THE DEVELOPMENT OF THE GUT FLORA (Table 1.3)

Non-immunological factors

EXPOSURE

One of the most important factors involved in the development of the infant flora is exposure; an infant cannot be colonized by an organism to which it has not been exposed. During birth, the infant is exposed to the mother's vaginal and faecal flora and this is thought to be an important source of the infant microflora of the skin, nose, mouth and conjunctiva.[112] After delivery, the environment and delivery personnel are also sources of microorganisms.[133] Little is known about the sources from which the newborn acquires its faecal flora. It has been suggested that the *E. coli* serotypes are acquired from the mother[12] but a study by Gothefors *et al.*[64] showed that in 17 out of 29 mother–infant pairs the dominant *E. coli* serotype of the infant either appeared first in the infant and then in the mother, or there were no serotypes in common. Gothefors[61] also showed that neither the breasts nor the vagina of the mother had any *E. coli* to colonize the newborn, which contradicted the findings of Mata and Urrutia[100] in Mayan women.

Table 1.3   Factors affecting development of the gut flora

External	Environment and exposure to microorganisms	
	Diet	
Maternal	Placental transfer of immunoglobulins	
	Colostrum and milk	
Host	Non-specific	Gastric acidity
		Mucus
		Peristalsis
		Microbial interactions
		Lysozyme
		Bile salts
		Hepatic barrier
	Specific	Secretory antibodies, mainly sIgA
		Systemic antibodies, IgM, IgG, IgA and IgE
		Cell-mediated immunity

DIET

Apart from the immunological benefits of breast milk which will be discussed later, there are certain properties of cows' milk-based formulae that directly affect the development of infant flora. The higher buffering capacity and lower lactose content of cows' milk preparations seem to favour the growth of Enterobacteriaceae rather than lactobacilli, which are found to predominate in the stools of breast-fed babies.[31] The acidic environment produced by these lactobacilli is thought to discourage the growth of Enterobacteriaceae, including the most common enteric pathogens. Other adverse effects of cows' milk formula on the gastrointestinal tract are shown in Table 1.4 and have been discussed in detail by Eastham and Walker.[49] The foreign protein element, particularly the casein, represents a vast antigenic challenge to the neonatal gut resulting in local (IgA) and systemic (IgG and IgM) antibody production. Hypersensitivity reactions to cows' milk protein are not uncommon, and may cause diarrhoea and malabsorption.

Table 1.4   Adverse effects of milk formula ingestion on the gastrointestinal tract

Cause	Symptom
High butterfat, curds	Intestinal obstruction
High osmolality	Slow gut motility
Foreign protein	Hypersensitivity

GASTRIC BARRIER

Many bacteria from the environment and normal flora of the mouth are swallowed with saliva. Most are killed on reaching the acid contents of the stomach, except in people with achlorhydria.[48] The stomach of the newborn infant may be, with respect to gastric acidity, similar to that of an achlorhydric adult.[104] However, in a study of infants aged from 12 hours to 3 months a state of achlorhydria was noted in only one infant.[2] Changes in gastric acidity in the infant that may take place during the early stages of development probably play an important role in the development of the gastrointestinal flora at this time.

MICROBIAL INTERACTIONS

Colonization of the gut with bacteria is an important factor in the development of the normal intestinal morphology and lymphoid structure and function, as will be described later. Microbes in the gastrointestinal tract are also important for nutritional and digestive functions, as well as metabolic functions such as re-cycling of bile acids. Growth of pathogenic organisms appears to be limited by mechanisms such as competition for substrates, alteration in microenvironment (e.g. pH) or production of antibacterial substances such as colicines. In addition, the release of short-chain fatty acids produced by bacteria into the lumen of the gastrointestinal tract may be a factor regulating the numbers of enteric pathogens, as it is known that short-chain fatty acids can express antimicrobial activity against these organisms.[17,95] The importance of the indigenous flora in adults is demonstrated during antibiotic therapy, which frequently results in the establishment and overgrowth of pathogenic organisms and consequently diarrhoea. In extreme cases this may be life threatening, as in *C. difficile*-mediated disease (see Chapter 16).

SECRETIONS

Enzymes such as lysozyme and lactoperoxidase, present in the secretions of the gastrointestinal tract, have been shown to have antibacterial activity *in vitro*, although their role in controlling the normal flora *in vivo* is not known. However there is sufficient lactoperoxidase in the saliva of babies which, together with the thiocyanate present and hydrogen peroxide produced by oral streptococci, could possibly have an inhibitory effect on *E. coli*.[63] Mucins in the mucous coat are also thought to be an important component of the gut defences. They have a similar molecular structure to components on the epithelial surface, which act as receptors for microorganisms. They appear to provide competitive inhibition for the attachment of these flora to the epithelial surface.[146]

PERISTALSIS

Motility is an important factor in controlling proliferation of microorganisms within the small intestine. Organisms held in the mucous coat can be readily dislodged by the peristaltic movement, and without attachment to the epithelial surface the organisms cannot proliferate and cause damage. In cases such as 'blind loop syndrome', when motility is disrupted, stagnation within the small intestine results in a massive bacterial overgrowth, and disruption of gastrointestinal function.[126]

Immunological factors

A detailed description of the ontogeny and functions of the immune system is given in the next chapter, but its importance in the development of normal flora justifies a brief description here. The existence of a separate immune system of secretions was first suggested by Hanson[71] and since then several studies [13,76,160] have established the local immunologic system as a unique protective process present in all epithelial surfaces in direct contact with the environment. This local system is independent of systemic immune responses and is stimulated by antigen at mucosal surfaces.

GUT ASSOCIATED LYMPHOID TISSUE (GALT)

The structure of this tissue and the routes of migration of the lymphoid cells are described in detail in Chapter 2. Lymphocytes in the lamina propria of the gut or at other epithelial surfaces secrete primarily IgA.[39,65] The role of the normal gut flora in the development of this system is very important.

The newborn infant is virtually devoid of a functionally differentiated immune system in the gut during the first week of life[70] due to lack of antigenic stimulation *in utero*. Also in germ-free animals the structure of the gut is quite different from normal adults; there is poor development of musculature, long thin villous structure and shorter crypts, as well as a profound reduction in all lymphoid tissues.[117] After parturition in infants, and after septic exposure in adult germ-free animals, there is a fairly rapid development of the intestinal mucosa, with plasma cell infiltrate and early local production of IgM followed by IgA production by 2–4 weeks *postpartum*.[138] Observations in germ-free mice selectively colonized with *Proteus morganii* or a group of seven commensal organisms suggest a role for the normal gut flora in stimulating clonal expansion of antigen sensitive cells and the process of B cell differentiation with the effect that Peyer's patch cells become preferentially committed to IgA expression.[35] Dissemination of these antigen-specific memory B cells yields a persistent population at sites distant from antigenic challenge, resulting in cross-priming along mucosal follicles.[57]

IMMUNOGLOBULIN A

This immunoglobulin is secreted by local plasma cells as a dimer which contains an extra polypeptide J chain.[86,159] This dimeric IgA binds to a polypeptide called secretory component (SC) which is produced by the epithelial cells of the overlying mucous surface. The sIgA molecule is particularly suited to the gut environment in that it is more resistant than other immunoglobulins to the proteolytic enzymes present. Disulphide bonds may form between the sIgA molecule and the mucin glycoproteins, ensuring a tight association with the mucous coat. A transfer system has been shown to exist in the rat in which dimeric IgA molecules are actively transported from blood to bile.[115] It seems to depend on the presence of a J chain in the molecule and the presence of SC on the surface of the hepatic cell. This mechanism results in a selective secretion of sIgA antibodies into the gut. The immune tissues in the gut may react to some components of the normal flora by mounting a low level immune response, whereas other organisms do not stimulate this response unless there is some disruption of the mucosal surface.[117] A state of partial tolerance seems to exist towards many of the commensal microorganisms,[55] but the gut immune tissues can respond to newly introduced organisms with pathogenic potential. Specific antibodies to a variety of organisms and food antigens have been demonstrated in the gut.[139] The functions of these antibodies will be discussed in more detail later.

CELL-MEDIATED IMMUNITY (CMI)

The intraepithelial lymphocytes found in the lamina propria are mainly T cells.[67] These are a subpopulation of T cells derived from GALT and therefore are likely to be primed by intraluminal antigens.[117] As well as helper functions, gut T cells also appear to have important suppressive functions which may affect the balance between immunity and tolerance to gut antigens.[36] Cytotoxic T cell activity and secretion of various lymphokines may be important in defence against some infectious agents such as nematodes but may also be responsible for the villous atrophy and crypt hyperplasia seen in these diseases which may result in malabsorption.[117]

Maternal factors

ANTIBODIES ACQUIRED IN UTERO

Mammals vary in the amount of immunity tranferred passively to the infant during fetal development.[24] In humans, IgG antibodies are selectively transferred to the fetus across the placenta, so that infants are born with high IgG levels in their serum. This is an important second line of defence in the gut if there is damage to the mucosal surfaces or the local defence mechanisms fail.

ROLE OF BREAST MILK

The factors in colostrum and milk which have antimicrobial activity *in vitro* are listed in Table 1.5, although their importance *in vivo* is not always clear. The role of breast milk in controlling the normal gut flora and preventing infections in infants has been a controversial issue since artificial feeds became more popular in the early part of this century. There is now good evidence[40,41,100,156,158] that colostrum and breast milk are important in the defence of the neonate against infections acquired via the gut, particularly gastroenteritis due to organisms such as *E. coli* and *Shigella* sp.

Table 1.5 Factors with antimicrobial activity, in colostrum and milk

Non-specific	Bifidus factor
	Lactoperoxidase
	Lysozyme
	Lactoferrin
	Complement components
Specific	sIgA and other immunoglobulins
	Lymphocytes and macrophages

Non-specific factors in milk

These will only be briefly discussed in the context of this chapter. The interested reader is referred to an extensive review of the non-specific antimicrobial activity of milk.[127]

BIFIDUS FACTOR

It has been suggested that there is a growth promoting factor in milk for lactobacilli.[31] The prevalence of lactobacilli in the stools of breast-fed infants has been mentioned above.

LACTOPEROXIDASE

Although this enzyme is present in large quantities in bovine milk[129] and guinea-pig milk,[150] the levels in human milk are lower than those in infants' saliva and the significance of lactoperoxidase in controlling the microbial flora has been questioned.[63]

LYSOZYME

This enzyme is present in large quantities in human milk (400 µg/ml) and is apparently more active than egg white lysozyme.[128] It can kill a variety of gram-positive and gram-negative organisms *in vitro*. Other lysozymes are also thought to interact with complement and antibody to lyse bacteria[1,163] although this activity has not been confirmed by other workers.[74]

COMPLEMENT

The presence of the nine components of complement has been demonstrated in human milk although some are at very low levels.[111] The significance of the role of complement in milk is not known. The IgA antibodies do not fix complement by the classical pathway, but sIgA aggregates or bacterial endotoxins may activate the alternative pathway and so enhance the phagocytosis of organisms.

LACTOFERRIN

Human milk contains 1–6 mg/ml of lactoferrin, an iron binding protein which has been shown to have a bacteriostatic effect *in vitro*.[99] This effect is thought to be due to the strong binding of iron, in the presence of bicarbonate, to this protein, so that the iron is unavailable to bacteria. An *in vivo* antibacterial function for lactoferrin has been suggested by the increased growth of *E. coli*, after oral challenge, in the small intestines of suckled guinea-pigs dosed with haematin, compared with undosed controls.[28] However, there are other possible explanations for these results and more direct evidence is still needed.[26] A bactericidal function of lactoferrin *in vitro* has also been described,[3] but its significance within the gut is unknown.

Specific factors in milk

IMMUNOGLOBULINS

The predominant immunoglobulin of human milk as with other secretions is sIgA, and this occurs in concentrations up to 100 mg/ml in early colostrum. Levels decline rapidly during the first week of lactation to a basal level of 1–2 mg/ml.[101] IgM and IgG antibodies also occur in colostrum and milk but these are only 10% and 3% respectively of the levels in serum.

Source of immunoglobulins in milk

Antibodies against enteric organisms have frequently been demonstrated in milk.[82,103] In rabbits, both the intramammary and the oral routes of immunization are effective in stimulating IgA antibodies in colostrum suggesting that precursor cells primed in the gut may migrate to the mammary gland.[108] A similar phenomenon was shown with a commensal strain of *E. coli* in humans.[59]

Roux *et al.*[134] have shown that mesenteric lymph node B cell blasts migrate to the mammary gland and are precommitted to IgA synthesis whereas peripheral node blasts do not. This localization appears to be hormonally controlled,[164] and provides a very effective mechanism of ensuring a constant supply to the breast-fed infant of antibodies to the organisms in the local environment. There is evidence that more than 70% of the IgA ingested in milk survives transit in the infant's gut and can be recovered from the faeces.[114] Some absorption of colostral IgA in the infant's gut may take place during the first 24–36 hours after birth,[114,162] but this absorption has not been found by other workers.[168] Whether or not small amounts of IgA are absorbed, the main action of the sIgA appears to be within the infant's gut. Specific antibodies have been found to a variety of organisms including *Clostridium tetani*, *Corynebacterium diphtheriae*, *Streptococcus pneumoniae*, *E. coli*, Salmonella, Shigella, *Haemophilus influenzae*, streptococci, staphylococci,[72,73,165] echovirus, Coxsackie virus, influenza, polio and rotaviruses,[165] and against microbial toxins such as *E. coli* and *Vibrio cholerae*,[152] and *Clostridium difficile*.[161]

FUNCTIONS OF sIgA IN MILK

Various activities of the specific antibodies of milk have been demonstrated *in vitro*. Since IgA antibodies do not have the strong bactericidal activity of IgG or IgM their main role is thought to be to limit attachment and proliferation of pathogenic organisms within the gut rather than to kill them. In support of this is the isolation of pathogenic organisms such as enteropathogenic *E. coli*, Shigella and Salmonella from the stools of healthy breast-fed infants. The role of antibodies in controlling commensal flora is less well understood. The presence of specific antibodies or antibacterial activity in the mother's milk to certain organisms such as *E. coli* does not appear to influence their isolation rate from the faeces of their infants[47,64] although there is a suggestion that less virulent strains may be selected.[64,116]

Anti-adhesive properties

Williams and Gibbons[166] have demonstrated that sIgA from the parotid gland inhibits bacterial adherence to epithelial cells, and a similar effect of colostrum has been shown on the adhesion of *E. coli* to the small intestine of the pig.[110] Anti-pili antibodies to adhesive *E. coli* strains have been found in human milk.[155] Antibodies in milk can cause the loss of the K88 plasmid, which is important for adhesion in porcine strains.[96]

Agglutination

Agglutinating antibodies have been demonstrated in colostrum and milk against many intestinal organisms.[102] Their relevance in the prevention of infection is not clear, but they may reduce the ability of an organism to colonize the gut epithelium.[32]

Opsonization and complement activation

The activity of sIgA as an opsonin has been investigated by several workers with conflicting results.[89] The demonstration of IgA receptors on neutrophils may be significant in solving this controversy.[14] Although artificial sIgA aggregates have been shown to activate complement *in vitro* by the alternative pathway,[37] sIgA : antigen complexes on the surface of red blood cells did not activate the alternative pathway. It is not yet known whether the conditions *in vivo* favour complement fixation or enhanced phagocytosis by sIgA.

Neutralization

Antibodies have been demonstrated in milk which are capable of neutralizing *E. coli* and *V. cholerae* enterotoxins[78] and *C. difficile* toxin[161] and these may be important *in vivo*. Virus neutralizing antibodies have also been demonstrated against a number of viruses.[165]

Bacteriostasis

A bacteriostatic system involving serum antibody (IgG) and lactoferrin was demonstrated *in vitro* against *E. coli* by Bullen *et al.*[28] A similar mechanism has since been demonstrated for sIgA isolated from human milk.[132,145] The antibody involved is thought to block the secretion of enterochelins by the bacteria. Enterochelins are normally produced by the organisms in iron deficient situations, they can compete for iron bound by the lactoferrin and are then actively taken up via a surface receptor on the organism. The inhibition by isolated sIgA and lactoferrin appears to be more effective against strains of pathogenic serotypes than commensal strains[149] although whole milk is equally active *in vitro* against both types of strain. This selective inhibition of pathogenic serotypes, if active *in vivo*, could be important in controlling growth of pathogens while allowing establishment of harmless commensal strains.

Cells of colostrum and milk

Human colostrum contains $0.5 - 10 \times 10^6$ viable cells/ml, and these consist mostly of macrophages (up to 90%), lymphocytes (1–15%), and a few polymorphonuclear leukocytes. When lactation becomes established the cell concentration drops to about one-fiftieth of that in colostrum, but because milk volume increases the total number remains large.[94] The macrophages of colostrum are large fat engorged cells — foamy macrophages — that are phagocytic for staphylococci, *E. coli*, *Candida albicans* and inert particles *in vitro*, and also produce C3, C4, lysozyme and lactoferrin.[60] Cultures of macrophages *in vitro* have been shown to release large quantities of sIgA over a period of 7 days; they may be important in storing this immunoglobulin.[123] Colostral macrophages have also been seen to interact with milk lymphocytes[140] and respond to lymphokines. A rat model of necrotizing enterocolitis suggests that the macrophages in milk are important in preventing necrotizing enterocolitis in susceptible infants.[122] The lymphocyte population of milk consists of approximately 50% T cells and 34% B cells.[45] The T cell population of milk responds to allogenic cells in a manner similar to peripheral blood lymphocytes but the response to mitogens is lower. Responses to specific antigens differ considerably,[118] with a greater responsiveness of milk T cells to gut antigens such as *E. coli* K1 and bronchial-associated antigens such as tuberculin (PPD) but a lower response to antigens such as tetanus toxoid. There may be an involvement of T cell migration in the common mucosal immune system.[119]

The B cell population of milk that originates from cells primed in the gut and at other mucosal sites, has been shown to differentiate into immunoglobulin secreting plasma cells *in vitro* and most of these secrete IgA.[109] Whether the cells of milk exert their effect entirely in the gut or whether they enter the neonate's tissues is not known.

With such a wide variety of factors controlling normal flora it is not surprising that there is great variation in the microflora of the gut, on both a qualitative and quantitative basis, not only between individuals but also in each individual throughout the length of the gut. Variations in environment are obviously of primary importance and the higher exposure rate to organisms experienced in 'third world' countries with no clean water facilities puts a much greater strain on all the defence mechanisms that control the gut flora. The relative importance of each defence factor in influencing colonization is impossible to estimate; frequently when one system fails another will compensate, but clearly they all play some role in the final balance. The combined effect of the non-specific defences, together with secretory antibodies and effector lymphocytes with a wide range of specificities provides a constant controlling influence on the flora; there is also a vast potential of the gut to respond to the specific antigenic challenge of pathogenic organisms.

Infants, whose non-specific defences are not so effective in limiting colonization, and whose specific gut defences are not yet fully developed, are very susceptible to infections acquired via the gut. For this reason the antibodies present in mothers' milk are very important in protecting infants, particularly in countries where babies experience a large bacteriological challenge.[46] In these countries a bottle-fed infant should clearly be considered as an immunodeficient infant.

In some infants the development of the gastrointestinal flora appears to be abnormal and can result in diseases such as infant botulism and necrotizing enterocolitis which are discussed below.

INFANT BOTULISM

INTRODUCTION

Infant botulism results from the *in vivo* production of toxin by *Clostridium botulinum* that have colonized the infant's gut, and thus this disease differs from classical botulism in adults which usually results from the ingestion of preformed toxin. Up to 1981 more than 60 cases of infant botulism had been reported, the majority in the United States of America. Infant botulism is not a new disease, but a newly recognized disease. The first case of human infant botulism, proven retrospectively, is now thought to have occurred in California in 1931.[8] The first cases of overt infant botulism were reported by Pickett *et al.*,[121] who suggested that the toxin was produced *in vivo*. *C. botulinum* produces the most potent poison known to man. This gram-positive anaerobic, spore forming bacillus has seven serotypes designated A to G. All cases of infant botulism recognized to date have been associated with toxin type A or B, and in one case in New Mexico, type F.[43] The toxin blocks neuromuscular transmission by preventing release of acetylcholine from presynaptic terminals.

PATHOGENESIS

The disease is the result of the ingestion of spores of *C. botulinum* and their subsequent germination, establishment and release of toxin in the lumen of the infant gut. After absorption and distribution the toxin binds presynaptically to block neuromuscular transmission by preventing release of acetylcholine. A number of animal models have recently been developed which provide some indication of the pathogenesis of infant botulism. It has been shown that oral challenge of baby chickens with toxin-free preparations of *C. botulinum* spores caused a fatal botulism.[106] These workers also showed that in chickens, the site of germination and toxin release was the caecum. Intragastric challenge of mice with *C. botulinum* spores has shown that germination only occurred in the gut of animals between 7 and 13 days of age. In addition although toxin could be demonstrated in the colon of these animals they remained well.[154] Recent studies indicate that the toxin was not being absorbed from the colonic lumen of these animals.[105] The importance of the normal flora in preventing the establishment of *C. botulinum* after challenge was demonstrated in the mouse model by the use of germ-free animals. Normal adult mice were resistant to colonization by *C. botulinum* even after challenge of up to 10^5 spores, whereas germ-free adult mice could be colonized after challenge with as few as 10 spores. However, after adult germ-free mice were held in the routine animal holding room for 3 days where they would no doubt be exposed to many components of the normal microbial flora and would start to establish a normal gut flora, they became resistant to challenge with up to 10^5 *C. botulinum* spores.[107] By analogy with the mouse model one could argue that infants would be at risk of infant botulism when exposed to this organism at a time when the components of the normal gut flora that normally confer colonization resistance have not become fully established. It is also possible that the type of feed at this time may also be important, either as a direct result of possible protective components in normal breast milk or because of the type of flora that develops in the presence of different milk feeds (see p. 311). Recent analysis of cases of infant botulism indicates that breast-feeding affords relative protection against infant botulism.[4]

CLINICAL AND DIAGNOSTIC FEATURES

The clinical spectrum of infant botulism ranges from transient carriage of *C. botulinum* associated with inapparent infection to cases of sudden infant death.[4,5,7] Mild cases of the disease have been considered as cases of 'failure to thrive'.[81] One of the first indications of disease, which is frequently overlooked is constipation. Normally the first noticeable signs are lethargy and listlessness with diminished spontaneous activity. There will often be dysphagia noticed as drooling from the mouth. Suck and gag reflexes as well as the appetite are diminished. The child's cry becomes feeble. Not infrequently, respiratory arrest occurs. In some cases the infant may present as 'floppy'.[4,81] Another indication of infant botulism is a characteristic pattern obtained at electromyography.[81,121] Diagnosis of infant botulism is only established by the identification of *C. botulinum* in faecal samples or specimens obtained at autopsy.[6] From a specimen of suitable size it should also be possible to detect *C. botulinum* toxin.

TREATMENT AND CONTROL

Supportive care with special attention paid to pulmonary hygiene and nutrition is the accepted method of treatment for infant botulism. With respect to nutrition it is worth noting that tube feeding has been successfully used in most patients and that this may stimulate peristalsis. An additional advantage is that the mother's expressed breast milk may be used. Oral feeding should only recommence on return of the gag reflex and the infant's ability to swallow. If apnoea and brachycardia occur, mechanical ventilation will be required until normal respiration is established. Urine retention, due to bladder atony induced by the toxin may result in infection which can be reduced by the use of appropriate measures such as Credé's method. The use of cathartic agents or bulk laxatives to reduce the concentration of intestinal *C. botulinum* and its toxin have rarely proved efficacious. In addition, botulinal antitoxin is not required for the successful management of infant botulism. In fact, of the only two recorded cases of the use of botulinal antitoxin in infant botulism, one of the infants had an immediate anaphylactic reaction to the horse antitoxin despite having received only one-tenth of the planned dose, and having been pretreated with epinephrine.[81] The use of antibiotics for the treatment of infant botulism also has yet to be determined. By analogy with the situation in pseudomembranous colitis it would appear that the use of vancomycin or metronidazole may prove useful areas for research, as these antibiotics have been used successfully to treat *C. difficile*-mediated gastrointestinal disease in adults (see Chapter 16). However if 'normal' gut flora protect against colonization by *C. botulinum* then it is possible that due to the disruption of the infant's flora by these antibiotics during treatment the infant would be susceptible to reinfection with *C. botulinum* in the immediate post-treatment phase until the gut flora has returned to normal. In addition, antibiotics may increase the concentration of intestinal botulinum toxin due to induced cell lysis, and so exacerbate the disease. Infants with infant botulism may excrete large numbers of *C. botulinum* which could be infectious by faecal-oral transmission. It is therefore recommended that the usual precautions employed for faecal pathogens are taken. Parents should be instructed in the need for hand-washing and careful diaper disposal as infants may continue to excrete *C. botulinum* months after becoming asymptomatic. The best method of control is prevention and one can decrease the risk of infant botulism by minimizing exposure to the organism, and in this respect it is inadvisable to feed honey, which frequently has *C. botulinum* spores present, to any child of 1 year of age or younger.[27]

NECROTIZING ENTEROCOLITIS

INTRODUCTION

Necrotizing enterocolitis (NEC), a serious condition of newborn infants, presents with vomiting, abdominal distension, bloody stools and pneumatosis intestinalis. At laparotomy or necropsy there is evidence of ischaemic necrosis of the bowel wall with sloughing of the intestinal mucosa. The disorder most commonly affects the terminal ileum but may extend to one or more areas of the large or small bowel. The associated mortality rate has ranged from around 30%[44] to 70%[15] of affected infants. Although recognized since 1891[58] there has been a recent upsurge of NEC in neonatal nurseries around the world, with a corresponding increase in interest in the aetiology of the disease. Many predisposing and associated factors have been proposed (Table 1.6), and much interest has been shown in the possible

Table 1.6 Factors associated with NEC

Perinatal asphyxia[148]	Bottle feeding[19]
Infant respiratory distress syndrome[98]	Low apgar score[136]
Recurrent apnoea[151]	Premature birth[136]
Umbilical vessel catheterization[131]	Hyperosmolar feeds[18]
Anaemia[83]	Hirschsprung's disease[56]
Congenital heart disease[124]	Hypoxia[10]
Low birth weight[18]	Hyperviscosity[68]

involvement of bacteria in this disease state, with a wide variety of implicated microorganisms (Table 1.7).

Table 1.7   Organisms associated with necrotizing enterocolitis

Coxsackie B₂ virus[80]	Enterobacter[125]
Enterovirus[88]	Clostridia[52,120]
E. coli[144]	C. butyricum[79,153]
Klebsiella[130]	C. perfringens[9,87]
Pseudomonas[75]	C. difficile[33,34]
Salmonella[147]	

EVIDENCE FOR MICROBIAL AETIOLOGY

There are a number of general observations that indicate that there may be a microbial aetiology for necrotizing enterocolitis. For example clusters of cases have been seen on both a temporal and geographical basis, and outbreaks have been associated with a single organism (Table 1.7). In addition some of these outbreaks have been limited by the use of strict control measures. Many of these aspects have been dealt with in detail in a thorough review by Kliegman.[84] Recent attention has been focused on the potential aetiological role of clostridia in NEC and discussion here will be limited to these more recent findings. A wide variety of gastrointestinal disease in man and animals are suggestive of a clostridial association with NEC. Necrotizing enteritis in neonatal pigs and a similar disease in neonatal lambs are caused by *C. perfringens* type C and B respectively;[91] and more recently *C. perfringens* type E iota toxin[90] and *C. spiroforme* (Borriello and Carmen, unpublished data) have been associated with both spontaneous and antibiotic associated enterotoxaemia in rabbits. *C. difficile* is now known to be implicated in ileocaecitis in hamsters and neonatal diarrhoea in young hares [42] as well as a range of gastrointestinal disorders in man, including pseudo-membranous colitis.[22,92] There are also a number of gastrointestinal diseases in adults that exhibit pathological changes similar to those found in NEC. 'Darmbrand disease' was a necrotizing enteritis, caused by *C. perfringens* type F, that was seen in postwar Germany. Histology revealed intestinal gas, oedema and necrosis.[169] Pig-bel, a similar disease, is seen among the highlanders of New Guinea and is caused by *C. perfringens* type C.[93] In addition, clostridial gas-gangrene of the intestine in adults has pathological characteristics that are similar to those to be found in cases of NEC.[137] Engel in 1974[52] was the first to comment on the possible aetiological role of clostridia in the pathogenesis of NEC. He reported three affected infants from whose blood clostridia were cultured. Since then, a number of reports have appeared that implicate *C. perfringens* in the disease. Pedersen *et al.*[120] showed that the histology of resected gut specimens from six of seven NEC patients was similar to that found in both gas-gangrene of the bowel and experimentally provoked pneumatosis cystoides intestinalis. In one infant *C. perfringens* type A was isolated postoperatively from the peritoneal cavity and abundant Gram-positive rods resembling clostridia were seen in resected ileum. In reviewing specimens from six patients with NEC who had undergone operation the previous year the same histological picture was seen in five of them. The presence of abundant Gram-positive rods, typical of clostridia, within the muscularis of 8 of 11 segments of resected necrotic intestine from 11 infants has been reported;[87] the infants who had positive blood or peritoneal fluid cultures for clostridia had the most severe clinical course, and three of the four infants positive for *C. perfringens* had fulminant disease, characterized by severe pneumatosis intestinalis and portal venous gas, early perforation and extensive bowel gangrene, resulting in a fatal outcome in all three cases. However in another study in which 7 of 51 infants with NEC harboured *C. perfringens*, there was no real difference in outcome with respect to mortality between the NEC infants with or without *C. perfringens*;[85] in this study it was also noted that there were large Gram-positive clostridia-like organisms in the intestinal lumen, mucosal and submucosal layers, and lining 'gas bubbles' in surgical specimens from three infants. Analysis of mucosa from five affected infants described by Tait and Kealy[157] also showed Gram-positive rods on the surface and inside the necrotic mucosa of all the specimens. However, in this study, the presence of these organisms in the cyst-like spaces was rare. The review of 83 cases of sporadic necrotizing enteritis by Arseculeratne[9] gave support for a pathogenic role for *C. perfringens*, and in addition showed that strains of *C. perfringens* from cases of necrotizing enteritis had significantly higher histidine decarboxylase activity than strains from control sources. It was inferred that the resultant histamine production could act as a promotion factor for a type I hypersensitivity reaction.

In contrast to these findings which implicate *C. perfringens*, others failed to show a correlation between the presence of faecal *C. perfringens* and NEC.[79,142] The absence of *C. perfringens* in the stools of infants with NEC has also been noted in a number of recent cases, some of which proved fatal (Borriello 1981, unpublished data). *C. butyricum* has been implicated by Howard *et al.*[79] and Sturm et al.,[153] and *C. difficile* by Cashore *et al.*[33,34] The work of Howard *et al.*[79] was criticized by Gothefors and Blenkharn[62] and this author would support their criticisms. In addition, no association between faecal carriage of *C. butyricum* and NEC was noted by Smith *et al.*[142] However, Sturm *et al.*[153] reported the isolation of a penicillin-resistant cytotoxigenic strain of *C. butyricum* from the peritoneal and cerebrospinal fluid of a neonate with NEC. The report of *C. difficile*[33,34] has been more difficult to evaluate, because although *C. difficile* were not cultured, a toxin characteristic of *C. difficile* could be detected in 5 of 15 infants with confirmed or suspected NEC. However, this toxin could not be detected in any of 38 previously-studied NEC infants from three different geographic areas. In addition, no difference in the presence of faecal *C. difficile* or stool cytotoxin has been demonstrated between NEC infants and control infants.[142] Thus the aetiology of infantile necrotizing enterocolitis is far from resolved and the role of clostridia in its aetiology is still unclear.

DIAGNOSIS

Diagnosis requires a high index of suspicion, especially if the infant has any of the predisposing factors associated with NEC (Table 1.6). The classic symptoms and signs of the disease include abdominal distension, vomiting, bile-stained gastric residuals, diarrhoea or constipation and either gross or occult blood in the stool. Radiological features include pneumatosis intestinalis, which is highly characteristic, hepatic portal venous gas, and free intra-abdominal gas. In 1981 Fenton et al.[54] advocated the use of proctoscopy with an ordinary auroscope as a method to aid in the diagnosis of NEC. They concluded that the finding of colitis on proctoscopy, together with bloody diarrhoea and abdominal distension in the appropriate clinical setting were sufficient criteria on which to base a diagnosis of NEC.

TREATMENT

Treatment should include bowel rest with cessation of oral feeds. Broad spectrum antibiotics should be administered and anaerobic coverage should be considered especially in cases of intra-abdominal sepsis and intestinal perforation. The child should be fully investigated including cultures of blood, urine, stool and cerebrospinal fluid, close monitoring of blood pressure and urine output, and regular abdominal X-ray examinations to detect perforation. Supportive care includes maintenance of adequate haematocrit, pH, Po_2 and Pco_2 values, elevating the head of the bed, and employing mechanical ventilation for apnoea or shock. If the illness is prolonged nutritional support with total parenteral alimentation should be started. Recognition of NEC late in the disease process, or failure to respond to treatment may result in the need for surgical intervention, which is directed to the management of complications. Details of surgical management are beyond the scope of this author and the interested reader is directed to a publication of Lister and Meio[97] and appropriate paediatric surgery texts.

CONTROL AND PREVENTION

It is essential druing an outbreak of necrotizing enterocolitis to institute strict measures to prevent cross infection. The implementation of infectious disease control measures has helped to interrupt clusters of cases.[20] It is also claimed that orally administered aminoglycosides may be efficacious in both the management,[11] and prevention of this disease.[23,50,66] Although a reduced number of NEC cases in high-risk infants has been demonstrated after treatment with kanamycin or gentamicin (Table 1.8), no reduction of cases could be shown by Rowley and Dahlenburg[135] with oral gentamicin (Table 1.8). In addition the routine use of aminoglycosides on a prophylactic basis for the prevention of NEC, may lead to the emergence of resistant strains. For example, in the study by Boyle

Table 1.8 Aminoglycoside prophylaxis for the prevention of necrotizing enterocolitis in high risk infant groups.

| Aminoglycoside regimen | Number of infants out of total studied developing NEC | | Ref. no. |
	Control group	Experimental group	
Kanamycin 15 mg/kg/day	5/40	0/35	50
Kanamycin 15 mg/kg/day	9/50	3/49	23
Gentamicin 2.5 mg/kg/6h for 1 week	4/22	0/20	66
Gentamicin 2.5 mg/kg/6h for 1 week	6/50	3/50	135
Total	24/162	6/154	

and coworkers,[23] oral kanamycin produced a significant increase ($P < 0.05$) in the prevalence of infants with kanamycin-resistant Gram-negative enteric flora. However, the nursery population of kanamycin-resistant Gram-negative enteric flora did not alter during the 9-month study. There has also been a report of the emergence of a multiple-antibiotic resistant strain of *Staphylococcus epidermidis* coincident with the use of prophylactic oral kanamycin.[38] Other preventive measures could include the use of fresh breast milk and the avoidance of hyperosmolar feeds. The important protective factors in human breast milk have been discussed previously, and from the description of these properties it would not be surprising if breast-fed infants were at lower risk of developing NEC than those infants receiving formula preparations. However, there are few data available to confirm the protective effect of breast milk. This may be due to the fact that in many cases the milk has been pasteurized or frozen.

With this in mind it is important to note that in the rat model of *Klebsiella pneumoniae*-associated NEC[122] fresh milk, but not frozen and thawed milk, was protective. This protection appeared to be dependent on the presence of functional leukocytes, and macrophages in particular. It is hoped that when the aetiology and pathogenesis of NEC are better defined, guidelines for the effective prevention and control of this disease will be more specific.

REFERENCES

1 Adinolphi M., Glynn A. A., Lindsay M. and Milne C. M. (1966) Serological properties of IgA antibodies to *E. coli* present in human colostrum. *Immunology* **10**, 517.
2 Agunod M., Yamaguchi N., Lopez R., Luhby A. L. and Glass G. B. J. (1969) Correlative study of hydrochloric acid, pepsin, and intrinsic factor secretion in newborns and infants. *Am. J. Dig. Dis.* **14**, 400.
3 Arnold R. R., Cole M. F. and McGhee J. R. (1977) A bactericidal effect for human lactoferrin. *Science* **197**, 263.
4 Arnon S. S. (1980) Infant botulism. *Annu. Rev. Med.* **31**, 541.
5 Arnon S. S. and Chin J. (1979) The clinical spectrum of infant botulism. *Rev. Infect. Dis.* **1**, 614.
6 Arnon S. S., Midura T. F., Clay S. A., Wood R. M. and Chin J. (1977) Infant botulism: epidemiological, clinical and laboratory aspects. *J. Am. Med. Assoc.* **237**, 1946.

7   Arnon S. S., Midura T. F., Damus K., Wood R. M. and Chin J. (1978) Intestinal infection and toxin production by *Clostridium botulinum* as one cause of Sudden Infant Death Syndrome. *Lancet* **i**, 1273.
8   Arnon S. S., Werner S. B., Faber H. K. and Farr W. H. (1979) Infant botulism in 1931: discovery of a misclassified case. *Am. J. Dis. Child.* **133**, 580.
9   Arseculeratne S. N., Panabokke R. G. and Navaratnam C. (1980) Pathogenesis of necrotising enteritis with special reference to intestinal hypersensitivity reactions. *Gut* **21**, 265.
10 Barlow B. and Santulli T. V. (1975) Importance of multiple episodes of hypoxia or cold stress on the development of enterocolitis in an animal model. *Surgery* **77**, 687.
11 Bell M. J., Kosloske A. M., Benton C. and Martin L. W. (1973) Neonatal necrotizing enterocolitis: Prevention of perforation. *J. Pediatr. Surg.* **8**, 601.
12 Bettelheim K. A., Breadon A., Faiers M. C., O'Farrell S. M. and Shooter R. A. (1974) The origin of O serotypes of *Escherichia coli* in babies after normal delivery. *J. Hyg. (Camb.)* **72**, 67.
13 Bienenstock J. (1974) The physiology of the local immune response and the gastrointestinal tract. *Progr. Immunol. II* **4**, 197.
14 Bienenstock J. and Befus A. D. (1980) Mucosal immunology (a review). *Immunology* **41**, 249.
15 Bill A. H. and Chapman N. D. (1962) The enterocolitis of Hirschsprung's disease. Its natural history and treatment. *Am. J. Surg.* **103**, 70.
16 Billroth quoted by Penner and Bernheim (1939) Acute postoperative enterocolitis. *Archs. Path.* **27**, 966.
17 Bohnhoff M. and Miller C. P. (1962) Enhanced susceptibility to *Salmonella* infection in streptomycin-treated mice. *J. Infect. Dis.* **111**, 117.
18 Book L. S., Herbst J. J., Atherton S. O. and Jung A. L. (1975) Necrotizing enterocolitis in low-birth-weight infants fed an elemental formula. *J. Pediatr.* **87**, 602.
19 Book L. S., Herbst J. J. and Jung A. L. (1976) Comparison of fast and slow-feeding rate schedules to the development of necrotizing enterocolitis. *J. Pediatr.* **89**, 463.
20 Book L. S., Overall J. C. Jr, Herbst J. J., Britt M. R., Epstein B. and Jung A. L. (1977) Clustering of necrotizing enterocolitis. Interruption by infection-control measures. *New Engl. J. Med.* **297**, 984.
21 Borriello S. P. (1981) Clostridial flora of the gastrointestinal tract in health and disease. PhD Thesis, University of London.
22 Borriello S. P. and Larson H. E. (1981) Antibiotic and Pseudomembranous Colitis. *J. Antimicrob. Chemother.* **7** Suppl. A, 53.
23 Boyle R., Nelson J. S., Stonestreet B. S., Peter G. and Oh W. (1978) Alterations in stool flora resulting from oral kanamycin prophylaxis of necrotizing enterocolitis. *J. Pediatr.* **93**, 857.
24 Brambell F. W. R. (1970) *The transmission of passive immunity from mother to young.* American Elsevier, New York.
25 Breslau (1866) Ueber entstehung und bedeutung der darmgase bei neugeborenen kindern. *Monatschr. F. Geburtsh. U. Frauenkr.* **28**, 1.
26 Brock J. H. (1980) Lactoferrin in human milk: its role in iron absorption and protection against enteric infection in the newborn infant. *Arch. Dis. Childh.* **55**, 417.
27 Brown L. W. (1979) Infant botulism and the honey connection (commentary). *J. Pediatr.* **94**, 337.
28 Bullen J. J., Rogers H. J. and Leigh L. (1972) Iron-building proteins in milk and resistance to *Escherichia coli* infection in infants. *Br. Med. J.* **1**, 69
29 Bullen C. L., Tearle P. V. and Stewart M. G. (1977) The effect of 'humanised' milks and supplemented breast-feeding on the faecal flora of infants. *J. Med. Microbiol.* **10**, 403.
30 Bullen C. L., Tearle P. V. and Willis A. T. (1976) Bifidobacteria in the intestinal tract of infants: An in-vivo study. *J. Med. Microbiol.* **9**, 325.
31 Bullen C. L. and Willis A. T. (1971) Resistance of the breast-fed infant to gastroenteritis. *Br. Med. J.* **3**, 338.

32 Cantey J. R. (1978) Prevention of bacterial infections of mucosal surfaces by immune secretory IgA. *Adv. Exp. Med. Biol.* **107**, 461.

33 Cashore W. J., Peter G., Lauermann M., Stonestreet B. S. and Oh W. (1981) Clostridia colonisation and clostridial toxin in neonatal necrotizing enterocolitis. *J. Pediatr.* **98**, 308.

34 Cashore W. J., Stonestreet B. S., Lauermann M., Bartlett J. G., Oh W. and Peter G. (1979) Colonisation with clostridia species of infants with neonatal necrotizing enterocolitis. In Current Chemotherapy and Infectious Disease, Proceedings of 11th Int. Congr. Chemoth. and 19th Int. Conf. Antimicrob. Agents Chemoth. 1197.

35 Cebra J. J., Gearhart P. J., Halsey J. F., Hurwitz J. L. and Shahin R. D. (1980) Role of environmental antigens in the ontogeny of the secretory immune response. *J. Reticuloendothel. Soc.* **28**, 61s.

36 Challacombe, S. J. and Tomasi T. B. (1980) Systematic tolerance and secretory immunity after oral immunisation. *J. Exp. Med.* **152**, 1459.

37 Colten H. R. and Bienenstock J. (1974) Lack of C3 activation through classical or alternate pathways by human secretory IgA anti-blood group A antibody. *Adv. Exp. Med. Biol.* **45**, 305.

38 Conroy M. M., Anderson R. and Cates K. L. (1978) Complications associated with prophylactic oral kanamycin in pre-term infants. *Lancet* **i**, 613.

39 Craig S. W. and Cebra J. J. (1971) Peyer's patches: An enriched source of precursors for IgA producing immunocytes in the rabbit. *J. Exp. Med.* **134**, 188.

40 Cunningham A. S. (1977) Morbidity in breast-fed and artificially-fed infants. *J. Pediatr.* **90**, 726.

41 Cunningham A. S (1979) Morbidity in breast-fed and artificially-fed infants, II. *J. Pediatr.* **95**, 685.

42 Dabard J., Dubos F., Martinet L. and Ducluzeau R. (1979) Experimental reproduction of neonatal diarrhoea in young gnotobiotic hares simultaneously associated with *Clostridium difficile* and other *Clostridium* strains. *Infect. Immun.* **24**, 7.

43 Davis D., De La Torre L., Kazemier A. *et al.* (1980) Type F infant botulism — New Mexico. *Morbid. Mortal. Wkly Rep.* **29**, 85.

44 De Luca F. G. and Wesselhoeft C. W. (1974) Neonatal necrotizing enterocolitis. *Am. J. Surg.* **127**, 410.

45 Diaz-Jouanen E. P. and Williams R. C. (1974) T and B lymphocytes in human colostrum. *Clin. Immunol. Immunopathol.* **3**, 248.

46 Dolby J. M., Honour P. and Rowland M. G. M. (1980) Bacteriostasis of *Escherichia coli* by milk. V. The bacteriostatic properties of milk of West African mothers in the Gambia: *in vitro* studies. *J. Hyg. (Camb.)* **85**, 347.

47 Dolby J. M., Honour P. and Valman H. B. (1977) Bacteriostasis of *Escherichia coli* by milk. 1. Colonization of breast-fed infants by milk resistant organisms. *J. Hyg. (Camb.)* **78**, 85.

48 Drasar B. S., Shiner M. and McLeod G. M. (1969) Studies on the intestinal flora I. The bacterial flora of the gastrointestinal tract in healthy and achlorhydric persons. *Gastroenterology* **56**, 71.

49 Eastham E. J. and Walker W. A. (1979) Adverse effects of milk formula ingestion on the gastrointestinal tract. An update. *Gastroenterology* **76**, 365.

50 Egan E. A., Mantilla G., Nelson R. M. and Eitzman D. V. (1976) A prospective controlled trial of oral kanamycin in the prevention of neonatal necrotizing enterocolitis. *J. Pediatr.* **89**, 467.

51 Ellis-Pegler R. B., Crabtree C. and Lambert H. P. (1975) The faecal flora of children in the United Kingdom. *J. Hyg. (Camb.)* **75**, 135.

52 Engel R. (1974) Report of 68th Ross Conference on Pediatric Research p. 66.

53 Escherich T. (1886) *Die Darmbakterien des Säuglings*, Stuttgart, F. Enke.

54 Fenton T. R., Walker-Smith J. A. and Harvey D. R. (1981) Proctoscopy in infancy with reference to its use in necrotising enterocolitis. *Arch. Dis. Childh.* **56**, 121.

55   Foo M. C. and Lee A. (1972) Immunological response of mice to members of the autochthonous intestinal flora. *Infect. Immun.* **6**, 525.

56   Frantz I. D., L'Heureux P., Engel R. R. and Hunt C. E. (1975) Necrotizing enterocolitis. *J. Pediatr.* **86**, 259.

57   Fuhrman J. A. and Cebra J. J. (1981) Special features of the priming process for a secretory IgA response. B cell priming with cholera toxin. *J. Exp. Med.* **153**, 534.

58   Genersich A. (1891) Bauchfellentzündung beim neugebornen folge von perforation des ileums. *Virchows. Arch. Anat.* **126**, 485.

59   Goldblum R. M., Ahlstedt S., Carlsson B., Hanson L. A., Jodal U., Lidin-Janson G. and Sohl-Akerlund A. (1975) Antibody-forming cells in human colostrum after oral immunization. *Nature* **257**, 797.

60   Goldman A. S. and Smith C. W. (1973) Host resistance factors in human milk *J. Pediatr.* **82**, 1082.

61   Gothefors L. (1975) Studies of antimicrobial factors in human milk and bacterial colonisation of the newborn. Umea University Medical Dissertations.

62   Gothefors L. and Blenkharn I. (1978) *Clostridium butyricum* and necrotising enterocolitis. *Lancet* **i**, 52.

63   Gothefors L. and Marklund S. (1975) Lactoperoxidase activity in human milk and in saliva of newborn infants. *Infect. Immun.* **11**, 1210.

64   Gothefors L., Carlsson B., Ahlstedt S., Hanson L. A. and Winberg J. (1976) Influence of maternal gut flora and colostral and cord serum antibodies on presence of *Escherichia coli* in faeces of newborn infant. *Acta Paediatr. Scand.* **65**, 225.

65   Gowans J. L. and Knight E. J. (1964) The route of recirculation of lymphocytes in the rat. *Proc. R. Soc. Lond. B* **159**, 257.

66   Grylack L. J. and Scanlon J. W. (1978) Oral gentamicin therapy in the prevention of neonatal necrotising enterocolitis A controlled double-blind trial. *Am. J. Dis. Child.* **132**, 1192.

67   Guy-Grand D., Griscelli C. and Vassalli P. (1974) The gut-associated lymphoid system: nature and properties of the large dividing cells. *Eur. J. Immunol.* **4**, 435.

68   Hakanson D. O. and Oh W. (1977) Necrotizing enterocolitis and hyperviscosity in the newborn infant. *J. Pediatr.* **90**, 458.

69   Hall I. C. and O'Toole E. (1935) Intestinal flora in newborn infants. *Am. J. Dis. Child.* **49**, 390.

70   Haneberg B. and Aarskog D. (1975) Human faecal immunoglobulins in healthy infants and children and in some with diseases affecting the intestinal tract or the immune system. *Clin. Exp. Immunol.* **22**, 210.

71   Hanson L. A. (1961) Comparative immunological studies of the immune globulins of human milk and of blood serum. *Int. Arch. Allergy* **18**, 241.

72   Hanson L. A., Carlsson B., Ahlstedt S., Svanborg-Eden C. and Kaijser B. (1975) Immune defence factors in human milk. In '*Milk and Lactation*', *Modern Problems in Pediatrics* **15**, 63.

73   Hanson L. A. and Winberg J. (1972) Breast milk and defence against infection in the newborn. *Arch. Dis. Childh.* **47**, 845.

74   Heddle R. J., Knop J. K., Steele E. J. and Rowley D. (1975) The effect of lysozyme on the complement-dependent bactericidal action of different antibody classes. *Immunology* **28**, 1061.

75   Henderson A., Maclaurin J. and Scott J. M. (1969) Pseudomonas in a Glasgow baby unit. *Lancet* **ii**, 316.

76   Heremans J. F. (1975) The secretory immune system. A critical appraisal. In *The Immune System and Infectious Diseases* 4th Int. Convoc. Immunol. (Karger, Basel) p. 376.

77   Hewitt J. H. and Rigby J. (1976) Effect of various milk feeds on numbers of *Escherichia coli* and *Bifidobacterium* in the stools of newborn infants. *J. Hyg. (Camb.)* **77**, 129.

78   Holmgren J., Hanson L. A., Carlsson B., Lindblad B. S. and Rahimtoola J. (1976) Neutralising antibodies against *Escherichia coli* and *Vibrio cholerae* enterotoxins in human milk from a developing country. *Scand. J. Immunol.* **5**, 867.

79 Howard F. M., Flynn D. M., Bradley J. M., Noone P. and Szawatkowski M. (1977) Outbreak of necrotising enterocolitis caused by *Clostridium butyricum*. *Lancet* **ii**, 1099.
80 Johnson F. E., Crnic D. M., Simmons M. A., Lilly J. R. (1977) Association of fatal Coxsackie B$_2$ viral infection and necrotizing enterocolitis. *Arch. Dis. Childh.* **52**, 802.
81 Johnson R. O., Clay S. A., Arnon S. S. (1979) Diagnosis and management of infant botulism. *Am. J. Dis. Child.* **133**, 586.
82 Kenny J. F., Boesman M. I. and Michaels R. H. (1967) Bacterial and viral coproantibodies in breast-fed infants. *Pediatrics* **39**, 202.
83 Kitterman J. A. (1975) Necrotizing enterocolitis in the newborn. Proceedings of the Sixty-eighth Ross Conference on Pediatric Research, Ross Laboratories, Columbus, Ohio, p. 35.
84 Kliegman R. M., (1979) Neonatal necrotizing enterocolitis: Implications for an infectious disease. *Pediatr. Clin. North Am.* **26**, 327.
85 Kleigman R. M., Fanaroff A. A., Izant R. and Speck W. T. (1979) Clostridia as pathogens in neonatal necrotizing enterocolitis. *J. Pediatr.* **95**, 287.
86 Koshland M. E. (1975) Structure and function of the J chain. *Adv. Immunol.* **20**, 41.
87 Kosloske A. M., Ulrich J. A. and Hoffman H. (1978) Fulminant necrotising enterocolitis associated with clostridia. *Lancet* **ii**, 1014.
88 Lake A. M., Lauer B. A. and Clark J. C (1976) Enterovirus infections in neonates. *J. Pediatr.* **89**, 787.
89 Lamm M. E. (1976) Cellular aspects of immunoglobulin A. *Adv. Immunol.* **22**, 223.
90 LaMont J. T., Sonnenblinck E. B. and Rothman S. (1979) Role of clostridial toxin in the pathogenesis of clindamycin colitis in rabbits. *Gastroenterology* **76**, 356.
91 Lancet editorial: (1977) Clostridia as intestinal pathogens. *Lancet* **ii**, 1113.
92 Larson H. E., Price A. B., Honour P. and Borriello S. P. (1978) *Clostridium difficile* and the aetiology of pseudomembranous colitis. *Lancet* **i**, 1063.
93 Lawrence G. and Walker P. D. (1976) Pathogenesis of enteritis necroticans in Papua New Guinea. *Lancet* **i**, 125.
94 Lawton J. W. M. and Shortridge K. F. (1977) Protection factors in human breast milk and colostrum. *Lancet* **i**, 253.
95 Lee A. and Gemmell E. (1972) Changes in the mouse intestinal microflora during weaning: role of volatile fatty acids. *Infect. Immun.* **5**, 1.
96 Linggood M. A., Ellis M. L. and Porter P. (1979) An examination of the O and K specificity involved in the antibody-induced loss of the K88 plasmid from porcine enteropathogenic strains of *E. coli. Immunology* **38**, 123.
97 Lister J. and Meio I. B. (1979) Surgical management of neonatal necrotizing entereocolitis. *J. R. Soc. Med.* **72**, 176.
98 Lloyd J. R. (1969) The aetiology of gastrointestinal perforations in the newborn. *J. Pediat. Surg.* **4**, 77.
99 Masson P. L., Heremans J. F., Prignot J. and Wauters J. (1966) Immunohistochemical localization and bacteriostatic properties of an iron-binding protein from bronchial mucus. *Thorax* **21**, 538.
100 Mata L. J. and Urrutia J. J. (1971) Intestinal colonization of breast-fed children in a rural area of low socioeconomic level. *Ann. N.Y. Acad. Sci.* **176**, 93.
101 McClelland D. B. L., McGrath J. and Samson R. R. (1978) Antimicrobial factors in human milk. *Acta Paediatr. Scand.* Suppl. 271, 1.
102 McClelland D. B. L., Samson R. R., Parkin D. M. and Shearman D. J. C. (1972) Bacterial agglutination studies with secretory IgA prepared from human gastrointestinal secretions and colostrum. *Gut* **13**, 450.
103 Michael J. G., Ringenback R. and Hottenstein S. (1971) The antimicrobial activity of human colostral antibody in the newborn. *J. Inf. Dis.* **124**, 445.
104 Miller R. A. (1941) Observations on the gastric acidity during the first month of life. *Arch. Dis. Childh.* **16**, 22.
105 Mills D. C. and Sugiyama H. (1979) Comparative sensitivities of infant and adult mice to botulinum toxin. 79th Ann. Meet. Am. Soc. Microbiol. Los Angeles Abstract, p. 11.

106   Miyazaki S. and Sakaguchi G. (1978) Experimental botulism in chickens: the cecum as the site of production and absorption of botulinum toxin. *Jpn. J. Med. Sci. Biol.* **31**, 1.

107   Moberg L. J. and Sugiyama H. (1979) Microbial ecologic basis of infant botulism as studied with germfree mice. *Infect. Immun.* **25**, 653.

108   Montgomery P. C., Cohn J. and Lally E. T. (1973) The induction and characterization of secretory IgA antibodies. *Adv. Exp. Med. and Biol.* **45**, 453.

109   Murillo G. J. and Goldman A. S. (1970) The cells of human colostrum II Synthesis of IgA and β1c. *Pediatr. Res.* **4**, 71.

110   Nagy L. K., Bhogal B. S. and Mackenzie T. (1976) The effect of colostrum or past colibacillosis on the adhesion of *E. coli* to the small intestine of the pig. *Res. Vet. Sci.* **21**, 303.

111   Nakajima S., Baba A. S. and Tamura N. (1977) Complement system in human colostrum. *Int. Arch. Allergy Appl. Immunol.* **54**, 428.

112   Nolte W. A. (1977) *Oral Microbiology* 3rd edn. C. V. Mosby Co., St. Louis.

113   Nothnagel H. (1881) Die Normal in den menschlichen Darmentleerungen vorkommenden niedersten (pflanzlichen) Organismen. *Ztschr. f. Klin. Med.* **3**, 275.

114   Ogra S. S., Weintraub D. and Ogra P. L. (1977) Immunologic aspects of human colostrum and milk. III Fate and absorption of cellular and soluble components in the gastrointestinal tract of the newborn. *J. Immunol.* **119**, 245.

115   Orlans E., Peppard J., Reynolds J. and Hall J. (1978) Rapid active transport of immunoglobulin A from blood to bile. *J. Exp. Med.* **147**, 588.

116   Orskov F. and Sorensen K. B. (1975) *Escherichia coli* serogroups in breast-fed and bottle-fed infants. *Acta Path. Microbiol. Scand.* Sect. B. **83**, 25.

117   Ottaway C. A., Rose M. L. and Parrott D. M. F. (1979) The Gut as an Immunological System. In *International Review of Physiology, Gastrointestinal Physiology III*, vol. 19 p. 323, R. K. Crane (ed.). Univ. Park Press, Baltimore.

118   Parmely M. J., Beer A. E., and Billingham R. E. (1976) *In vitro* studies on the T-lymphocyte population of human milk. *J. Exp. Med.* **144**, 358.

119   Parmely M. J., Reath D. B., Beer A. E. and Billingham R. E. (1977) Cellular immune responses of human milk T-lymphocytes to certain environmental antigens. *Transplant Proc.* **9**, 1477.

120   Pedersen P. V., Hansen F. H., Halveg A. B., Christiansen E. D., Justesen T. and Høgh P. (1976) Necrotising enterocolitis of the newborn — is it gas-gangrene of the bowel? *Lancet* **ii**, 715.

121   Pickett J., Berg B., Chaplin E. and Brunstetter-Shafer M. (1976) Syndrome of botulism in infancy: clinical and electrophysiologic study. *N. Engl. J. Med.* **295**, 770.

122   Pitt J., Barlow B. and Heird W. C. (1977) Protection against experimental necrotizing enterocolitis by maternal milk. I. Role of milk leukocytes. *Pediatr. Res.* **11**, 906.

123   Pittard III W. B., Polmar S. H. and Fanaroff A. A. (1977) The breast milk macrophage: a potential vehicle for immunoglobulin transport. *J. Reticuloendothel. Soc.* **22**, 597.

124   Polin R. A., Pollock P. F., Barlow B., Wigger H. J., Slovis T. L., Santulli T. V. and Heird W. C. (1976) Necrotizing enterocolitis in term infants. *J. Pediatr.* **89**, 460.

125   Powell J., Bureau M. A., Paré C., Gaildry M., Cabana D. and Patriquin H. (1980) Necrotizing Enterocolitis. Epidemic following an outbreak of *Enterobacter cloacae* Type 3305573 in a neonatal intensive care unit. *Am. J. Dis. Child.* **134**, 1152.

126   Reilly R. W. and Kirsner J. B. (1959) Blind loop syndrome. *Gastroenterology* **37**, 491.

127   Reiter B. (1978*a*) Review of non-specific antimicrobial factors in colostrum. *Ann. Rech. Vét.* **9**, 205.

128   Reiter B. (1978*b*) Review of the progress of Dairy Science: Antimicrobial systems in milk. *J. Dairy Res.* **45**, 135.

129   Reiter B., Pickering A., Oram J. D. and Pope G. S. (1963) Peroxidase-thiocyanate inhibition of Streptococci in raw milk. *J. Gen. Microbiol.* **33**, xii.

130   Roback S. A., Foker J., Frantz I. F., *et al.* (1974) Necrotizing enterocolitis. *Arch. Surg.* **109**, 314.

131 Rogers A. F. and Dunn P. M. (1969) Intestinal perforation, exchange transfusion and PVC. *Lancet* **ii**, 1246.

132 Rogers H. J. and Synge C. (1978) Bacteriostatic effect of human milk on *Escherichia coli*: the role of IgA. *Immunology* **34**, 19.

133 Rotimi V. O. and Duerden B. I. (1981) The development of the bacterial flora in normal neonates. *J. Med. Microbiol.* **14**, 51.

134 Roux M. E., McWilliams M., Phillips-Quagliata J. M., Weisz-Carrington P. and Lamm M. E. (1977) Origin of IgA-secreting plasma cells in the mammary gland. *J. Exp. Med.* **146**, 1311.

135 Rowley M. P. and Dahlenburg G. W. (1978) Gentamicin in prophylaxis of neonatal necrotising enterocolitis. *Lancet* **ii**, 532.

136 Santulli T. V., Heird W. C., Wigger J., Blanc W. A., Schullinger J. N., Gongaware R. D., Barlow B. and Berdon W. E. (1975) Acute necrotizing enterocolitis in infancy: a review of 64 cases. *Pediatrics* **55**, 376.

137 Sawyer R. B., Sawyer K. C. and List J. E. (1970) Infectious emphysema of the gastrointestinal tract in the adult. *Am. J. Surg.* **120**, 579.

138 Selner J. C., Merrill D. A. and Claman H. N. (1968) Salivary immunoglobulin and albumin: Development during the neonatal period. *J. Pediatr.* **72**, 685.

139 Shearman D. J. C., Parkin D. M. and McClelland D. B. L. (1972) The demonstration and function of antibodies in the gastrointestinal tract. *Gut* **13**, 483.

140 Smith C. W. and Goldman A. S. (1970) Interactions of lymphocytes and macrophages from human colostrum. *J. Reticuloendothel. Soc.* **8**, 91.

141 Smith H. W. and Crabb W. E. (1961) The faecal bacterial flora of animals and man: its development in the young. *J. Path. Bact.* **82**, 53.

142 Smith M. F., Borriello S. P., Claydon G. S. and Casewell M. W. (1980) Clinical and bacteriological findings in necrotising enterocolitis: A controlled study. *J. Infect.* **2**, 23.

143 Snyder M. L. (1940) The normal faecal flora of infants between two weeks and one year of age. *J. Inf. Dis.* **66**, 1.

144 Speer M. E., Taker L. H., Yow M. D., *et al.* (1976) Fulminant neonatal sepsis and necrotizing enterocolitis associated with a 'nonenteropathogenic' strain of *Escherichia coli*. *J. Pediatr.* **89**, 91.

145 Spik G., Cheron A., Montreuil J. and Dolby J. M. (1978) Bacteriostasis of a milk-sensitive strain of *Escherichia coli* by immunoglobulins and iron-binding proteins in association. *Immunology* **35**, 663.

146 Springer G. F. (1970) Importance of blood-group substances in interactions between man and microbes. *Ann. N.Y. Acad. Sci.* **169**, 134.

147 Stein H., Beck J., Solomon A. *et al.* (1972) Gastroenteritis with necrotizing enterocolitis in premature babies. *Br. Med. J.* **2**, 616.

148 Stein M., Schreiner R. L., Ballantine T. V. N., Grosfeld J. L. and Gresham E. L. (1978) Necrotizing enterocolitis in the newborn: analysis of 32 cases. *J. Indiana State Med. Assoc.* **71**, 393.

149 Stephens S., Dolby J. M., Montreuil J. and Spik G. (1980) Differences in inhibition of the growth of commensal and enteropathogenic strains of *Escherichia coli* by lactotransferrin and secretory immunoglobulin A isolated from human milk. *Immunology* **41**, 597.

150 Stephens S., Harkness R. A. and Cockle S. M. (1979) Lactoperoxidase activity in guinea-pig milk and saliva: correlation in milk of lactoperoxidase with bactericidal activity against *Escherichia coli*. *Br. J. Exp. Pathol.* **60**, 252.

151 Stevenson J. K. and Stevenson D. K. (1977) Necrotizing enterocolitis in the neonate. *Surg. Ann.* **9**, 147.

152 Stoliar O. A., Pelley R. P., Kanieki-Green E., Klaus M. H. and Carpenter C. C. J. (1976) Secretory IgA against enterotoxins in breast milk. *Lancet* **i**, 1258.

153 Sturm R., Staneck J. L., Stauffer L. R. and Neblett W. W. III. (1980) Neonatal necrotizing enterocolitis associated with penicillin-resistant, toxigenic *Clostridium butyricum*. *Pediatrics* **66**, 928.

154 Sugiyama H. and Mills D. C. (1978) Intraintestinal toxin in infant mice challenged intragastrically with *Clostridium botulinum* spores. *Infect. Immun.* **21**, 59.

155 Svanborg Edén C., Carlsson B., Hanson L. A., Jann B., Jann K., Korhonen T. and Wadström T. (1979) Anti-pili antibodies in breast milk. *Lancet* **ii**, 1235.

156 Svirsky-Gross S. (1958) Pathogenic strains of coli (O,111) among prematures and the use of human milk in controlling the outbreak of diarrhoea. *Ann. Paediatr.* **190**, 109.

157 Tait R. A. and Kealy W. F. (1979) Neonatal necrotising enterocolitis *J. Clin. Pathol.* **32**, 1090.

158 Tassovatz B. and Kotsitch A. (1961) Le lait de femme et son action de protection contre les infections intestinales chez le nouveauné. *Ann. Pediatr.* **8**, 285.

159 Tomasi T. B. and Bienenstock J. (1968) Secretory immunoglobulins. *Adv. Immunol.* **9**, 2.

160 Tomasi T. B., Tan E. M., Solomon A. and Prendergast R. A. (1965) Characteristics of an immune system common to certain external secretions. *J. Exp. Med.* **121**, 101.

161 Wada N., Nishida N., Iwaki S., Ohi H., Miyawaki T., Taniguchi N. and Migita S. (1980) Neutralizing activity against *Clostridium difficile* toxin in the supernatants of cultured colostral cells. *Infect. Immun.* **29**, 545.

162 Walker W. A. (1977) Development of intestinal host defence mechanisms and the passive protective role of human milk. Mead Johnson Symposium on Perinatal and Developmental Medicine **11**, 39.

163 Wardlaw A. C. (1962) The complement-dependent bacteriolytic activity of normal human serum. *J. Exp. Med.* **115**, 1231.

164 Weisz-Carrington P., Roux M. E., McWilliams M., Phillips-Quagliata J. M. and Lamm M. E. (1978) Hormonal induction of the secretory immune system in the mammary gland. *Proc. Natl Acad. Sci. USA* **75**, 2928.

165 Welsh J. K. and May J. T. (1979) Anti-infective properties of breast milk. *J. Pediatr.* **94**, 1.

166 Williams R. C. and Gibbons R. J. (1972) Inhibition of bacterial adherence by secretory immunoglobulin A; a mechanism of antigen disposal. *Science* **177**, 697.

167 Willis A. T., Bullen C. L., Williams K., Fogg C. G., Bourne A. and Vignon M. (1973) Breast Milk substitute: A Bacteriological Study. *Br. Med. J.* **4**, 67.

168 Yap P. L., Pryde A., Latham P. J. and McClelland D. B. L. (1979) Serum IgA in the neonate. Molecular size, concentration and effect of breast feeding. *Acta Paed. Scand.* **68**, 695.

169 Zeissler J. and Rassfeld-Sternberg (1949) Enteritis necroticans due to *Clostridium welchii* type F. *Br. Med. J.* **1**, 267.

2 Immunological aspects of the intestinal lymphoid system

G. N. Cooper

Introduction   27
Immunoglobulins of the intestine   28
Transport of immunoglobulins to the intestinal lumen   31
   Transport of monomeric Igs   31
   Transport of polymeric Igs   32
Cellular aspects of the intestinal immune system   33
   Morphology of the gut-associated lymphoid tissue (GALT)   33
   Development and normal functions of the intestinal lymphoid system   36
Immune responses in the intestinal lymphoid system   37
   Cell-mediated immunity   40
Summary   41
References   42

INTRODUCTION

The studies of Besredka,[9] Davies[33] and others more than 50 years ago signalled the existence of specific defence mechanisms that operate within the intestinal tract, often independently of those associated with the internal, circulatory system. Despite this, it is only within the past 20 years that immunologists have developed any lasting interest in the general field of mucosal immunity or, in particular, the local defence mechanisms of the alimentary tract attributable to the intestinal lymphoid system. There are still many features of this system that are the subjects of speculation and hypothesis but in recent times sufficient evidence has accumulated to establish beyond doubt that the gut-associated lymphoid tissue (GALT) has a major bearing on the health and well-being of all vertebrate animals.

Most of the information available on the GALT has been derived from studies in laboratory animals, particularly rodents. Because of differences in anatomical structures, reproductive and digestive physiology of the gut, and age-related changes of the GALT amongst mammalian species, direct extrapolation from one species to another may not always be possible; thus, it must be left to the reader's discretion, and future discoveries, to determine how much of the information presented in this chapter is directly relevant to man. Nevertheless, the GALT of all mammalian species shares a number of common properties and character-istics and it is reasonable to assume that, despite quantitative or even qualitative differences, there must be many similarities in ontogeny and function.

The most obvious common property is that, with the exception of the mesenteric lymph nodes, the GALT of all vertebrates is separated from the external environment by a single layer of cells; this covering sheet is permeable and thus the activity of the GALT is profoundly influenced by immunogenic materials that have almost direct access to it. Furthermore, because of the vast area exposed to the 'external' milieu, the intestinal surface and internal tissues are vulnerable to potentially harmful microorganisms and macromolecules derived from permanent or casual microbial residents, and dietary or other materials that are ingested. Whatever the animal species, it is to be expected that part of the GALT's function is to provide an effective, specific back-up to the innate mech-anical, physiological and chemical defences that protect the intestinal surfaces and tissues from these agents. The basic properties of the specific defence system are the primary concern in this chapter.

IMMUNOGLOBULINS OF THE INTESTINE

Though it is known that phagocytic cells are extruded from the intestinal surface, there is no evidence that they retain their functions in the unfriendly environment of the intestinal lumen. It must therefore be assumed that if immune mechanisms contribute to surface protection, it is probably by means of specific immune globulins. While it has been known for many years that antibodies appear in the faeces after dysentery infection,[33] the importance of mucosal antibody as a specific defence mechanism was first established experimentally for influenza virus infections of the respiratory tract;[37] about the same time, studies on *Vibrio cholerae* infections suggested that the same might apply within the intestine.[17]

During the 1950s, immunochemical techniques were developed for detecting, isolating and characterizing the immunoglobulins (Igs) of body fluids and secretions. In 1959, after identification of the IgM and IgG classes, a third Ig (now known as IgA) was recognized as a minor component of serum.[48] Later a form of IgA was found in several external human secretions in far higher concentrations than in serum; it was distinguishable from serum IgA on the basis of sediment-ation characteristics.[49,73] This 'secretory' IgA (sIgA), has been found to be the predominant class in the secretions of most mammalian species.

In man, the sIgA in all secretions is found as an 11S dimer (MW 390 000 daltons) unlike serum IgA which is a 7S monomer (MW 170 000 daltons). As shown diagrammatically in Fig. 2.1, sIgA contains two extra polypeptides.

The J (joining)-chain is covalently bound to the Fc regions of the molecule and is thought to be necessary for maintenance of the polymeric structure; this J poly-peptide is also present in IgM molecules where it presumably serves the same purpose. The second additional component in sIgA is a 4.2 S glycopeptide (MW

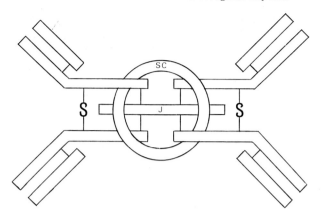

Fig. 2.1 Diagrammatic representation of secretory IgA molecule indicating two IgA monomers linked through the J-chain and incorporation of Secretory Component (SC) in this region of the molecule

58 000 daltons) that is described as the secretory piece (SP) or secretory component (SC); it is bound covalently and non-covalently to the α-chains of the molecule and is believed to exert a stabilizing effect on the polymer, rendering it relatively resistant to enzymic degradation. Two subclasses of IgA (IgA_1 and IgA_2) have been identified in man; both occur in serum but the IgA_2 subclass predominates in secretions. In some animal species, e.g. rodents, serum IgA is often found in the dimeric form and can only be distinguished from sIgA by the absence of SC.[74] A secretory form of IgM has also been identified; SC is, however, bound only by non-covalent forces and thus the molecule is far less stable than sIgA.[13]

The concentrations of Igs in intestinal secretions of man and other animals are shown in Table 2.1. It can be seen that sIgA is not the only Ig class present in the intestinal lumen and also that wide differences exist between and even within species. However, it is normally found that while the IgA:IgG ratio in serum is never less than 1:10, in intestinal secretions it is usually 1:1 or greater. Though IgD and IgE are rarely found in normal intestinal secretions, significant concentrations of IgE have been found in patients suffering from inflammatory conditions of the intestine. In patients suffering from IgA-deficiency syndromes, the total Ig concentration of intestinal secretions is usually little different from normal due to a compensating increase in IgM levels.[29]

Table 2.1 Immunoglobulin concentrations in intestinal secretions

| Species | Reference | Ig concentration (mg per 100 ml) | | |
		IgG	IgM	IgA
Human	42	10	20	31
	15	30	–	30
Rabbit	35	10	2.4	15
Mouse	7	99	524	172
Pig	12	110	20	700

Table 2.2 records the concentrations of the three major Igs present in serum, lymph and gut of rats. The results indicate that the secretions collected by saline

Table 2.2 Immunoglobulin concentrations in serum and materials derived from the intestinal regions of adult UNSW rats*

Material	Ig concentrations (mg per 100 ml)			
	Total	IgG	IgM	IgA
Serum	1340	1250	70	23
Thoracic duct lymph	592	210	22	160
Intestinal surface mucus†	62	31.3	7.9	22.8
Intestinal secretions (saline wash-out)†	34	4.9	0.7	28.4

* Jackson, Cooper and Manning, unpublished observations. † Small intestine preparations concentrated to 1 ml.

washout (or intubation) do not properly reflect the levels of Igs present in the gut. Distortions may arise because of collection methods, contamination with other secretions and, most importantly, the presence of proteolytic enzymes which inevitably weight the values in favour of sIgA; the tenfold drop in IgG and IgM concentrations between the surface mucus and the fluid secretions underlines this point. Other complicating factors are discussed elsewhere.[71]

Thus, when considering the Ig, or antibody content of the intestine, it is convenient to distinguish three compartments as shown in Fig. 2.2. The concentrations of Ig in the fluid secretions and surface mucus can be determined directly but those in the interstitial tissues cannot; however, as suggested by Hall et al.,[45] the concentrations of the latter are probably similar to those in the mesenteric/thoracic duct lymph.

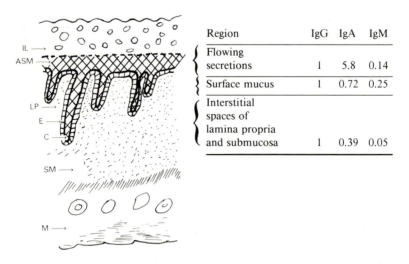

Region	IgG	IgA	IgM
Flowing secretions	1	5.8	0.14
Surface mucus	1	0.72	0.25
Interstitial spaces of lamina propria and submucosa	1	0.39	0.05

Fig. 2.2 Diagrammatic representation of longitudinal section of the small intestine indicating the three regions in which the actual and relative concentrations of the major immunoglobulins differ markedly.
IL, intestinal lumen; ASM, adherent surface mucus; E, epithelium; C, crypts; LP, lamina propria; SM, submucosa; M, muscle layers

Based on the actual Ig concentrations (Table 2.2) and the IgG:IgA:IgM ratios (Fig. 2.2) four features of the intestinal immune system of the rat become evident. First, it is likely that transfer from the blood capillaries accounts for much of the IgG, and possibly IgM, present in the interstitial spaces of the intestinal lamina propria and submucosa, but the marked difference between the IgG:IgA ratios in serum and lymph indicates that much IgA is synthesized within the intestinal tissues. It has been found that the IgA in thoracic duct lymph is polymeric but does not contain SC.[55] Second, there can be little doubt that the Igs present in the surface mucus, which covers the villus tips and almost fills the crypts, are derived from the interstitial spaces of the lamina propria by transepithelial passage. The relative increase in IgA and IgM concentrations compared with IgG between the thoracic duct lymph and surface mucus implies that the mechanisms of transport across the epithelium may be different and favour the secretion of polymeric Igs. Third, it is important to recognize that despite the relative increase in concentrations of IgA, IgG is the predominant Ig of the interstitial spaces and surface mucus, indicating that in both locations IgG antibodies may contribute significantly to humoral immunity through classical mechanisms, such as phagocytosis or complement-mediated effects.[16] Finally, the surface mucus must serve as a major source of the Igs present in the intestinal secretions. It is to be expected that antibodies of the IgA class are the major contributors to any defensive reactions that occur within the secretions.

TRANSPORT OF IMMUNOGLOBULINS TO THE INTESTINAL LUMEN

Although the 'classical' means of humoral defence based on phagocytosis and complement-mediated reactions probably serves as the major protective barrier against microorganisms or other biologically-active agents which penetrate the intestinal epithelium, there is much evidence to suggest that antibodies located within the two intraluminal compartments provide an immune barrier which prevents access of such agents to the mucosal surfaces. However, naturally, maintenance of Igs (antibodies) within the lumen requires different transport mechanisms; the quantities transported are almost certainly governed by their concentrations in the lamina propria, and their molecular size.

Transport of monomeric Igs

Using immunohistochemical techniques, Brandtzaeg and Baklien[13] demonstrated the presence of IgG between the epithelial cells at the villus tips of the small intestine. It is deduced that IgG is passively transuded into the surface mucus at sites where the integrity of the epithelium is most likely to be jeopardized, that is where cells are excluded and lost into the intestine. The mechanism is apparently similar for other mucosal surfaces. Thus in normal hosts, the concentrations of IgG in intestinal surface mucus, and other mucus secretions, should represent a constant, small proportion of the serum levels. After intravenous injection of labelled IgG, the serum:secretion ratio of the labelled IgG has been found to be approximately 40:1, irrespective of the source of the secretion. However, during inflammation associated with a mucosal surface, when the extravascular concentrations of IgG may be increased or the epithelial surface damaged, greater amounts of IgG would exude into the surface secretions.[13] IgE and possibly IgD are also transported to the external surfaces by the same mechanisms.[13]

Transport of polymeric Igs

There is an active and selective mechanism of transport for IgA and IgM across the intestinal and other glandular secretory surfaces; it accounts for the preponderance of sIgA in normal surface secretions and IgM in secretions from patients with IgA-deficiency disease. In contrast to IgG, both these Igs are found in direct association with the secretory cells at the base of the crypts of the small intestine or those of other glandular epithelia, and it is through these cells that Ig secretion occurs. Incorporation of J-chain during assembly of the dimeric IgA, or polymeric IgM, gives rise to a configuration in the Fc region of the molecules that serves as a receptor site for SC.[13] As the Ig molecules are secreted from plasma cells they probably become non-covalently bound to SC which is synthesized by the epithelial cells and concentrated at the baso-lateral aspects of the epithelial cell membrane. Pinocytosis or facilitated diffusion permits uptake of the Ig–SC complex into the epithelial cells where, in the case of sIgA, covalent bonding of the two components occurs. The final event is secretion of the Ig–SC complex along the normal secreting pathways of the cells.[14,32]

In 1970 it was first suggested that antibodies may also enter the intestine by way of bile.[57] The significance of this was not recognized till several years later when Jackson and his colleagues[52,53,54,59] clearly established the existence of a 'hepato-biliary' pump in rodents that was responsible for the rapid removal of polymeric IgA from the blood. The IgA that appeared in bile was of the sIgA class and it was calculated that in the rat, between 10 and 20 mg of it is secreted into the duodenum daily by this route. Subsequent studies have shown that antibodies induced by intraintestinal or Peyer's patch injection of antigens are also secreted through the bile.[25,46] As with the glandular surface secretory mechanisms, it appears that SC, synthesized by the hepatic parenchymal cells[72] serves as the mediator of the transport of IgA from blood to bile.[11,39]

In the rat, the amount of IgA entering the blood daily from the thoracic duct is 20–50 times greater than that present in the circulation.[45] This suggests that much of the IgA in bile is derived from the intestinal tissues. Thoracic duct cannulation in rats leads to a significant decrease in sIgA concentration in bile (Manning and Jackson, unpublished data).

Though the bile of normal rats and chickens contains very little IgM, during the early stages of immune responses appreciable concentrations of specific IgM antibodies are secreted by this route for 2–3 days. Therefore this Ig also may be actively secreted by the hepato-biliary system in the same manner as sIgA. Bile contains low concentrations of IgG which are probably derived by passive exudation across the biliary tree; in hyperimmunized animals this Ig may also serve as an additional source of antibody in bile. Although the biliary transport system is now well-established for rodents, its contribution to the Ig content of the intestinal secretions of man is not yet known.

CELLULAR ASPECTS OF THE INTESTINAL IMMUNE SYSTEM

In contrast to the internal secretory tissues of the lymphoreticular system — the lymph nodes and spleen — the gut lymphoid tissue of man and animals is predominantly concerned with production and secretion of polymeric Igs, particularly those of the sIgA class, including specific antibodies induced by oral or intraintestinal immunization.

Morphology of the gut-associated lymphoid tissue (GALT)

In normal animals and man GALT is the largest component of the lymphoid system and, in terms of cell numbers, makes up approximately 25% of the gut tissues. It occurs as well-defined nodular aggregates in the tonsils, Peyer's patches, appendix and sacculus rotundus and also as non-organized collections of follicles and cells distributed diffusely throughout the submucosa, lamina propria and epithelial layer of the large and small intestine. The chyle-filled lacteals of the mesentery drain from the intestine into the mesenteric lymph node chain; though the morphology and immunological behaviour of these tissues differ in many respects from the superficial GALT, they warrant inclusion as components of the system as they are often exposed to antigens derived from the gut lumen.

The tonsils, appendix and sacculus rotundus participate in immune responses, but the Peyer's patches, the lamina propria, the mesenteric lymph nodes and the epithelial compartment are the sites of the greatest immunological interest, and are described in detail.

INTEREPITHELIAL LYMPHOID TISSUE

Between 10 and 20% of the cells of the intestinal epithelial surface have the morphology of lymphocytes; they are often called theliolymphocytes. It has been estimated that if they were massed together they would form an organ of the size of the pancreas.[38] These cells are located between the columnar epithelial cells, usually immediately above the basement membrane. Many contain well-defined organelles characterized as lysosome-like bodies, ribosomes and mitochondria. This morphological heterogeneity suggests that these cells may undergo blast transformation, mitosis and degeneration and thus may be a self-perpetuating population of cells indigenous to the epithelium; they also move with epithelial cells to the villus tips and are shed into the intestinal lumen.[21] Though mitosis may help maintain the normal theliolymphocyte population, it is believed that they are supplemented by blood-borne lymphoblasts which pass across the lamina propria into the interepithelial compartment. All evidence points to the fact that the theliolymphocytes are thymus-derived (T cells).[34]

LAMINA PROPRIA

The large numbers of plasma cells underlying the epithelium are easily seen, but the lymphocyte population is equivalent in numbers, and during the course of a number of intestinal diseases considerable changes occur in the relative numbers of these two populations.[79] Irrespective of the animal species the duodenal and jejunal regions are richest in plasma cells and the colon is poorest.[28] Throughout the intestine, plasma cells containing IgA are most abundant, usually amounting to 80% of the total. The ratio of IgA-:IgG-:IgM-containing cells has usually been found to be 10:1.6:1, while smaller numbers of IgE- and IgD-containing cells are also found.[4] Significant changes in these ratios have been reported in sections from patients suffering from a number of gastrointestinal diseases.[78] Both B cells and T cells have been found amongst the lymphocyte populations and it has been suggested that an appreciable number of the latter class may possess suppressor functions (Clancy, personal communication).

PEYER'S PATCHES

Embryologically these discrete nodular aggregates appear on the antimesenteric border of the jejunum and ileum. In man they first become obvious about the 24th week of gestation; their size and number increase after birth and by puberty approximately 240 may be identified. Thereafter, there is a gradual loss by involution.[27] Though structurally similar in other mammalian species, the numbers, size and occurrence of age-related changes differ considerably. Thus in rats they do not become obvious until after birth and generally number no more than 10 to 12.

Four recent regions have been identified on both structural and functional grounds;[64,65,77] these are illustrated in Fig. 2.3. The covering epithelium is quite distinctive; the normal columnar epithelium is replaced by a thin membrane consisting of cells containing numerous micro-folds (M cells). These interdigitate with each other forming a lattice-like network which forms tight junctions with the surrounding columnar epithelium.

Immediately beneath the membrane, the 'dome' region is found to contain numerous medium and large lymphocytes, predominantly of T cell origin, and macrophages that often contain bacterial debris. Membranous processes of the lymphocytes are regularly seen in close proximity to the bases of M cells and are often separated by an electron dense substance that suggests an exchange of macromolecular material in this region. Underlying the dome is the 'corona', a region of densely packed small lymphocytes intermingled with macrophages.

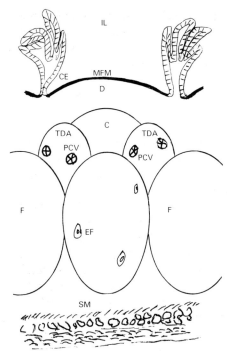

Fig. 2.3 Diagrammatic representation of longitudinal section of a Peyer's patch. IL, intestinal lumen; CE, columnar epithelium; MFM, microfold cell membrane; D, dome; C, corona; TDA, thymus-dependent area; PCV, postcapillary venules; R, follicles; EF, efferent lymphatics; SM, submucosa

This region merges with the 'follicles' which contain large germinal centres composed of blast cells and cells undergoing mitosis; the cells in these regions are of B cell origin. The 'thymus-dependent region' is adjacent to the corona, immediately above the follicles. It contains large numbers of small lymphocytes (T cells) and post-capillary venules are obvious within it. The lymphatic system consists only of efferent vessels originating in the follicles, which transfer materials and cells directly to the mesenteric lymph nodes via the lacteals. The follicles resemble those found in other lymphoid tissues, but they do not carry a mantle of small lymphocytes nor are dendritic reticulum cells present. Moreover, very few cells containing Igs are to be seen within these tissues.

MESENTERIC LYMPH NODES

This large chain of lymph nodes lies in the direct pathway of drainage from the superficial GALT; the lacteals carry the macromolecular products of digestion — chylomicra — microorganisms, antigens, lymphocytes and plasma cells from the Peyer's patches, lamina propria and submucosa to their cortical sinuses. Unless trapped within the nodes, these materials pass to the major lymph trunks and thence to the blood via the thoracic duct. These lymph nodes normally have an abundance of large, secondary cortical follicles, well-defined paracortical regions and large numbers of plasma cells in the medulla. In contrast to the lamina propria, IgA-containing cells are less numerous than those containing IgG and

IgM; there is, in fact, little to distinguish these lymph nodes from those taken from other regions of the body. More detailed descriptions of the lymph nodes are to be found elsewhere.[81]

Development and normal functions of the intestinal lymphoid system

Studies of the GALT and other lymphoid tissues of germ-free rodents have revealed that they are poorly developed and generally restricted to relatively small accumulations of small lymphocytes; plasma cells are few in number and usually are found to be confined to IgM-production. However, after presentation of specific antigens intraintestinally,[24,31] or after acquisition of an intestinal microflora,[30] the GALT develops and within 3–4 weeks displays the characteristics of normal GALT. The GALT of human and other animal fetuses is also poorly developed and only expands during the early stages of extrauterine life. The full development of the GALT is probably antigen-dependent and associated with the establishment of the natural gut-associated microflora. The wide range of the latter must present a vast array of antigenic specificities at the epithelial surface. Their presence probably maintains the processes of cell differentiation and maturation sufficient to account for the large, seemingly constant populations of plasma cells within the intestinal lamina propria and submucosa. Dietary and other ingested materials may further supplement these processes.

If this view is correct, two obvious predictions can be made. First, the GALT will be constantly primed to respond to a great many antigens but may fail to respond normally when confronted with a specificity not likely to have been encountered previously; this point will be considered in a later section. Second, the GALT will serve as a continual source of antibodies of many different specificities. Because of the large excess of IgA-forming plasma cells present in the intestinal lamina propria and submucosa they should be primarily of the IgA class.

The appearance of 'natural' antibodies in the serum of animals is connected with the acquisition and development of the intestinal microflora. These antibodies are maintained at relatively constant, but low, levels throughout the life of the animal; they react specifically with a wide range of microbial and other antigens and, in serum, have been found in association with all three major classes of Igs. The surface mucus of the normal rat intestine also contains these antibodies and the bile has been found to contain appreciably greater levels than serum; the latter have been found to be of the sIgA class (Jackson and Cooper, unpublished data). Most of the natural antibodies produced within the GALT are of the IgA class and those which enter the serum via the thoracic duct are rapidly secreted through the hepato-biliary system. Maintenance of natural antibody production is dependent upon the continued presence of a particular antigenic specificity within the intestinal lumen.[40] The amount of any individual antigen within the intestinal lumen, and the extent of this uptake may exercise some primary control over natural antibody production, but the striking constancy of the concentration of all these antibodies indicates that the GALT has the capacity for rigorous control and regulation of antibody production. It is possible that this is exercised by suppressor T cell populations present in these tissues, which regulate responses to naturally acquired — or deliberately presented — antigenic materials.

Natural antibodies of the IgM and IgG classes within serum and extravascular tissues constitute an important first line of defence against microbial invasion, exerting their influence through the classical pathways of phagocytosis and complement-mediated lysis. However as antibodies of these classes are only minor products of the GALT, there are presumably other, perhaps fundamentally more important, roles for those of the IgA class. It is likely that the naturally-occurring sIgA antibodies of the flowing secretions and surface mucus of the intestine, through complexing with luminal antigens, restrict their access to, and passage through, the mucosal surface. However it is certain that some antigens, even if only in minute quantities, do get absorbed into the intestinal tissues. Reaction of these antigens with natural IgG or IgM antibodies in this region could lead to complement activation and generation of the mediators of acute inflammatory responses. Such responses could, if unchecked, jeopardize the integrity and normal functions of the intestinal surface and its underlying tissues. IgA antibodies appear to block certain complement-mediated reactions[56,61] while polymeric IgA has been found to interfere with the phagocytic and digestive capacities of polymorphonuclear cells;[75] it is therefore possible that naturally-induced IgA antibodies control or restrict inflammatory reactions in the vicinity of the mucosal surface. In a similar context, Andre *et al.*[2] have found that oral feeding of antigen induces tolerance in the systemic immune system; this is attributable to circulating IgA-antigen complexes. It is therefore possible that complexes of natural IgA antibodies and antigens absorbed from the intestine limit systemic immune responses which would otherwise cause the appearance of potentially harmful levels of IgG (or IgM) antibodies in the intestinal tissues.

IMMUNE RESPONSES IN THE INTESTINAL LYMPHOID SYSTEM

The GALT of man and animals is capable of mounting specific humoral immune responses to antigens derived from the intestinal lumen and these augment the natural defence mechanisms of the region. Some aspects of the responses are poorly understood, but these are sometimes ignored by those who favour simple unifying concepts rather than a holistic explanation of a system that cannot be anything else but complicated. Thus the dogma that places Peyer's patches as the essential generators of immune responses[68] cannot account for the findings of the elegant studies by Ogra *et al.*[63] which demonstrated that local IgA synthesis occurred only in sites of antigen contact that were devoid of these tissues. A second area of uncertainty relates to the routes of uptake and localization of antigen. It is clear that some protein antigens — ferritin and horse radish peroxidase — are primarily taken into the Peyer's patches, and these tissues are also, probably, a major portal of entry for many living microorganisms.[8] The M cells of the dome epithelium are specifically involved; antigen enters the surface pits, passes into their tubulo-vascular network then becomes enclosed in vesicles which serve as carriers across the cell, discharging the material into the M cell lattice cavities by reverse pinocytosis.[65] Antigen is thus presented in close proximity to T cells and may also be taken up by macrophages in the dome region. At present there is little quantitative information on the extent of antigen-uptake by this route, or on the amounts sequestered in the Peyer's patches or transferred to the mesenteric lymph nodes and the general circulation.

When hamsters were orally immunized with bovine serum albumin none of it was found in Peyer's patches, but was detected in the macrophages of the intestinal lamina propria and throughout the peripheral lymphoid tissues.[10] This might suggest that, for some antigens, direct absorption across the epithelial surfaces may also occur. Intercellular passage of microorganisms and other particulate materials also appears to occur through the villus tips of the small intestine, a phenomenon described as 'persorption';[67] submucosal entrapment is apparently limited because materials entering by this route can be found in the blood within a few minutes of per-oral administration. Some may eventually return to and sequester in the lamina propria.

Specific antibody synthesis in the intestinal tissues has been established.[6,18] However when antigen is derived from the intestinal lumen, often the immune responses of GALT are augmented by simultaneous responses in the mesenteric lymph nodes and spleen, which are responsible for the appearance of IgM and IgG antibodies frequently found in serum following intestinal immunization.[23,58,69] These responses have been attributed to transport of antigen from the local sites to the internal lymphoid tissues.

Local application of antigen leads to the appearance of specific IgA-antibody synthesizing plasma cells in the intestinal lamina propria.[47] There is a clear distinction between the IgA-oriented responses of the intestinal lamina propria and the IgM-IgG directed responses of the mesenteric lymph nodes and spleen.[69] With some antigens at least, Peyer's patches are the key sites for generation of immune responses within the intestinal tissues, despite the fact that they have limited capacity for in situ antibody formation.[68] It is now clear that on contact with antigen, precursors of IgA-antibody forming cells are produced within these tissues; these cells then migrate through the mesenteric lymph nodes, the blood and subsequently sequester in the lamina propria where they mature to IgA-producing plasma cells. It is likely that the precursor cells undergo part of the differentiation processes within the mesenteric lymph nodes[62] and the spleen.[19] It is not known whether the same movement between these compartments of the GALT occurs in the case of cells destined to produce antibodies of the other Ig-classes nor whether Peyer's patches are the only sources of these cells. It is likely, for instance, that some may be derived from the submucosal follicles and move directly to the lamina propria.

The classic studies of Gowans and Knight[43] first drew attention to the fact that approximately 50% of the small lymphocyte population continually traverses the lymphoid system by way of trafficking through the blood and lymphatics; this recirculating pool of T cells is of fundamental importance in many functions of the immune system.[41] The GALT is an integral part of the traffic system, receiving small lymphocytes from blood capillaries in the lamina propria and the post-capillary venules of the Peyer's patches. In these regions they may come in contact with antigens, thereupon becoming participants in immune responses either locally or in other tissues that may be in their migration pathway. Additionally, however, the GALT acts as an independent, open-ended migratory system in which cells are continually transferred from one region to another, are lost through the epithelium and replaced by others generated within it. The migratory and differentiation pathways taken by the specifically-induced precursor cells of the Peyer's patches are identical to those taken by similar cells in the non-immunized animal;[50] in the latter case, covert antigenic stimulation almost certainly accounts for their development and the appearance of IgA-synthesizing cells in the lamina propria. The mechanisms which promote homing of these cells to the intestinal tissues are far from clear; it may be, in part, antigen-dependent but may also reflect some non-antigenic, possibly physiological, properties of the small intestine.[50]

One of the intriguing questions that remains to be answered concerns the extraordinary class commitment of the intestinal tissues, and those associated with other glandular secretory surfaces, to IgA production. The foregoing sections underline this in respect of the highly favoured IgA antibody formation when antigen is given via the intestine. This commitment is also seen in terms of memory cell formation. For instance, large numbers of these cells, committed to IgA-antibody production on subsequent exposure to antigen, appear in extraintestinal tissues following a single intestinal injection of antigen.[70] Though there is no direct supporting evidence, it has been speculated that the phenomenon may relate to the method of antigen presentation. It has been noted that there are certain compartments of the GALT — tonsils[51] and mesenteric lymph nodes[69] — in which humoral responses favour IgM and IgG antibody production. These tissues obviously behave as peripheral lymphoid tissues where dendritic processes of reticular cells play an important role in antigen display. These cells and processes do not occur in Peyer's patches or submucosal lymphoid follicles where macrophages appear to be the only likely vehicles for presenting antigen to the lymphocytic cells.

With regard to the nature of the differentiation and maturation processes that occur in the IgA-committed precursor cells once they are induced by antigen contact, it has been suggested that these cells are first induced to IgM-antibody formation and that later they switch to IgA production either directly or with an intermediate stage of IgG production.[50] Helper T cells, known to be present in Peyer's patches,[36] may directly cause the switch.[76] Others have suggested that class commitment is both antigen and thymus-independent; and that T cells function by forcing the maturation of immature B cells — IgM-antibody formers — to plasma cells which synthesize antibodies of the IgA or IgG classes.[80] Large numbers of cells, which can be induced to IgM-antibody production, appear in the spleen within 6–24 hours of Peyer's patch injection of a specific antigen;[26] this suggests that the cells produced early in the intestinal immune response are IgM-formers and their maturation to IgA-producing plasma cells occurs once they reach the lamina propria. However it must be questioned whether T cells are essential for maturation.[1] It is interesting to note that though the serum of athymic (nude) mice is low in IgA levels, their lamina propria has normal populations of IgA-forming plasma cells[80] and their bile contains almost normal levels of sIgA (Jackson, personal communication). In addition, sIgA antibodies specific for the lipopolysaccharide (LPS) somatic antigens of several Gram-negative organisms appear in intestinal secretions and bile following intraintestinal[25] or Peyer's patch injection[46] of the whole organisms; this class of antigen is presumed to be capable of antibody formation without T cell assistance. These observations suggest that the peculiar environment of the Peyer's patch (and the intestinal lamina propria or submucosa) may force a direct IgM to IgA switch without involvement of helper T cells.

The nature of secondary antibody responses in the intestinal tissues has not been explored in detail. However most evidence suggests that these tissues do not display the memory responses characteristic of lymph nodes and the spleen (see Chapter 12). In most instances responses to second or repeated doses of antigen given intraintestinally are no greater and no more prolonged than those which occur after the first dose. The one exception so far reported has concerned immunization of dogs with cholera toxoid; no response was observed following a first series of intestinal injections whereas after a second course given some weeks later, a brief but significant IgA-antitoxin response occurred.[66] These observations may be explained in terms of the constantly-primed state of the GALT arising from continual exposure to antigens of microbial and dietary origin;[20] thus, it is possible that the normal, IgA-directed responses of the GALT to many antigens are in fact secondary-type reactions. However when confronted with an antigen carrying a specificity not likely to have been experienced previously, priming occurs first, and later exposures to the same specificity induce the characteristic IgA-directed response. It might be argued on teleological grounds that because of the continued presentation of many different antigens, it would be most unlikely for the GALT to discriminate to the extent of favouring excess memory development or prolonged antibody production against a specific antigen that has been deliberately introduced into the intestinal lumen.

Cell-mediated immunity

At present little is definitely known about this limb of the defence system except that the intraepithelial lymphocytes may be involved. These cells are probably generated in Peyer's patches and traverse the same routes as the activated B cell populations.[44] They appear to be the only lymphocytes of the GALT which possess direct and antibody-mediated cytotoxic activities.[3] T cells from Peyer's patches have also been shown to participate in graft-versus-host reactions,[60] again indicating the potential of these tissues for generating cells possessing effector T cell functions. Little is known of the roles these cells may play within the intestine, though it seems reasonable to assume that they are primarily concerned with surveillance mechanisms, perhaps in the control of fortuitously-developing neoplastic cells and in macrophage-mediated defence against invading microorganisms.

SUMMARY

Immunity to potentially harmful microorganisms and macromolecules which may attach to or penetrate the intestinal surface is dependent upon local defence mechanisms that are largely attributable to functions of the intestinal lymphoid system. These functions are shared by other components of the lympho-reticular tissues that are associated with glandular secretory surfaces and are distinctive in terms of their pre-emption to production and secretion of polymeric antibodies, particularly those of the sIgA class. While many features of the development and behaviour of the intestinal lymphoid system have been clarified over the past 10 years, other features remain within the realms of speculation. Despite this qualification, it is now possible to construct a reasonable working model which accounts for both cellular and humoral aspects of the intestine's local defence system. Figure 2.4 presents this model in as simple a form as possible.

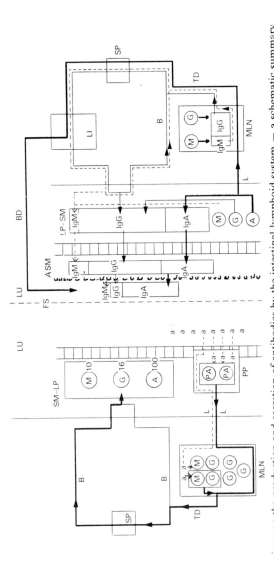

Fig. 2.4 Current views on the production and secretion of antibodies by the intestinal lymphoid system – a schematic summary.

(a) *Antigen uptake and cell traffic.* Antigen (a) enters Peyer's patches (PP) from the lumen (LU) and induces IgA-antibody precursor cells (PA); these cells move from the PP along the route shown by the solid line via the lacteals (L), the mesenteric lymph node (MLN) and the thoracic duct (TD). They enter the blood (B) pass through the spleen and 'home' to the intestinal lamina propria and submucosa (SM-LP) where they mature to IgA-antibody producing cells (A). It is possible that some antigen follows the route of the broken line, enters the MLN and induces IgM- and IgG-antibody producing cells (M) (G), a proportion of which also traverse the lymph and blood, appearing later in the SM-LP; the majority remain within the MLN.

(b) *Routes of secretion of the major immunoglobulins.*

→ IgA ⟶ IgG ⋯⟩⋯ IgM

○⋯ cells producing immunoglobulins M,G or A

⋯⋯ Immunoglobulin content (and relative proportions in mesenteric lymph node (MLN), lamina propria and submucosa (LP-SM), adherent surface mucus (ASM) and flowing secretions (FS) of the intestinal lumen (LU).

Note that whilst IgG and probably most IgM that enters ASM and FS is derived from the LP-SM by transepithelial passage, a proportion of the IgA formed in the LP-SM passes via the lacteals (L) through the MLN and enters the blood (B) via the thoracic duct (TD); it is removed in the liver (LI) and enters the LU via the bile duct (BD) and may contribute to the IgA content of the FS.

Most of the IgG and IgM is produced in the MLN (and other peripheral lymphoid tissues) and enters the LP-SM by exudation from the blood. IgM and

REFERENCES

1 Abney E. R., Cooper M. D., Kearney J. F., Lawson A. R. and Parkhouse R. M. (1978) Sequential expression of immunoglobulin on developing mouse B lymphocytes: a systematic survey that suggests a model for the generation of immunoglobulin isotype diversity. *J. Immunol.* **120**, 2041.

2 Andre C., Heremans J. F., Vaerman J. P. and Cambiaso C. L. (1975) A mechanism for the induction of immunological tolerance by antigen feeding: antigen-antibody complexes. *J. Exp. Med.* **142**, 1509.

3 Arnaud-Battandier F., Bundy B. M., O'Neill M., Bienenstock J. and Nelson D. L. (1978) Cytotoxic activities of gut mucosal lymphoid cells in guinea pigs. *J. Immunol.* **121**, 1059

4 Baklien K. and Brandtzaeg P. (1976) Immunohistochemical characterization of local immunoglobulin formation in Crohn's disease of the ileum. *Scand. J. Gastroent.* **11**, 447.

5 Bankhurst A. D., Lambert P. H. and Miescher P. A. (1975) Studies on the thymic dependence of the immunoglobulin classes of the mouse. *Proc. Soc. Exp. Biol. and Med.* **148**, 501.

6 Batty I. and Warrack G. H. (1955) Local antibody production in the mammary gland, spleen, uterus, vagina and appendix of the rabbit. *J. Path. Bact.* **70**, 355.

7 Bazin H., Maldague P., Schonne E., Crabbe P. A., Bauldon H. and Heremans J. F. (1971) The metabolism of different immunoglobulin classes in irradiated mice. V. Contribution of the gut to serum IgA levels in normal and irradiated mice. *Immunology* **20**, 571.

8 Berg R. D. and Garlington A. W. (1979) Translocation of certain indigenous bacteria from the gastrointestinal tract to the mesenteric lymph nodes and other organs in a gnotobiotic mouse model. *Infect. Immun.* **23**, 403.

9 Besredka A. (1923–24) Local immunity in infectious diseases. *Trans. R. Soc. Trop. Med. Hyg.* **17**, 346.

10 Bienenstock J. and Dolezel J. (1971) Peyer's patches: lack of specific antibody-containing cells after oral and parenteral immunization. *J. Immunol.* **106**, 938.

11 Birbeck M. S., Cartwright P., Hall J. G., Orlans E. and Peppard J. (1979) The transport by hepatocytes of immunoglobulin A from blood to bile visualized by autoradiography and electron microscope. *Immunology* **37**, 477.

12 Bourne F. J., Honour J. W. and Pickup J. (1971) Natural antibodies to *Escherichia coli* in the pig. *Immunology* **20**, 433.

13 Brandtzaeg P. and Baklien K. (1976) Immunohistochemical studies of the formation and epithelial transport of immunoglobulins in normal and diseased human intestinal mucosa. *Scand. J. Gastroenterol.* **11**, Suppl. 36, 1.

14 Brown W. R., Isobe K., Nakane P. K. and Pacini B. (1977) Studies on translocation of immunoglobulins across intestinal epithelium. IV. Evidence for binding of IgA and IgM to secretory component in intestinal epithelium. *Gastroenterology* **73**, 1333.

15 Bull D. M., Bienenstock J. and Tomasi T. B. Jr. (1971) Studies on human intestinal immunoglobulin A. *Gastroenterology* **60**, 370.

16 Burrows W. (1975) The function of antibody in local immunity in the small bowel. *Immunochemistry* **12**, 621.

17 Burrows W. and Havens I. (1948) Studies on immunity to Asiatic cholera. V. The absorption of immune globulin from the bowel and its excretion in the urine and faeces of experimental animals and human volunteers. *J. Infect. Dis.* **82**, 231.

18 Burrows W. and Ware L. L. (1953) Studies on immunity to Asiatic cholera. VII. Prophylactic immunity to experimental enteric cholera. *J. Infect. Dis.* **92**, 164.

19 Cebra J. J., Kamat R., Gearhart P., Robertson S. M. and Tseng J. (1977) The secretory IgA system of the gut. In: *Immunology of the Gut*, Ciba Foundn Symposium vol. **46**, pp. 5 and 26.

20 Cebra J. J., Emmons R., Gearhart P. J., Robertson S. M. and Tseng J. (1978) Cellular parameters of the IgA response. *Adv. Exp. Med. Biol.* **107**, 19.

21 Collan Y. (1972) Characteristics of nonepithelial cells in the epithelium of normal rat ileum. *Scand. J. Gastroenterol.* (Suppl.) **7**, 1.

22 Cooper G. N., Halliday W. H. and Thonard J. D. (1967) Immunological reactivity associated with antigens in the intestinal tract of rats. *J. Path. Bact.* **93**, 223.

23 Cooper G. N. and Thonard J. C. (1967) Serum antibody responses to intestinal implantation of antigens in rats. *J. Path. Bact.* **93**, 213.

24 Cooper G. N., Thonard J. C., Crosby R. L. and Dalbow M. H. (1968) Immunological responses in rats following antigenic stimulation of Peyers patches; II Immunological changes in germ free rats. *Aust. J. Exp. Biol. Med. Sci.* **46**, 407.

25 Cooper G. N. and Jackson G. D. F. (1981) Immune responses of rats to live *Vibrio cholerae*; secretion of antibody in bile. *Parasit. Immunol.* **3**, 127.

26 Cooper G. N. and Turner K. (1969) Development of IgM memory in rats after antigenic stimulation of Peyer's patches. *J.R.E. Soc.* **6**, 419.

27 Cornes J. S. (1965) Number, size and distribution of Peyer's patches in the human small intestine. 1. The development of Peyer's patches. *Gut* **6**, 225.

28 Crabbe P. A., Carbonara A. O. and Heremans J. F. (1965) The normal human intestinal mucosa as a major source of plasma cells containing gamma-a-immunoglobulin. *Lab. Invest.* **14**, 235.

29 Crabbe P. A. and Heremans J. F. (1967) Selective IgA deficiency with steatorrhea. A new syndrome. *Am. J. Med.* **42**, 319.

30 Crabbe P. A., Bazin H., Eyssen H. and Heremans J. F. (1968) The normal microbial flora as a major stimulus for proliferation of plasma cells synthesizing IgA in the gut. *Int. Arch. Allergy* **34**, 362.

31 Crabbe P. A., Nash D. R., Bazin H., Eyssen H. and Heremans J. F. (1969) Antibodies of the IgA type in intestinal plasma cells of germfree mice after oral or parenteral immunization with ferritin. *J. Exp. Med.* **130**, 723.

32 Crago S. S., Kulhavy R., Prince S. J. and Mestecky J. (1978) Secretory component of epithelial cells as a surface receptor for polymeric immunoglobulins. *J. Exp. Med.* **147**, 1832.

33 Davies A. (1922) An investigation into the serological properties of dysentery stools. *Lancet* **ii**, 1009.

34 Douglas A. P. and Weetman A. P. (1975) Lymphocytes and the gut. *Digestion* **13**, 344.

35 Eddie D. S., Schulkind M. L. and Robbins J. B. (1971) The isolation and biologic activities of purified secretory IgA and IgG anti-*Salmonella typhimurium* 'O' antibodies from rabbit intestinal fluid and colostrum. *J. Immunol.* **106**, 181.

36 Elson C. O., Heck J. A. and Strober W. (1979) T-cell regulation of murine IgA synthesis. *J. Exp. Med.* **149**, 632.

37 Fazekas de St Groth S., Donnelley M. and Graham D. M. (1951) Studies in experimental immunology of influenza. VIII. Pathotopic adjuvants. *Aust. J. Exp. Biol. Med. Sci.* **29**, 323.

38 Ferguson A. (1972) Immunological roles of the gastrointestinal tract. *Scott. Med. J.* **17**, 111.

39 Fisher M. M., Nagy B., Bazin H. and Underdown B. J. (1979) Biliary transport of IgA: role of secretory component. *Proc. Natl Acad. Sci. USA* **76**, 2008.

40 Foo M. C., Lee A. and Cooper G. N. (1974) Natural antibodies and the intestinal flora of rodents. *Aust. J. Exp. Biol. Med. Sci.* **52**, 321.

41 Ford W. L. and Gowans J. L. (1969) The traffic of lymphocytes. *Seminars in Haematology* **6**, 67.

42 Girard J. P. and de Kalbermatten A. (1970) Antibody activity in human duodenal fluid. *Europ. J. Clin. Invest.* **1**, 188.

43 Gowans J. L. and Knight E. J. (1964) The route of recirculation of lymphocytes in the rat. *Proc. R. Soc. (Biol.)* **159**, 257.

44 Guy-Grand D., Griscelli C. and Vassalli P. (1974) The gut-associated lymphoid system: nature and properties of the large dividing cells. *Europ: J. Immunol.* **4**, 435.

45 Hall J., Orlans E., Peppard J. and Reynolds J. (1978) Lymphatic physiology and secretory immunity. *Adv. Exp. Med. Biol.* **107**, 29.

46 Hall J., Orlans E., Reynolds J., Dean C., Peppard J., Gyure L. and Hobbs S. (1979) Occurrence of specific antibodies of the IgA class in the bile of rats. *Int. Archs. Allergy Appl. Immun.* **59**, 75.

47 Heremans J. F. and Bazin H. (1971) Antibodies induced by local antigenic stimulation of mucosal surfaces. *Ann. N.Y. Acad. Sci.* **190**, 268.

48 Heremans J. F., Heremans M. Th. and Schultze H. E. (1959) Isolation and description of a few properties of the β2A-globulin of human serum. *Clin. Chim. Acta* **4**, 96.

49 Heremans J. F., Vaerman J. P., Carbonara A. O., Rodhaim J. A. and Heremans M. Th. (1963) γ1A-Globulin (β2A-Globulin): its isolation properties, functions and pathology. *Protides. Biol. Fluids, Proc. Colloq.* **10**, 108.

50 Husband A. J., Monie H. J. and Gowans J. L. (1977) The natural history of the cells producing IgA in the gut. In: *Immunology of the Gut*. Ciba Foundation Symposium. **46**, 29, 26.

51 Ishikawa T., Wicher K. and Arbesman C. E. (1972) Distribution of immunoglobulins in palatine and pharyngeal tonsils. *Int. Arch. Allergy and Appl. Immunol.* **43**, 801.

52 Jackson G. D. F., Lemaitre-Coelho I. and Vaerman J. P. (1977) The clearance of MOPC-315-tumour immunoglobulin A from the serum of BALB/c mice. *Proc. Biochem. Soc. Trans.* **5**, 1576.

53 Jackson G. D. F., Lemaitre-Coelho I. and Vaerman J. P. (1977) Transfer of MOPC-315 IgA to secretions in MOPC-315 tumour-bearing and normal BALB/c mice. *Prot. Biol. Fluids* **25**, 919.

54 Jackson G. D. F., Vaerman J. P. and de Steenwinkel F. (1977) Clearance of I.V.-injected MOPC-315 IgA from normal BALB/c mouse serum. *Prot. Biol. Fluids* **25**, 927.

55 Kaartinen M., Imir T., Klockars M., Sandholm M. and Makela O. (1978) IgA in blood and thoracic duct lymph: concentration and degree of polymerization. *Scand. J. Immunol.* **7**, 229.

56 Kearney R. and Halliday W. J. (1970) Immunity and paralysis in mice. Serological and biological properties of two distinct antibodies to type III pneumococcal polysaccharide. *Immunology* **19**, 551.

57 Keclik M., Wolf R. H., Felsenfeld O. and Smetana H. F. (1970) Immunoglobulins and antibodies in gall-bladder bile. *Am. J. Gastroenterol.* **54**, 19.

58 Kenrick K. G. and Cooper G. N. (1978) Antibodies in the intestinal secretions of rats. Primary and secondary responses to polymeric flagellin. *Aust. J. Exp. Biol. Med. Sci.* **56**, 441.

59 Lemaitre-Coelho I., Jackson G. D. F. and Vaerman J. P. (1977) Rat bile as a convenient source of secretory IgA and free secretory component. *Europ. J. Immunol.* **7**, 588.

60 MacDonald T. T. and Carter P. B. (1978) Mouse Peyer's patches contain T-cells capable of inducing the graft-versus-host reaction (GVHR). *Transplantation* **26**, 162.

61 McLeod Griffiss J. (1975) Bactericidal activity of meningococcal antisera. Blocking by IgA of lytic antibody in human convalescent sera. *J. Immunol.* **114**, 1779.

62 McWilliams M., Phillips-Quagliata J. M. and Lamm M. E. (1977) Mesenteric lymph node B lymphoblasts which home to the small intestine are precommitted to IgA synthesis. *J. Exp. Med.* **145**, 866.

63 Ogra P. L., Wallace R. B., Umana G., Ogra S. S., Kerr-Grant D. and Morag A. (1974) Implications of secretory immune system in viral infections. *Adv. Exp. Med. Biol.* **45**, 271.

64 Owen R. L. and Jones A. L. (1974) Epithelial cell specialization within human Peyer's patches: an ultrastructural study of intestinal lymphoid follicles. *Gastroenterology* **66**, 189.

65 Owen R. L. and Nemanic P. (1978) Antigen processing structures of the mammalian intestinal tract: an SEM study of lymphoepithelial organs. *Scanning Electron Microscopy* **2**, 367.

66 Pierce N. F. and Reynolds H. Y. (1975) Immunity to experimental cholera. II. Secretory and humoral antitoxin response to local and systemic toxoid administration. *J. Infect. Dis.* **131**, 383.

67 Raettig H. (1970) Mechanisms of oral immunization with inactivated microorganisms. *Progr. Immunobiol. Standard.* **4**, 337.

68 Robertson S. M. and Cebra J. J. (1976) A model for local immunity. *La Ricerca in Clinica e in Laboratoria* **VI**, Suppl., 3.

69 Robertson P. W. and Cooper G. N. (1972) Immune responses in intestinal tissues to particulate antigens. Plaque forming and rosette forming cell responses in rats. *Aust. J. Exp. Biol. Med. Sci.* **50**, 703.

70 Robertson P. W. and Cooper G. N. (1973) Immune responses in intestinal tissues to particulate antigens. Development of cells forming different classes of antibody in primary and secondary responses. *Aust. J. Exp. Biol. Med. Sci.* **51**, 575.

71 Samson R. R., McClelland D. B. L. and Shearman D. J. (1973) Studies on the quantitation of immunoglobulin in human intestinal secretions. *Gut* **14**, 616.

72 Socken D. J., Jeejeebhoy K. N., Bazin H. and Underdown B. J. (1977) Identification of secretory component as an IgA receptor on rat hepatocytes. *J. Exp. Med.* **150**, 1538.

73 Tomasi T. B. and Zigelbaum S. (1963) The selective occurrence of γ1A globulins in certain body fluids. *J. Clin. Invest.* **42**, 1552.

74 Vaerman J. P., Andre C., Bazin H. and Heremans J. F. (1973) Mesenteric lymph as a major source of serum IgA in guinea pigs and rats. *Europ. J. Immunol.* **3**, 580.

75 Van Epps D. E., Reed K. and Williams R. C. Jr. (1978) Suppression of human PMN bactericidal activity by human IgA paraproteins. *Cell. Immunol.* **36**, 363.

76 Vitetta E. S., Grundke-Iqbal I., Holmes K. V. and Uhr J. W. (1974) Cell surface immunoglobulin: VII Synthesis shedding and secretion of immunoglobulin by lymphoid cells of germ-free mice. *J. Exp. Med.* **139**, 862.

77 Waksman B. H. and Ozer H. (1976) Specialized amplification elements in the immune system. The role of nodular lymphoid organs in the mucous membranes. *Progr. Allergy* **21**, 1.

78 Weibel E. R. (1975) Quantitation in morphology: possibilities and limits. *Beitr. Path. (Anat.)* **155**, 1.

79 Whitehead R. and Skinner J. M. (1978) Morphology of the gut associated lymphoid system in health and disease: a review. *Pathology* **10**, 3.

80 Weisz-Carrington P., Schrater A. F., Lamm M. E. and Thorbecke G. J. (1979) Immunoglobulin isotypes in plasma cells of normal and athymic mice. *Cell Immunol.* **44**, 343.

81 Yoffey J. M. and Courtice F. C. (1970) *Lymphatics, Lymph and the Lymphomyeloid Complex.* Academic Press, London.

3 Salmonellosis, campylobacter enteritis and shigella dysentery

B. Rowe and R. J. Gross

Salmonellosis	47
Epidemiology	49
Pathogenesis	52
Clinical features	53
Treatment	53
Laboratory investigations	54
Campylobacter enteritis	55
Epidemiology	56
Pathogenesis	57
Clinical features	58
Treatment	59
Laboratory investigations	59
Shigella dysentery	60
Epidemiology	62
Pathogenesis	64
Clinical features	65
Treatment	66
Laboratory investigations	67
References	72

SALMONELLOSIS

Members of the genus *Salmonella* are characterized by their biochemical reactions. On this basis they are divided into four subgenera (Table 3.1), although the great majority of clinical isolates belong to subgenus I. Within these subgenera they are divided into serotypes according to their somatic 'O' and flagella 'H' antigens. On this basis about 2000 serotypes have been recognized and are included in the internationally accepted Kauffmann-White scheme. There is disagreement concerning the taxonomic status of these serotypes. Many authorities regard them all as species, while others accept only three species, *S. typhi*, *S. cholerae-suis* and *S. enteritidis*, and regard all others as serotypes or 'vars' of these. *S. typhimurium* might thus be written as *S. enteritidis* var

47

Table 3.1 Salmonella subgenera

Subgenus	Occurrence Humans	Animals	No. serotypes (approx.)	Biochemical reactions Dulcitol	Lactose	β galactosidase	Salicin	D-tartrate	Mucate	Malonate	Gelatin	KCN
I	Important cause of disease	Important cause of disease in a wide range of animals	1100	+	-	-	-	+	+	-	-	-
II	Rare	Common in reptiles e.g. tortoises, terrapins	350	+	-	-/×	-	-/×	+	+	+	-
III (Arizona)	Rare	Found in reptiles, can cause disease in poultry	370	-	+/×	+	-	-/×	d	+	+	-
IV	Rare	Rare	40	-	-	-	+	-/×	-	-	+	+

/ = or. × = late and irregularly positive. d = different reactions.

typhimurium. These disagreements are of little interest to clinicians and in this chapter we shall continue to use the familiar species names for all serotypes.

The many serotypes of *Salmonella* can be divided into three groups according to their host specificity: (a) Those primarily adapted to man, including the enteric fever organisms *S. typhi* and *S. paratyphi A*, *B* and *C*. Infections with these organisms are considered in Chapter 6; (b) Salmonella serotypes primarily adapted to particular animal hosts, such as *S. cholerae-suis* in pigs, *S. dublin* in cattle, *S. pullorum* and *S. gallinarum* in poultry, *S. abortus-equi* in horses and *S. abortus-ovis* in sheep. Human infections with these serotypes are rare. However, of the serotypes in this group, *S. dublin* and *S. cholerae-suis* are the most common cause of human infections and have a tendency to cause septicaemia; (c) The numerous remaining serotypes have no particular host specificity. They may all infect humans, although in practice the great majority of human infections are due to only a small number of serotypes.

Human infections with salmonellas in categories (b) and (c) usually originate from the animal reservoir and are usually transmitted in contaminated foods and sometimes in water. Nevertheless, cycles of infection resulting from direct person to person transmission, or infections direct from animals or the environment, also occur. While the disease is most commonly expressed as an acute enteritis, septicaemia may also occur and tends to be more frequently associated with particular serotypes.

Epidemiology

Enteritis due to *Salmonella* is a worldwide problem. In developed countries, where mass production of foods and intensive rearing of food animals occurs, the problem is even greater. The true scale of the problem cannot be accurately determined since even in countries with good clinical laboratory services many cases are mild and are therefore not investigated. In England and Wales laboratories reported 10 856 cases of bacterial food poisoning during 1980. *Salmonella* accounted for 9540 of these and caused 439 outbreaks, most of which were related to meals taken at receptions, in restaurants and hotels. Of 20 outbreaks reported in hospitals, however, 17 were probably due to cross-infection rather than food-poisoning.[67] These figures indicated a slight reduction in the number of *Salmonella* infections compared with the previous record year, but fluctuations had occurred throughout the previous decade and it is too early to know whether this indicates a trend. In the United States the most recent figures available are those for 1979, which proved to be a record year with 31 123 isolations of *Salmonella* from human sources being reported to the Centers for Disease Control, an increase of 8% over the previous year.[16]

In England and Wales 37 deaths were reported as a result of salmonellosis other than enteric fever in 1980.[67] This corresponds to a case-fatality rate of 0.39%. In 1978 the World Health Organization reported a similar case-fatality rate of 0.41% for salmonella outbreaks observed in the US since 1962.[102] The case-fatality rate therefore remains low on the whole, although occasional outbreaks with a high rate may occur among particularly susceptible individuals.

Statistics from many countries show that children under 5, and particularly those less than 1 year of age, have the highest incidence of salmonellosis. Among individuals under 20 years of age in the US males are more likely to be affected than females, while the reverse is true among those over 20 years of age.[16] The differences, however, are small. In England and Wales male children are affected more frequently than females but there is little or no difference in incidence between the sexes among adults.[67]

The order of prevalence of the various serotypes of *Salmonella* varies from time to time and place to place. Nevertheless, certain serotypes, such as *S. typhimurium* and *S. enteritidis*, predominate throughout the world. Although these serotypes are commonly isolated from animals, human foods and environmental sources, they are relatively uncommon in animal feeds. Their frequency in human infections is therefore difficult to account for in terms of the well-known cycle of infections involving foods, feeds, environment, animals and man. It has been suggested that such serotypes have a special host-parasite relationship which enables them to establish prolonged intestinal carriage and to be directly transmitted from animal to animal. The animal reservoir is therefore maintained without the need for the constant introduction of organisms by way of contaminated animal feeds.

In contrast, certain serotypes which were previously rare may suddenly rise to prominence and then spread internationally within the space of a few years. In such cases careful investigation usually reveals the source and manner of spread of the organism. For example, *S. agona* was rarely isolated in Britain or the USA before 1969 but following the introduction of contaminated fishmeal from Peru[18] this organism became the third most common serotype in the USA in 1976.[99] *S. agona* is now frequently isolated from pigs and their environment, from pork products and from poultry. In this case the cycle of infection seems to be related to the recycling of animal wastes for addition to animal feeds.[50] A more recent example is that of *S. hadar*. This organism was rarely isolated in England and Wales before 1971 but by 1980 it was reported to be the second most prevalent serotype after *S. typhimurium*.[67] In the case of *S. hadar* no connection with imported animal feeds was established. Nevertheless, between 1971 and 1974 the organism became established among the stock of a large turkey breeder. Breeding stock was subsequently distributed to numerous rearing units throughout the country and widespread human infections soon followed. The recent practice of recycling dried poultry manure as a source of protein for animal feeds may help to maintain the cycle of infection.[82]

Phage-typing schemes exist for some of the more common serotypes of *Salmonella* and these enable more detailed epidemiological studies to be undertaken. When the organisms are drug-resistant, genetic studies of the drug-resistance plasmids can be combined with phage-typing to allow the study of individual clones of bacteria. For example, studies in Britain have shown that certain phage-types of *S. typhimurium* are associated with poultry, while others are more commonly isolated from bovine sources. Isolates of the bovine-associated phage-types have a high incidence of multiple drug-resistance, whereas multiple drug-resistance is rare among the poultry-associated phage-types. It has been possible to show that various clones of multiple-resistant *S. typhimurium* have become disseminated in cattle herds throughout the country, have entered the human food chain and become significant causes of human infection. Salmonellosis in young cattle can be a severe disease with important economic consequences. Antibiotics are therefore frequently used in both treatment and prophylaxis of bovine salmonellosis and this widespread use of antibiotics undoubtedly encourages the persistence of the resistant strains.[83] Serious outbreaks of salmonellosis due to multiply-resistant strains have also occurred in developing countries during the last 10 years and have frequently been accompanied by a high incidence of septicaemia. A multiply-resistant clone of *S. typhimurium* phage type 208 spread throughout the Middle East after 1969 and another clone belonging to phage type 66/122 has spread in Asia and the Middle East since 1978.[77] Similarly, a multiply-resistant clone of *S. wien* has become disseminated throughout southern Europe and caused many infections in paediatric units between 1970 and 1979. As far as is known the food chain was not involved in the spread of this multiply-resistant strain and the infection was transmitted from person to person. Unlike the situation with *S. typhimurium* in Britain, the predisposing selective pressure probably resulted from the use of antibiotics in human medical practice.[57]

Attempts to control the spread of salmonella infection depend on an understanding of its epidemiology. It can be deduced from studies of outbreaks like those mentioned above that a cycle of infection exists. Animal feed ingredients of animal origin, such as bone and fishmeal, are often contaminated with *Salmonella*. Food animals that consume feeds prepared using these ingredients become infected, often as healthy carriers, and excrete the organisms. Their excrement contaminates the environment by way of effluent and by its use as fertilizer. At the abattoir their gut contents cross-contaminate meat intended for human consumption. Humans infected by meat products also excrete the organisms and further contaminate the environment and human foods, and may set up cycles of infection spread directly from person to person. The cycle is completed when contaminated offal, waste products and dried poultry manure are recycled for use in animal feeds, or when infection is introduced into previously uninfected animal stock from the contaminated environment. This is clearly a simplified account. Contaminated milk may also be an important source of infection if untreated and contaminated water may occasionally cause outbreaks, although these are rare. Other non-food items, such as pharmaceutical products of animal origin, may occasionally be contaminated and cause outbreaks.[51]

Many measures can contribute to the control of the salmonella problem. Proper food handling and preparation, including refrigeration and thorough cooking, can prevent the transmission of infection even when the raw materials are contaminated. Good nursing technique may reduce the spread of infection in hospitals. Nevertheless, at present much attention is being devoted to the possibility of breaking the cycle of infection by the introduction of compulsory heat treatment of materials for use in animal feeds. Such measures have considerably reduced the salmonella problem in Denmark[71] and provision is made for a similar approach in England and Wales and in the new Protein Processing Order.

Pathogenesis

It is generally accepted that the dose of organisms required to initiate clinical salmonellosis in a healthy individual is high compared with *Shigella*.[25] This is consistent with the usual food-borne route of infection in salmonellosis which contrasts with the ease with which *Shigella*, a low dose organism, is transmitted directly from person to person. However, other factors such as the age and immune status of the host and the presence of underlying debilitating disease may significantly alter the infective dose. Outbreaks of infection may therefore result from the person to person spread of infection among particularly susceptible patients, such as the very young or the very old. Even in healthy individuals outbreaks occasionally occur in which small infective doses appear to have led to large numbers of clinical cases of salmonellosis. For example, an outbreak caused by chocolate contaminated with *S. eastbourne* occurred in the USA and Canada in late 1973 and early 1974. The chocolate contained an average of only 2.5 organisms/g and in this case it may be that the organisms were protected from the lethal action of gastric acids by the fat in the chocolate.[21]

In experimental animals, those salmonellas that survive the passage through the gastric acid and that are not carried away by peristaltic action adsorb onto the epithelial cells of the small intestine and the colon, although the adsorptive mechanism is unknown. They then penetrate the epithelial cells and migrate through them to arrive in the lamina propria where they give rise to an inflammatory response. Those strains which cause only enteritis do not usually penetrate any further than this.[34] The net secretion of water and the consequent diarrhoea probably depends in part on this inflammatory response, but evidence exists that at least some salmonellas produce enterotoxins which may also contribute to the disease process. Sakazaki and his colleagues in 1974 used the rabbit ligated ileal loop model to demonstrate enterotoxin production; among 12 strains they identified 8 different serotypes.[84] In 1976 Sandefur and Peterson used a skin permeability factor assay in rabbits (a test previously developed as an assay for cholera toxin and the heat-labile enterotoxin of *E. coli*) and detected two factors: a rapidly acting, heat-stable factor and a slow acting, heat-labile factor. The latter resembled the cholera toxin and the heat-labile enterotoxin of *E. coli* in its action on Chinese hamster ovary (CHO) cells in tissue culture and was neutralized by cholera antitoxin.[86] Other authors have described enterotoxins detected using an infant mouse model which has been widely used to detect the heat-stable enterotoxin of *E. coli*.[48] Cholera toxin and the heat-labile enterotoxin of *E. coli* cause diarrhoea by a mechanism involving the adenylate cyclase-cAMP system (see Chapter 5). Experimental evidence shows that salmonella infection also causes ileal secretion by stimulating adenylate cyclase. The mechanism of this stimulation is unclear but differs from that of cholera toxin in that it is inhibited by indomethacin. This suggests that prostaglandins may play a part in salmonella-induced activation of adenylate cyclase.[35] Nevertheless, it is not yet clear to what extent enterotoxins are involved in salmonella diarrhoea and much work remains to be done before this question can be resolved.

Clinical features

Diarrhoea is the most common clinical feature of salmonellosis in humans. The incubation period may be 6–48 hours, but is more commonly between 12 and 24 hours, and is followed by the abrupt onset of diarrhoea and vomiting, often accompanied by fever, headache and abdominal pain. The acute stage usually ends after about 48 hours but in some cases the diarrhoea may be severe and prolonged with frequent passage of watery stools, sometimes with mucus and blood. In severe cases dehydration results and may lead to hypotension, cramps and impaired renal function. Symptoms are often more severe in the very young and the aged, although subclinical infections may also occur in these age groups. Indeed asymptomatic excretion is more common among infants and young children than in other age groups. In adults, permanent excreters of salmonellae other than *S. typhi* and *S. paratyphi* are rare. Most adult carriers stop excreting the organism within 3 months of infection, while infants may continue to excrete for more than a year.[73]

Any serotype of salmonella may occasionally penetrate the intestinal mucosa and cause septicaemia, although certain serotypes appear to be more capable than others of causing such complications. In such cases the symptoms resemble those of enteric fever (see Chapter 6).

For a detailed summary of the clinical manifestations of more than 7000 cases of salmonellosis the reader is referred to the study of Saphra and Winter.[87]

Treatment

Most cases of salmonella food poisoning are mild and the symptoms subside without the need for specific treatment. Patients with severe diarrhoea or vomiting may become dehydrated, especially the very young and the aged. In such cases the correction of fluid and electrolyte balance is all important.

Although salmonellas are usually sensitive to many antibiotics *in vitro*, infections frequently do not respond readily to treatment with antimicrobial agents. There is little evidence that antibiotic treatment shortens the illness and studies have shown that such treatment may result in persistence of the organism.[6] Indiscriminate use of antibiotics also encourages the dissemination of drug-resistant organisms. For these reasons antibiotics should not be given to patients with uncomplicated salmonella infections or to carriers of non-typhoid salmonellas. Most authorities advise that patients with septicaemia due to non-typhoid salmonellas should be given antimicrobial treatment in the same way as those with enteric fever.

Laboratory investigations

For a detailed consideration of the methods employed in the isolation, identification and serotyping of salmonellas from clinical specimens, the book by Edwards and Ewing is recommended.[26] Only a brief outline will be given here.

ISOLATION

Stools are preferable to rectal swabs and should be collected as early as possible in the course of the illness and before treatment has begun. The specimens should be examined as soon as possible after collection. The choice of plating media for the isolation of *Salmonella* will depend on the strategy adopted in the laboratory for the isolation of all members of the Enterobacteriaceae, since numerous selective media are available. Bismuth sulphite (Wilson-Blair) agar is a highly selective medium that is particularly efficient for the isolation of *S. typhi*. Most laboratories will also use a relatively non-selective medium such as MacConkey agar, or eosin methylene blue agar, since one of these is essential for the isolation of *Shigella*.

Other moderately selective media which might be considered include Shigella-Salmonella (SS), deoxycholate citrate (DCA), hektoen enteric and xylose lysine deoxycholate (XLD). The stool specimens should be streaked directly onto whichever plating media are chosen and should be subcultured into an enrichment medium such as selenite F broth or Rappaport's medium before plating once again onto the chosen media.

IDENTIFICATION

Colonies suspected of being *Salmonella* should be picked from the selective plating media by laboratory staff who are familiar with the colonial morphology of *Salmonella* growing on the media used. Such colonies are then identified by means of biochemical tests. Numerous schemes for the biochemical identification of the Enterobacteriaceae have been described and will not be considered here. Suffice it to say that biochemical identification is essential; members of the Enterobacteriaceae cannot be identified by serotyping alone because there is widespread sharing of antigens between the various genera and species.

SEROTYPING

The serotyping scheme for *Salmonella* is well developed and widely used. Strains are serotyped according to their somatic 'O' and flagella 'H' antigens and on this basis they are placed in the internationally used Kauffmann-White scheme. Both 'O' and 'H' antigens are usually identified first by using slide agglutination techniques and then positive reactions are confirmed using tube agglutination. Specific antisera are widely available from commercial sources. Strains of *Salmonella* are usually 'biphasic'; that is to say most strains are capable of producing two antigenically distinct flagellae. For proper serotyping both 'phases' must be identified. To achieve this it is necessary to change the phase of the organism under examination by growing it in semisolid agar containing the homologous 'H' antiserum — this inhibits the motility of organisms in the original phase but allows the passage through the agar of organisms in the alternate phase. These can then be subcultured and retested. A small section of the Kauffmann-White scheme is shown in Table 3.2.

Table 3.2   Extract from the Kauffmann-White serotyping scheme

Serotype	Somatic 'O' antigen	Flagella 'H' antigen Phase I	Phase II
	Group A		
S. paratyphi A	1, 2, 12	a	–
S. kiel	1, 2, 12	g,p	–
	Group B		
S. paratyphi B	1, 4, 5, 12	b	1, 2
S. typhimurium	1, 4, 5, 12	i	1, 2
S. heidelberg	1, 4, 5, 12	r	1, 2
S. ruki	4, 5, 12	y	e,n,x
	Group C		
S. cholerae-suis	6, 7	c	1, 5
S. braenderup	6, 7	e,h	e,n,z_{15}

PHAGE TYPING

Certain serotypes are common all over world. For example, in some countries in some years isolations of *S. typhimurium* outnumber isolations of all other serotypes of *Salmonella* combined. The epidemiological value of serotyping alone may therefore be limited in some situations. Phage-typing schemes have been developed for most of the common serotypes and those for *S. typhi, S. paratyphi A* and *B* and *S. typhimurium* are employed internationally. For a detailed description, the review of Guinée and Leeuwen is recommended.[40]

CAMPYLOBACTER ENTERITIS

The organisms now known as *Campylobacter* were first described by MacFadyean and Stockman in 1913.[54] In 1919 they were placed in the genus *Vibrio* by Smith and Taylor and given the specific name of *V. fetus* because of their association with abortion in sheep and cattle.[93] The fundamental differences between *V. fetus* and the true vibrios were pointed out by Sebald and Veron in

1963 and the recognition of a new genus, *Campylobacter*, was proposed.[88] The genus is divided into the catalase-negative species, *C. sputorum* and *C. bubulus*, which are not known to be pathogenic to man, and the catalase-positive species *C. fetus*, *C. jejuni* and *C. coli* (Table 3.3). The last two species were first recognized in 1957 by King[47] who described them as a thermophilic group of 'related vibrios' and it is these that are associated with enteritis is man.

Table 3.3 Classification of the genus *Campylobacter* (based on Newell, 1982)[63]

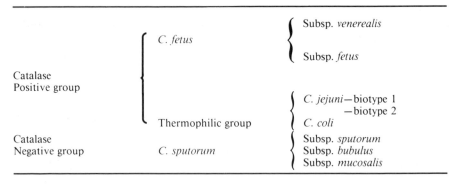

	C. fetus	Subsp. *venerealis*
		Subsp. *fetus*
Catalase Positive group		
		C. jejuni—biotype 1
		—biotype 2
	Thermophilic group	*C. coli*
Catalase Negative group	*C. sputorum*	Subsp. *sputorum*
		Subsp. *bubulus*
		Subsp. *mucosalis*

Because of their exacting growth requirements, the importance of campylobacters as a cause of human enteritis went unnoticed for many years after their first description. Dekeyser and his colleagues in 1972[23] used a filtration technique to isolate campylobacters from the stools of two patients in Brussels and further studies in the same city showed that these organisms were present in about 5% of children with diarrhoea.[9] The development of selective media for the isolation of campylobacters from stools led to a rapid increase in the number of laboratories able to detect these organisms and it was soon established that they were an important cause of acute diarrhoea both in children and adults in many different countries. During 1980 the Communicable Disease Surveillance Centre received reports of 9505 campylobacters, 11 473 salmonellas and 2905 shigellas from England and Wales.[19] Reports from the tropics suggest that campylobacter infections may be even more common than in temperate regions but their importance as a cause of diarrhoeal disease in tropical regions is yet to be established.[8,24,5]

Epidemiology

Surveys show that campylobacter infections are common throughout the world accounting for up to 20% of diarrhoea cases during the peak season in some areas. There is little difference in overall attack rate between the sexes, but closer analysis suggests that there is a higher incidence in males under 15 years old and in females over 65.[10] Estimates of the age-related incidence vary depending on the method of reporting. Reports to the Communicable Disease Surveillance Centre for England and Wales suggest that the under 5 years age group is most affected.[103] If, however, results are expressed in terms of the percentage of positive faecal specimens obtained from patients with diarrhoea in each age group, it is usually found that young adults give the highest isolation rate.[10] Surveys in Europe[103] and the USA[4] suggest that there is a seasonal variation in the incidence of campylobacter enteritis with a distinct peak in the summer months. In contrast, a survey in Hong Kong showed a peak in the cooler months of the year,[58] while a study of Japan showed little seasonal variation.[45]

Campylobacter enteritis resembles salmonellosis in that it is a zoonosis. The organisms may be found in a wide variety of warm-blooded vertebrate hosts. They may be transmitted directly from animals to man or by means of contaminated food or water. In addition, they may be transmitted from person to person. In a series of over 25 000 reports of campylobacter isolations in England and Wales, contact with sick dogs or cats was reported in 94 cases; campylobacter was isolated from the animals in 56 cases.[103] Poultry is frequently infected and careless handling of the uncooked carcasses has resulted in infections among housewives, butchers and workers in poultry processing plants. Campylobacters are often present in the faeces of healthy sheep and it has been suggested that the high incidence of campylobacter enteritis among Moroccans living in Brussels may result from their habit of keeping sheep in their households at times of religious feasting.[10] Campylobacters are also found in pigs, but the organisms belong to a biotype which is uncommon in human infections.[10] Food-borne outbreaks associated with shellfish and poultry have been reported in Japan[45] and the USA[4] and outbreaks associated with untreated water and tap water have been described in the USA[97] and Sweden.[60] Unpasteurized milk has been found to be an important vehicle of campylobacter infection in England.[74,46]

Campylobacters are excreted in the faeces of patients both during and after their illnesses. Nevertheless, the infectivity appears to be low and when spread of infection does occur it is usually from young children to other members of the family. No doubt such spread of infection results from the tendency of young children with diarrhoea to contaminate their surroundings. Adults are less likely to pass on their infections and, once the stools have returned to normal, adult patients can probably be regarded as noninfectious for practical purposes.

The distinction between *C. coli* and *C. jejuni* biotypes 1 and 2 has only recently been established and may be subject to further changes in the future. Few studies have distinguished between these organisms, but Skirrow and Benjamin in a survey in Worcester, England, found that 77% of human infections were due to *C. jejuni* biotype 1, 18% to *C. jejuni* biotype 2 and 5% to *C. coli*. *C. jejuni* biotype 1 also predominated in infections of cattle, sheep and dogs. In poultry, biotypes 1 and 2 were almost equally common, while in pigs *C. coli* predominated.[92]

Pathogenesis

Various animal species have been experimentally infected with campylobacters with differing results. In cattle there was fever and diarrhoea with the presence of mucus and sometimes blood in the faeces.[95] Diarrhoea also followed experimental infections in lambs[28] and dogs[53] while milder symptoms were observed using rhesus monkeys.[29] Adult and suckling mice, infant rabbits and hamsters showed no obvious symptoms, although the organisms could be recovered, indicating that colonization had occurred. Indeed, colonization of the intestine follows oral challenge with *C. jejuni* in all species examined. In gnotobiotic animals colonization is largely restricted to the colon[70] while in conventional animals the terminal ileum is involved.[95] In man the principle site of infection appears to be the jejunum and ileum. However, the passage of bright red blood in the stools as the disease progresses suggests that the colon may also be involved. In some cases this has been confirmed by sigmoidoscopy or colonoscopy.[49]

Using electron microscopy, organisms have been observed attached to the intestinal epithelium of colonized animals.[61] In addition, adhesion to and penetration of epithelial tissue culture cells has been reported.[64] Penetration has also been reported in experimental infections of cattle[95] and chick embryos.[22] However, using the Sereny test which demonstrates epithelial cell invasion in *Shigella* by means of its ability to cause keratoconjunctivitis of the guinea pig eye, *C. jejuni* strains are reported to give uniformly negative results.[39] Results so far therefore suggest that epithelial adhesion and invasion may be important pathogenic mechanisms in campylobacter enteritis, but many questions remain to be answered.

The possible role of enterotoxins in campylobacter enteritis is an even more controversial question. Some workers have detected heat-stable enterotoxin production in a few strains using the infant mouse test,[10] but others have failed to do so. The production of heat-labile enterotoxin has reportedly been detected using tissue culture tests,[38] but is unconfirmed by other workers.[10] Some authorities claim that the effects seen in tissue culture are cytotoxic and do not indicate the production of enterotoxin.

In most animal species oral challenge is followed by a period of 1–3 days during which the organism can be isolated from extraintestinal sites. These findings are in accord with those in human infections, since campylobacters can often be isolated from the blood of patients with enteritis.[10]

Clearly the relative importance of, and relationship between, epithelial cell adhesion and invasion, cytotoxin and enterotoxin require clarification. For the time being the pathogenic mechanisms of campylobacter enteritis remain unclear.

Clinical features

Campylobacter infections range from asymptomatic and mild cases to severe illness that may be life-threatening in the elderly or debilitated. In most cases, however, the disease consists of a self-limiting attack of acute diarrhoea lasting a few days. The incubation period is usually about 3–5 days but may be as long as 10 days in some cases. There may be a febrile prodromal period lasting from a few hours to a few days, with temperatures of 40° C being common. This may be accompanied by malaise, headache, dizziness, backache, myalgia, abdominal pain, and sometimes rigors. The abdominal pain eventually becomes colicky and the diarrhoea begins. The stools become liquid and foul smelling and may be bile stained. After 1 or 2 days fresh blood may appear in the stools and microscopic examination of acute specimens shows the presence of inflammatory cellular exudate. After 2 or 3 days the diarrhoea begins to subside although the abdominal pain persists. In the absence of chemotherapy the organism is likely to be excreted for about 2–5 weeks, although occasionally excretion may continue for much longer. In general, children are less severely affected than adults, but their illness may tend to be persistent or relapsing.

Treatment

In common with other diarrhoeal diaseases, campylobacter enteritis usually requires supportive and symptomatic treatment and the routine use of antimicrobial chemotherapy is not recommended. The decision to use chemotherapy should be taken on clinical grounds, but the choice of drug requires a knowledge of the *in vitro* susceptibility of the organism. Surveys have shown that aminoglycosides, erythromycin, tetracycline, chloramphenicol and furazolidone are the most active antibiotics, with gentamicin being the most active aminoglycoside. For uncomplicated enteritis erythromycin has the advantage of a relatively narrow spectrum of activity and low toxicity. Serum levels that enable the drug to act in the tissues can easily be achieved. For septicaemic patients, erythromycin has also been used successfully, but since a minority of strains are resistant, it is advisable to give gentamicin or chloramphenicol.

Laboratory investigations

ISOLATION

The isolation of campylobacters from faeces requires the use of selective media. Two such media are widely used. Skirrow's medium consists of a blood agar base containing vancomycin, polymyxin B and trimethoprim, while Butzler's medium consists of a thioglycollate agar containing bacitracin, novobiocin, cyclo-heximide, colistin and cefazolin.[10] Whichever medium is used it is necessary to incubate under reduced oxygen tension (5–7%). Selectivity is increased by incubating at 43° C.

IDENTIFICATION

The thermophilic or 'related' campylobacters yield flat, glossy and effuse colonies with a tendency to spread. Suspicious colonies should be shown to be oxidase positive, and microscopical examination should reveal slender (0.2–0.4 μm), gram negative, spiral or S-shaped organisms. Strains with these characteristics which grow at 43° C and which also show a rapid darting motility can be regarded as thermophilic campylobacters for routine purposes. The differentiation between *C. coli* and the two biotypes of *C. jejuni* can be made by means of tests for hippurate hydrolysis and H_2S production (Table 3.4). In addition, a distinct group of nalidixic acid-resistant thermophilic campylobacters (NARTC) can be differentiated.

Table 3.4 Differentiation of the catalase positive campylobacters (Skirrow and Benjamin 1982)[92]

	C. fetus	NARTC	*C. jejuni* biotype 1	*C. jejuni* biotype 2	*C. coli*
Growth at: 25.0° C	+	−	−	−	−
43.0° C	−	+	+	+	+
Nalidixic acid (30 μg disc)	R	R	S	S	S
Hippurate hydrolysis	−	−	+	+	−
H_2S production (FBP)	−	+	−	+	−

+ = growth. − = no growth. R = resistant (0 mm). S = sensitive (>6mm from disc).

SEROTYPING

Several different serotyping schemes for *C. jejuni* have been proposed. Methods used include enzyme linked immunoabsorbent assay (ELISA), fluorescent antibody, haemagglutination, slide and tube agglutination. None of these systems has yet gained international acceptance. A useful collection of papers may be found in the recent book edited by Newell.[63]

SHIGELLA DYSENTERY

Dysentery or 'bloody flux' was recognized by Hippocrates as a particular form of diarrhoea that could be identified by clinical observation. Throughout history, dysentery has frequently been a scourge of armies at war, since in wartime sanitary conditions are often poor and water and food supplies may be unsatisfactory. In these conditions epidemics may reach enormous proportions. Nevertheless, it was not until the late nineteenth century that the causative organisms were discovered. In 1875 Lösch isolated *Entamoeba histolytica* from patients with dysentery and reproduced the disease in dogs by injecting the amoebae into the rectum.[52] For the next 20 years it was thought that all dysentery was amoebic, but in 1898 Shiga isolated the bacillus named after him[90] and now known as *Shigella dysenteriae* 1. During the following 30 years many different types of dysentery bacilli were identified and the clinical and epidemiological distinction between amoebic and bacillary dysentery was established. Amoebic

Table 3.5   Classification and nomenclature of Shigella

Characters	Species and serotypes	Main synonyms
Subgroup A	*S. dysenteriae* 1	*S. shigae*
	S. dysenteriae 2	*S. schmitzii, S. ambigua*
Non-mannitol	*S. dysenteriae* 3	*S. largei* Q771; *S. arabinotarda A*
fermenters;	*S. dysenteriae* 4	*S. largei* Q1167; *S. arabinotarda B*
each	*S. dysenteriae* 5	*S. largei* Q1030
serologically	*S. dysenteriae* 6	*S. largei* Q454
distinct	*S. dysenteriae* 7	*S. largei* Q902
	S. dysenteriae 8	Serotype 599-52
	S. dysenteriae 9	Serotype 58
	S. dysenteriae 10	Serotype 2050-50
Serogroup B	*S. flexneri* 1a	V
	S. flexneri 1b	VZ
Usually	*S. flexneri* 2a	W
mannitol	*S. flexneri* 2b	WX
fermenters;	*S. flexneri* 3a	Z
members	*S. flexneri* 3b	
serologically	*S. flexneri* 4a	103*
related to each	*S. flexneri* 4b	103Z
other	*S. flexneri* 5	P119
	S. flexneri 6	Newcastle, Manchester or Boyd 88 bacillus†
	S. flexneri X variant	X
	S. flexneri Y variant	Y
Subgroup C	*S. boydii* 1	170
	S. boydii 2	P288
	S. boydii 3	D1
Usually	*S. boydii* 4	P274
mannitol	*S. boydii* 5	P143
fermenters;	*S. boydii* 6	D19
each	*S. boydii* 7	Lavington 1; *S. etousae*
serologically	*S. boydii* 8	Serotype 112
distinct	*S. boydii* 9	Serotype 1296/7
	S. boydii 10	Serotype 430
	S. boydii 11	Serotype 34
	S. boydii 12	Serotype 123
	S. boydii 13	Serotype 425
	S. boydii 14	Serotype 2770-51
	S. boydii 15	Serotype 703
Subgroup D	*S. sonnei*	Duval's bacillus; *B. ceylonensis* A
Mannitol-		
fermenter, late		
lactose and		
sucrose		
fermenter		

* Mannitol negative biotypes are sometimes known as *S. rabaulensis* or *S. rio.* † See Table 3.7.

dysentery tends to run a chronic course, frequently with liver abscess complications. Furthermore, although certain geographical areas, notable in the tropics, have a high endemicity, epidemics generally do not occur. In contrast, bacillary dysentery is usually of short duration, extraintestinal involvement is uncommon and epidemics frequently occur.

In the modern classification the genus *Shigella* consists of four species, or subgroups; *S. dysenteriae*, *S. flexneri*, *S. boydii* and *S. sonnei* (Table 3.5).

Epidemiology

Bacillary dysentery has a global distribution but the highest incidence occurs in areas where standards of hygiene and sanitation are poor. Notably these areas are in the developing countries of the tropics where bacillary dysentery frequently combines with malnutrition to cause high morbidity and mortality. In some such areas as many as 50% of children die from diarrhoea before reaching 7 years of age.

The reservoir of infection for *Shigella* is man, and reports of human infections originating from animals are epidemiological curiosities. Food-borne outbreaks occur in the tropics and occasionally in developed countries.[20] Food may be infected from the faeces of food-handlers and in some situations flies may act as vectors. Water-borne disease is said to be particularly important in the rainy seasons of tropical countries when drinking water may be contaminated with sewage. In developed countries, water-borne outbreaks of shigellosis are occasionally reported and may occur when some defect in the water distribution system allows cross-connection between drinking water and sewerage pipes.[2] Outbreaks have resulted from swimming in sewage contaminated water but this is probably rare.[75]

In developed countries with good sewage disposal it is unlikely that flies act as vectors. The spread of *Shigella* infection is generally from person to person by faecal-oral transmission. Cases of dysentery in the acute phase constitute the main risk because the liquid stools are teeming with *Shigella* and easily contaminate environmental surfaces, especially in toilets. The solid stools of symptom-free excreters in the recovery phase are less likely to produce significant environment contamination. *Shigella* organisms can survive for several weeks in cool, humid environments such as toilets.[44] This may explain why the main seasonal peak occurs in the winter in the developed countries of the temperate zones, while in the tropics the seasonal peak is usually in the warm months and may be related to fly prevalence.

In north-west Europe and North America common-source outbreaks are rare, although shigellosis remains endemic. Infant schools and day-care centres for children are the main centres of infection and although the usual epidemiological pattern is of low grade endemicity occasional brisk epidemics are not uncommon in such institutions.[101] Children frequently bring the infection home from school and thence to parents and siblings who may then introduce the infection to other groups, thus maintaining the endemic cycle.[96] Institutions for the mentally-subnormal are also important foci of bacillary dysentery and the control and eradication of the disease is even more difficult to achieve than in schools.

Despite the high incidence of infection in primary school children and in the preschool age groups attending nursery classes, it is rare in the developed countries to find infants infected with *Shigella*.[42] This must be contrasted with the developing countries where shigella infections are common in infants at the time of weaning. It is likely that during this period the infant is more at risk of infection from gross environmental contamination as well as from infected food.

S. sonnei and *S. flexneri* are the most common causes of bacillary dysentery but the different shigella subgroups show a variable distribution and incidence throughout the world. In tropical countries many different types of *Shigella* are found and epidemics due to more than one type are common. In Britain there has been a marked change in the epidemiology of *Shigella*. Between the two world wars both *S. flexneri* and *S. sonnei* were endemic, but by 1940 *S. sonnei* had become predominant. *S. sonnei* reached a peak of almost 99% of all Shigella infections in England and Wales between 1960 and 1970 but has now fallen back to around 70% of all infections. At the same time the total number of *Shigella* infections reported has declined from around 40 000 per year between 1950 and 1960 to less than 3000 in 1980.[67] This decline has been due to a fall in the incidence of indigenous infections due to *S. sonnei*, while infections due to other *Shigella* subgroups are usually acquired abroad and have remained fairly constant in number in recent years (Fig. 3.1). In the United States, *S. sonnei* is also predominant and accounted for 62% of *Shigella* infections in 1976.[15] As *S. sonnei* becomes predominant there is a change in the seasonal pattern of bacillary dysentery since *S. sonnei* tends to have its seasonal peak in the autumn and winter, whereas *S. flexneri* tends to have its peak in the warmer months.

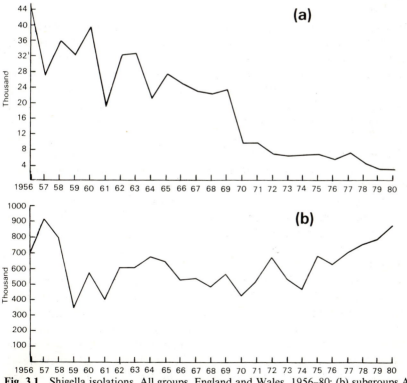

Fig. 3.1 Shigella isolations. All groups, England and Wales, 1956–80; (b) subgroups A, B and C, England and Wales, 1956–80

Shiga's bacillus (*S. dysenteriae* 1) was the cause of severe and extensive epidemics in Japan during the last 10 years of the nineteenth century and before World War I this organism caused serious outbreaks in Europe and the Americas. Since 1925, however, such outbreaks have been uncommon. In Asia, India and the Middle East dysentery due to Shiga's bacillus has remained an endemic disease and occasionally epidemics still occur. During World War II, outbreaks affected British troops in the Middle East and infections occurred in United States troops in Vietnam. In 1963 an outbreak of severe dysentery due to Shiga's bacillus occurred in Somalia.[11]

During 1969 and 1970 there was a serious pandemic due to Shiga's bacillus originating in Guatemala and spreading to most Central American countries.[32,56] The epidemic strain possessed plasmid-mediated multiple drug resistance and the epidemic was characterized by high attack rates with high morbidity and mortality, especially in children. It has been reported that there were 120 000 cases and 13 000 deaths. Returning travellers imported infections into the USA and in 1970–72 there were 140 cases, mostly in the border states with Mexico. In contrast, there were only 11 isolates between 1965 and 1968 and only 10 cases in 1976.[100] A severe epidemic of Shiga dysentery began in Bangladesh in 1972 and showed many similarities to the Central American outbreak.[72] The epidemic strain possessed multiple drug resistance and many of the patients had serious clinical disease. Since late 1979 further extensive outbreaks of dysentery due to Shiga's bacillus have occurred in Central Africa and again the epidemic strain was multiply resistant.[31] Although epidemic dysentery due to Shiga's bacillus had been absent from these areas for a prolonged period, the outbreaks demonstrate that when a virulent strain is introduced into populations with poor standards of hygiene, serious pandemic disease may occur.

In western Europe sporadic cases of Shiga's dysentery are almost always in persons returning from abroad. In England and Wales less than 10 cases are reported each year, and most of these have a history of recent travel to Asia (especially the Indian subcontinent) or less frequently the Middle East or Africa.[78]

S. boydii and *S. dysenteriae* serotypes other than Shiga's bacillus are unusual in England and Wales[79] and the USA[15] but are not uncommonly reported in Asia and the Middle East. For many geographical areas, reliable epidemiological data are not available.

Pathogenesis

Shigella are pathogens of man and other primates and although there have been occasional reports of infections in dogs, other animals are resistant to infection. Laboratory animals such as mice, rabbits and guinea-pigs may be infected orally but only after conditioning by starvation and treatment with gastric antacids, together with antiperistaltic agents at the time of challenge.

In man the lesions of bacillary dysentery are usually limited to the rectum and large intestine but in severe cases a part of the terminal ileum may be involved. The typical lesion is acute inflammation with ulceration limited to the epithelium; the bacteria rarely spread deeper than the lamina propria and bloodstream involvement is uncommon. Infections due to *S. sonnei* rarely extend beyond the epithelial inflammatory stage, but infections with Shiga's bacillus or *S. flexneri* strains frequently produce ulceration.

In the investigation of the pathophysiology of dysentery, rhesus monkeys were challenged orally and these studies showed that penetration of the colonic epithelial cells and intraepithelial multiplication are the essential prerequisites for the production of disease.[33] In monkeys with classical dysentery the only physiological defect was in the colon, whilst in those animals with simple diarrhoea there was a net jejunal secretion, although ileal transport remained normal. Bacterial invasion was not seen in the ileum or jejunum and the results suggested that a bacterial enterotoxin might also be involved.[76]

The invasive properties of *Shigella* have been investigated using the ability to produce kerato-conjunctivitis in the guinea-pig eye (Sereny test), and to invade cells in tissue culture.[68] In addition, recent work has demonstrated that strains of *S. dysenteriae* 1 and *S. flexneri* 2a produce toxins that are lethal to mice, enterotoxic for rabbit ileal loops and cytotoxic for HeLa cells.[66] The demonstration of related toxins from *S. dysenteriae* 1 and *S. flexneri* might imply that the enterotoxin has a role in the pathogenesis of bacillary dysentery. It was intially suggested that the enterotoxin of *S. dysenteriae* 1 did not stimulate adenylate cyclase as does the cholera enterotoxin and the heat labile enterotoxin of *Escherichia coli* but it has now been shown that under optimal assay conditions adenylate cyclase is stimulated by Shiga enterotoxin.[17] Further work is needed and in any case there is little doubt that epithelial invasion and multiplication are the main virulence factors.

Clinical features

For man the infecting dose of *Shigella* varies from 10 to 100 organisms and this contrasts with the high infecting dose (10^5) required for salmonella food-poisoning.[25] Children are more susceptible to *Shigella* infection than adults and in an epidemic children are more likely to suffer with diarrhoea, whereas adults often become symptomless carriers.[89] Age-sex correlations show that, except in women of childbearing age, infection is less frequent amongst females.[96]

The incubation period is usually between 2 and 3 days, but may be as brief as 12 hours. The onset of symptoms is usually sudden and frequently the initial symptom is abdominal colic. In all but the very mild cases there is pyrexia which is accompanied by general prostration in severe cases. In a typical case of bacillary dysentery there are numerous stools of small volume containing blood and mucus. In a mild case the frequency of stools is about eight in 24 hours, whereas in severe cases as many as 30 stools may be passed. In some cases the typical dysentery stools do not occur; instead, watery stools may be produced and these may vary from mild diarrhoea to a fulminating cholera-like disease with profound loss of fluid. In a typical case of dysentery the symptoms last about 4 days but exceptionally continue for 10 to 14 days.

S. sonnei infection usually causes a mild disease with short-lived diarrhoea. The disease associated with *S. flexneri* tends to be more severe, whilst *S. boydii* and *S. dysenteriae* infections produce a wide range of severity. Shiga's bacillus has caused many epidemics of severe disease but even so some infections are mild. Host factors play an important part in determining the clinical course. Case fatality is usually low except when infection occurs in babies less than 3 months, in malnourished patients or in psychiatric hospitals.

Extraintestinal complications are rare but some patients develop a sterile polyarthritis and eye disorders such as conjunctivitis or iritis may develop. These complications usually appear about 10–14 days after the onset of dysentery and there is evidence to suggest that these are manifestations of autoimmune disease and are a form of Reiter's syndrome. A similar complex is seen following infection with *Yersinia enterocolitica* and patients with histocompatibility antigen HLA B27 seem particularly prone to these sequelae. Chronic complications following bacillary dysentery are rare but may include peripheral neuritis and intestinal stenosis.

During the acute stage of the disease the shigella organisms are excreted in large numbers in the faeces but during recovery the numbers fall, although the organisms may remain in the faeces for several weeks after the symptoms have subsided.[96]

Treatment

Most cases of shigellosis, especially those due to *S. sonnei*, are mild and do not require antibiotic therapy. Symptomatic treatment with the maintenance of hydration is all that is required. Treatment with a suitable antibiotic is necessary in the very young, the aged or the debilitated, and in severe infections. The evidence that antibiotic therapy reduces the period of excretion of the organisms seeems equivocal.

In many countries the incidence of antibiotic resistance amongst *Shigella* is high and is frequently plasmid-mediated and multiple.[36,62,96] Because of this it is necessary to determine the resistance pattern of the strain before giving antibiotics in treating a severe case of shigellosis. Routine treatment with antibiotics is to be avoided because it exerts a selective pressure which increases the incidence of plasmid-mediated resistance.

USE OF VACCINES

Various vaccines have been evaluated in laboratory studies with monkeys and in challenge trials on humans. Parenteral immunization with killed vaccines has failed to produce protection in experimental animals[30] or against natural disease.[43] A polyvalent oral vaccine of streptomycin-dependent strains of *S. flexneri* or *S. sonnei* when given in large scale trials to children and adults gave significant protection, but the application of the vaccine was limited because of the multiple high doses which were required.[59] These and other vaccines are discussed in more detail in Chapter 12.

Laboratory investigations

ISOLATION

Food and water

Because the minimum infecting dose of *Shigella* is small, its occurrence in food, milk and water may be significant even when only a small number of organisms are present. Reliable and effective enrichment methods are not available, however, and the true incidence of *Shigella* contamination of foodstuffs cannot be determined. The gram-negative (GN) broth of Hajna[41] has sometimes proved useful for the enrichment of *Shigella* and it is recommended that the investigation of foodstuffs should include an enrichment step using this medium. Subsequent steps in the isolation of *Shigella* from foodstuffs should follow the procedure recommended for the examination of faecal specimens.

Faecal specimens

Whenever possible freshly passed stools should be examined, although if this is not possible faecal swabs showing marked faecal staining may be used. The specimens should be collected during the acute stage of the disease and before any chemotherapy is started. Specimens should be examined as soon after collection as possible. Enrichment with GN broth may be advantageous but isolation is normally effected by direct plating. If the specimen includes blood and mucus these should be included in the portion to be examined.

Some strains grow poorly on inhibitory media and it is advisable to use both a relatively non-inhibitory medium, such as MacConkey or eosin methylene blue (EMB) agar, and an inhibitory medium, such as deoxycholate citrate agar (DCA) or Shigella-Salmonella (SS) agar. Instructions for the preparation of these media are given by Edwards and Ewing.[26] The stool specimens are streaked onto the chosen media and after overnight incubation at 37° C, non lactose-fermenting colonies are selected for further examination. It should be noted that even when stool specimens from acute dysentery are examined there may be only a scanty growth of *Shigella*.

IDENTIFICATION

Biochemical characteristics

The genus *Shigella* consists of non-motile organisms that conform to the

Table 3.6 Biochemical reactions of *Shigella*

Test or substrate	Result
β-galactosidase	d[a]
Simmons' citrate	−
Christensen's citrate	−
Sodium acetate	− or +[b]
Arginine decarboxylase	d
Lysine decarboxylase	−
Ornithine decarboxylase	d[c]
Gelatin	−
Gluconate	−
H₂S (TSI)	−
Indole	d[d]
KCN	−
Malonate	−
MR	+
VP	−
P.P.A.	−
Urease	−
Motility	−
Glucose; Acid	+
Gas	− or +[e]
Adonitol	−
Cellobiose	−
Dulcitol	d
Inositol	−
Lactose	d[f]
Mannitol	d[g]
Salicin	−
Sucrose	d[h]
Xylose	d

− or +; majority of strains negative. d different reactions.

[a] Strains of *S. dysenteriae* 1 and *S. sonnei* are positive; positive strains of *S. flexneri* 2a and *S. boydii* have been described.
[b] Some biotypes of *S. flexneri* 4a are positive, all other types are negative.
[c] Strains of *S. boydii* 13 and *S. sonnei* are positive.
[d] Strains of *S. dysenteriae* 1, *S. flexneri* 6 and *S. sonnei* are always negative. *S. dysenteriae* 2 is always positive.
[e] Some biotypes of *S. flexneri* 6 are positive; positive strains of *S. boydii* 13 and 14 have been described.
[g] Strains of *S. sonnei* are usually positive after several days incubation; positive strains of *S. flexneri* 2a and *S. boydii* 9 have been described.
[g] Strains of *S. dysenteriae* are negative; negative biotypes of *S. flexneri* 4a ('*S. rabaulensis*', '*S. rio*') and *S. flexneri* 6 (Newcastle biotype) occur; negative biotypes of *S. sonnei* occur rarely.
[h] Strains of *S. sonnei* are usually positive after several days incubation.

definition of the family Enterobacteriaceae.[26] Their biochemical reactions are summarized in Table 3.6. Members of the genus do not produce hydrogen sulphide in triple sugar iron (TSI) agar; they do not produce urease and they do not utilize citrate in Simmons' medium or in Christensen's medium. They do not decarboxylate lysine or deaminate phenylalanine. Salicin, adonitol and inositol are not fermented. Only *S. sonnei* strains commonly ferment lactose, usually after more than 24 hours incubation, although lactose-fermenting strains of *S. flexneri*

2a[98] and *S. boydi* 9[55] have been reported. In addition to these lactose-fermenting strains, *S. dysenteriae* 1 strains give positive results in tests for β-galactosidase activity. Fermentation of sucrose, like that of lactose, is restricted to strains of *S. sonnei* and usually requires several days incubation. Only *S. sonnei* and *S. boydii* 13 strains decarboxylate ornithine and only certain biotypes of *S. flexneri* 4a utilize sodium acetate. The production of gas from glucose ocurs only in certain biotypes of *S. flexneri* 6 (Table 3.7) although aerogenic strains of *S. boydii* 13[81] and *S. boydii* 14[12] have been described. The ability to produce indole varies with serotype but it is worth noting that strains of *S. dysenteriae* 1, *S. flexneri* 6 and *S. sonnei* are always negative.

Table 3.7 Biotypes of *S. flexneri* 6

	Glucose	Mannitol	Dulcitol
Boyd 88	A	A	– or (A)
Manchester	AG	AG	– or (AG)
Newcastle	A or AG	–	– or (A) or (AG)

Results in parentheses indicate delayed reactions. A, acid production. G, gas production.

The G + C content of *Shigella* DNA is 49–53%.[65] DNA reassociation studies indicate that most *Shigella* strains share 80% or more of their nucleotide sequences and a similar degree of relatedness exists between *Shigella* and *E. coli* strains. Strains of *S. boydii* 13 average only about 65% relatedness to other *Shigella* and *E. coli* strains.[7]

The biochemical identification of *Shigella* is complicated by the similarity of some strains of other genera. In particular strains of *Hafnia*, *Providencia*, *Aeromonas* and atypical *Escherichia coli* frequently cause difficulties.

Non lactose-fermenting or anaerogenic strains of *E. coli* are a common problem. In particular, members of the Alkalescens-Dispar (A-D) group are defined as nonmotile, anaerogenic biotypes of *E. coli*. These may be differentiated from *Shigella* by means of the Christensen's citrate and lysine decarboxylase tests in which *Shigella* are always negative. Some highly atypical strains have caused difficulties and Shmilovitz and his colleagues have suggested the recognition of an intermediate group to be known as Intermediate Shigella Coli Alkalescens Dispar (ISCAD).[91] Stenzel proposed the inclusion of such strains in (Shigella) subgroup D and suggested that this subgroup should be renamed *S. metadysenteriae*.[94] Further complications arise since some strains of *E. coli* share with *Shigella* the ability to cause bacillary dysentery and to cause keratoconjunctivitis of the guinea-pig eye in the Sereny test.[85] Nevertheless, the Enterobacteriaceae Subcommittee of the International Committee on Bacteriological Nomenclature advised that pathogenicity should not be a criterion in the classification of Enterobacteriaceae and strains with biochemical reactions which do not conform strictly to those of *Shigella* are classified as atypical *E. coli*.[13]

Serotyping scheme

The genus *Shigella* is divided into four subgroups on the basis of biochemical and antigenic characteristics (Table 3.5). Each subgroup is divided into a number of different serotypes which are distinguished by the presence of a specific somatic antigen. Antisera are used in slide agglutination tests for the identification of these specific antigens, although the results should be confirmed using tube agglutination techniques.

Within the subgroup *S. flexneri*, common or group antigens exist in addition to the specific or type antigens. Each group antigen occurs in more than one serotype and subserotypes are distinguished by the presence of particular group antigens (Table 3.8). In practice it is necessary in the identification of *S. flexneri* to be able to recognize group factors 7, 8 (X group factors), 3, 4 (Y group factors) and 6. When commercial antisera are used this is usually achieved by the provision of separate antisera for factors X and Y, while group factor 6 is included in antiserum for specific antigen III (Table 3.9). Variants of *S. flexneri* are occasionally found that lack specific antigen and therefore contain only group factor antigens. According to which group factors are present these may be identified either as X or Y variants.

Table 3.8 Shigella subgroup B. *Shigella flexneri*

Serotype	Sub-serotype	Specific antigen	Group antigens		
1	1a	I	1,2,	4,5,	9
	1b	IS	1,2,	4,5,6,	9
2	2a	II	1,	3,4,	
	2b	II	1,		7,8,9
3	3a	III	1,		6,7,8,9
	3b	III	1,	3,4	6
	3c	III	1,		6
4	4a	IV	1,	3,4,	B
	4b	IV	1,	3,4, 6	B
5	5*	V	1,		7,8,9
	5	V	1,	3,4	
6		VI	1,2,	4	
X variant			1,		7,8,9
Y variant			1,	3,4	

Subtypes of *S. flexneri* 5 are *sub-judice*.

The immunochemical and genetic basis of the complex antigenic structure of *S. flexneri* has been summarized by Petrovskaya and Bondarenko.[69] The lipopolysaccharide O antigen of most *S. flexneri* serotypes contains group antigens 3, 4 as a main primary structure. The type-specific antigens I, II, IV and V and the group antigens 7, 8 are all the result of phage conversion of the 3, 4 antigens resulting in the incorporation of α-glucosyl secondary side chains. Type-specific antigen III and group antigen 6 differ from the above antigens in that they

Table 3.9   Reactions of *S. flexneri* serotypes in diagnostic slide-agglutinating antisera

Serotype	Simplified antigenic formula	Antiserum (agglutinins)							
		1 (I)	2 (II)	3 (III.6)	4 (IV)	5 (V)	6 (VI)	X (7,8)	Y (3,4)
1a	I:2,4	+	–	–	–	–	–	–	–/+
1b	I:6:2,4	+	–	+	–	–	–	–	–/+
2a	II:3,4	–	+	–	–	–	–	–	–/+
2b	II:7,8	–	+	–	–	–	–	+	–
3a*	III:6:7,8	–	–	+	–	–	–	+	–
3b	III:6:3,4	–	–	+	–	–	–	–	+
3c	III:6.	–	–	+	–	–	–	–	–
4a	IV:3,4	–	–	–	+	–	–	–	–/+
4b	IV:6:3,4	–	–	+	+	–	–	–	–/+
5†	V:7,8	–	–	–	–	+	–	+	–
5	V:3,4	–	–	–	–	+	–	–	–/+
6	VI:2,4	–	–	–	–	–	+	–	–
X	–:7,8	–	–	–	–	–	–	+	–
Y	–:3,4	–	–	–	–	–	–	–	+

* Occasional variants may also react in Y antiserum. † The subtypes of *S. flexneri* 5 are still *sub-judice*.
  Note   Arabic numerals are used to designate serotypes but it is customary to use Roman numerals to designate type-specific antigens and Arabic numerals for group antigens.

contain acetyl groups. Nevertheless, these antigens are also formed as a result of phage conversion of the 3, 4 antigens. The lipopolysaccharide O antigen of *S. flexneri* 6 differs considerably from that of other *S. flexneri* serotypes and it does not contain the immunochemical determinants of the 3, 4 antigens. Strains of *S. flexneri* 6 therefore resemble strains of *S. boydii* immunochemically and Petrovskaya and Bondarenko recommend that they should be reclassified as such.

In strains of *S. sonnei* the somatic antigens may undergo a variation of form from *S. sonnei* I to *S. sonnei* II. This variation resembles the smooth to rough (S to R) variation which is common among the Enterobacteriaceae. Separate antisera are available for the identification of the two forms, although it is of little importance to distinguish between them since cultures often consist of a mixture of S and R forms.

In addition to the serotypes shown in Table 3.4, a number of provisional *Shigella* serotypes have been described.[27,37] They may be added to the serotyping scheme in the future but in the meantime they remain *sub-judice* and antisera for their identification are usually available only at reference laboratories.

Strains of *Shigella* occasionally occur which do not agglutinate with *Shigella* antisera in the unheated state. Such strains may become agglutinable after heating at 100° C for 30 minutes.

The serological identification of *Shigella* is complicated by the widespread sharing of antigens among the Enterobacteriaceae. In particular, most *Shigella* somatic antigens are identical to, or related to, one or other of the somatic antigens of *E. coli*.[26,80] It is therefore essential that serological and biochemical tests should be interpreted together.

Colicine typing of *S. sonnei*

Colicine typing is of value in epidemiological studies of *S. sonnei*. The current scheme is based on that of Abbott and Shannon and distinguishes 14 colicine types using 15 indicator strains.[1] In this method the organism under investigation is inoculated heavily in a broad streak across a blood agar plate and incubated at 37° C for 24 hours. The growth is then removed from the agar by scraping with a glass slide and the organisms remaining on the agar are killed with chloroform. The fifteen indicator strains are then inoculated onto the plate in streaks at right angles to the original line of growth. After incubation for a further 8–12 hours the patterns of inhibition of growth of the indicator strains can be examined and compared with a chart. It is important that colicine type strains should be maintained for use as controls and colicine types 3 and 11 should be included in every batch of tests.

Phage-typing

Phage-typing is not widely used for epidemiological studies of *Shigella*. Nevertheless, schemes have been described and those for *S. flexneri* and *S. sonnei* have received the most attention. For further information, the review of Bergan is recommended.[3]

REFERENCES

1   Abbott J. D. and Shannon R. (1958) A method for typing *Shigella sonnei*, using colicine production as a marker. *J. Clin. Pathol.* **11**, 71.
2   Baine W. B., Herron C. A., Bridson K., Barker W. H., Lindell S., Mallison G. F., Wells J. C., Martin W. T., Kosuri M. R., Carr F. and Volker E. (1975) Waterborne Shigellosis at a public school. *Am. J. Epidemiol.* **101**, 323.
3   Bergan T. (1979) In: *Methods in Microbiology*, p.178. Vol. 13, Eds. Bergan T. and Norris J. R., Academic Press, New York.
4   Blaser M. J., Feldman R. A. and Wells J. G. (1982) Epidemiology of endemic and epidemic campylobacter infections in the United States. In: *Campylobacter*, p.3. Ed. Newell D. G., MTP Press, Lancaster.
5   Bokkenheuser V. D., Richardson N. J., Bryner J. H. and Ziegenfuss R. (1978) Enteric Campylobacter infections in small children. *Abstr. Ann. Meet. Am. Soc. Microbiol.*, p. 287.
6   Bowmer E. J. (1964) The challenge of salmonellosis. Major public health problem. *Am. J. Med. Sci.* **247**, 467.
7   Brenner D. J., Fanning G. R., Miklos G. V. and Steigerwalt A. G. (1973) Polynucleotide sequence relatedness among *Shigella* species. *Int. J. System. Bacteriol.* **23**, 1.
8   Butzler J. P. (1973) Related vibrios in Africa (Letter). *Lancet* **ii**, 858.
9   Butzler J. P., Dekeyser P., Detrain M. and Dehaen F. (1973) Related vibrio in stools. *J. Pediatr.* **82**, 493.
i0   Butzler J. P. and Skirrow M. B. (1979) Campylobacter enteritis. *Clin. Gastroenterol.* **8**, 737.

11 Cahill K. M., Davies J. A. and Johnson R. (1966) Report on an epidemic due to *Shigella dysenteriae* type 1 in the Somalia interior. *Am. J. Trop. Med. Hyg.* **15**, 52.

12 Carpenter K. P. (1961) The relationship of the Enterobacterium A12 (Sachs) to *Shigella boydii* 14. *J. Gen. Microbiol.* **26**, 535.

13 Carpenter K. P. (1963) Report of the Subcommittee on Taxonomy of the *Enterobacteriaceae*. *Int. J. System. Bacteriol.* **13**, 69.

14 Centers for Disease Control (1977) *Salmonella Surveillance Annual Summary 1976*, U.S. Department of Health and Human Services.

15 Centers for Disease Control (1977) *Shigella Surveillance* No. 39, U.S. Department of Health Education and Welfare.

16 Centers for Disease Control (1981) *Salmonella Surveillance Annual Summary 1979*, U.S. Department of Health and Human Services.

17 Charney A. N., Gots R. E., Formal S. B. and Giannella R. A. (1976) Activation of intestinal mucosal adenylate cyclase by *Shigella dysenteriae* 1 enterotoxin. *Gastroenterology* **70**, 1085.

18 Clark G. McC., Kaufmann A. F., Gangarosa E. J. and Thompson M. (1973) Epidemiology of an international outbreak of *Salmonella agona*. *Lancet* **ii**, 490.

19 Communicable Disease Report (1980) *Quarterly Edition 4*, Public Health Laboratory Service, London.

20 Coultrip R. L., Beaumont W. and Siletchnik M. D. (1977) Outbreak of Shigellosis — Fort Bliss, Texas. *Morbid. Mortal. Wkly Rept* **26**, 107.

21 Craven P. C., Mackel D. C., Baine W. B., Barker W. H., Gangarosa E. J., Goldfield M., Rosenfeld H., Altman R., Lachapelle G., Davies J. W. and Swanson R. C. (1975) International outbreak of *Salmonella eastbourne* infection traced to contaminated chocolate. *Lancet* **i**, 788.

22 Davidson J. A. and Solomon J. R. (1982) Onset of resistance to pathogenic strains of *Campylobacter jejuni* in the chicken embryo. In: *Campylobacter*, p.178. Ed. Newell D. G., MTP Press, Lancaster.

23 Dekeyser P., Gossuin-Detrain M., Butzler J. P. and Sternon J. (1972) Acute enteritis due to related vibrio: first positive stool cultures. *J. Infect. Dis.* **1325**, 390.

24 De Mol P. and Bosmans E. (1978) Campylobacter enteritis in Central Africa (Letter). *Lancet* **i**, 604.

25 Dupont H. L. and Hornick R. B. (1973) Clinical approach to infectious diarrhoeas. *Medicine* **52**, 265.

26 Edwards P. R. and Ewing W. H. (1972) *Identification of Enterobacteriaceae*. Burgess Publishing Co., Minneapolis.

27 Ewing W. H., Reavis R. W. and Davis B. R. (1958) Provisional *Shigella* serotypes. *Can. J. Microbiol.* **4**, 89.

28 Firehammer B. D. and Myers L. L. (1982) Experimental *Campylobacter jejuni* infections in calves and lambs. In: *Campylobacter*, p.168. Ed. Newell D. G., MTP Press, Lancaster.

29 Fitzgeorge R. B., Baskerville A. and Lander K. P. (1982) Experimental *Campylobacter jejuni* infections of rhesus monkeys. In: *Campylobacter*, p.180. Ed. Newell D. G., MTP Press, Lancaster.

30 Formal S. B., Maenza R. M., Austin S. and LaBrec E. H. (1967) Failure of parenteral vaccines to protect monkeys against experimental shigellosis. *Soc. Exp. Biol. Med. Proc.* **125**, 347.

31 Frost J. A., Rowe B., Vandepitte J. and Threlfall E. J. (1981) Plasmid characterisation in the investigation of an epidemic caused by multiply resistant *Shigella dysenteriae* type 1 in Central Africa. *Lancet* **ii**, 1074.

32 Gangarosa E. J., Perera D. R., Mata L. J., Mendizabal-Morris C., Guzman G. and Reller L. B. (1970) Epidemic Shiga bacillus dysentery in Central America. II. Epidemiologic studies in 1969. *J. Infect. Dis.* **122**, 181.

33 Gemski G., Akio T., Washington O. and Formal S. B. (1972) Shigellosis due to *Shigella dysenteriae* 1 : Relative importance of mucosal invasion versus toxin production in pathogenesis. *J. Infect. Dis.* **126**, 523.

34 Gianella R. A., Formal S. B., Dammin D. J. and Collins H. (1973) Pathogenesis of salmonellosis: studies of fluid secretion, mucosal invasion and morphologic reaction in the rabbit ileum. *J. Clin. Invest.* **52**, 441.

35 Gianella R. A., Gots R. E., Charney M. D., Greenough W. B. and Formal S. B. (1975) Activation of adenylate cyclase and inhibition by indomethacin. *Gastroenterology* **69**, 1238.

36 Gross R. J., Rowe B., Cheasty T. and Thomas L. V. (1981) Increase in drug resistance among *Shigella dysenteriae, Sh. flexneri* and *Sh. boydii. Br. Med. J.* **283**, 575.

37 Gross R. J., Thomas L. V. and Rowe B. (1980) New provisional serovar (E10163) of *Shigella boydii. J. Clin. Microbiol.* **12**, 167.

38 Gubina M., Zajc-Satler J., Dragas A. Z., Zeleznik Z. and Mehle J. (1982) Enterotoxin activity of campylobacter species. In: *Campylobacter*, p.188. Ed. Newell D. G., MTP Press, Lancaster.

39 Guerrant R. L., Lahita R. G., Winn W. C. and Roberts R. B. (1978) Campylobacteriosis in man: pathogenic mechanisms and review of 91 bloodstream infections. *Am. J. Med.* **65**, 584.

40 Guinee P. A. M. and van Leeuwen W. J. (1978) Phage typing of *Salmonella*. In: *Methods in Microbiology*, p.157, Vol. **11**, Eds, Bergan T. and Norris J. R., Academic Press, London.

41 Hajna A. A. (1955) A new enrichment broth medium for Gram-negative organisms of the intestinal group. *Public Health Lab.* **13**, 85.

42 Haltalin K. C. (1967) Neonatal shigellosis. Report of 16 cases and review of the literature. *Am. J. Dis. of Child.* **114**, 603.

43 Higgins A., Floyd T. and Koder M. (1955) Studies in Shigellosis. III. A controlled evaluation of a monovalent shigella vaccine in a highly endemic environment. *Am. J. Trop. Med. Hyg.* **4**, 281.

44 Hutchinson R. I. (1956) Some observations on the method of spread of Sonne Dysentery. *Monthly Bulletin Ministry of Health and Public Health Laboratory Service* **15**, 110.

45 Itoh T., Saoito K., Yanagawa Y., Sakai S. and Ohashi M. (1982) Campylobacter enteritis in Tokyo. In: *Campylobacter*, p.5. Ed. Newell D. G., MTP Press, Lancaster.

46 Jones P. H. and Willis A. T. (1982) A large milk-borne outbreak of campylobacter enteritis in Luton. In: *Campylobacter*, p.276. Ed. Newell D. G., MTP Press, Lancaster.

47 King E. O. (1957) Human infections with *Vibrio fetus* and a closely related vibrio. *J. Infect. Dis.* **101**, 119.

48 Koupal L. R. and Diebel R. H. (1975) Assay, characterisation and localisation of an enterotoxin produced by salmonella. *Infect. Immun.* **11**, 14.

49 Lambert M. E., Schofield P. F., Ironside A. G. and Mandal B. K. (1979) Campylobacter colitis. *Br. Med. J.* **i**, 857.

50 Lee J. A. (1974) Recent trends in human salmonellosis in England and Wales: the epidemiology of prevalent serotypes other than *Salmonella typhimurium. J. Hyg.* **72**, 185.

51 Lipson A. and Meikle H. (1977) Porcine pancreatin as a source of salmonella infection in children with cystic fibrosis. *Arch. Dis. Childh.* **52**, 569.

52 Losch F. (1875) Massenhafte Entwicklung von Amoeben im Dickdarn. *Virchows Archives* **65**, 196.

53 Macartney L., McCandlish I. A. P., Al-Mashat R. R. and Taylor D. J. (1982) Natural and experimental enteric infections with *Campylobacter jejuni* in dogs. In: *Campylobacter*, p.172. Ed. Newell D. G., MTP Press, Lancaster.

54 MacFadyean F. and Stockman S. (1913) Report of the Departmental Committee Appointed by the Board of Agriculture and Fisheries to Enquire into Epizootic Abortion, Vol. 3, HMSO, London.

55 Manolov D. G., Trifonova A. and Ghinchev R. (1962) A new lactose-fermenting species of the *Shigella* genus. *J. Hyg. Epidemiol. Microbiol. Immunol.* **6**, 422.

56 Mata L. J., Gangarosa E. J., Caceres A., Perera D. R. and Mejicanos M. L. (1970) Epidemic Shiga bacillus dysentery in Central America. I. Etiologic investigations in Guatemala 1969. *J. Infect. Dis.* **122**, 170.

57 McConnell M. M., Smith H. R., Leonardopoulos J. and Anderson E. S. (1979) The value of plasmid studies in the epidemiology of infections due to drug-resistant *Salmonella wien*. *J. Infect. Dis.* **139**, 178.

58 McGechie D. B., Tesh T. B. and Bamford V. W. (1982) Campylobacter enteritis in Hong Kong and Western Australia. In: *Campylobacter*, p.19. Ed. Newell D. G., MTP Press, Lancaster.

59 Mel D., Gangarosa E. J. Badovanovic M. L., Arsic B. L. and Litvinjenko S. (1971) Studies on vaccination against bacillary dysentery. 6. Protection of children by oral immunisation with streptomycin dependent Shigella strains. *Bull. WHO* **45**, 457.

60 Mentzing L. O. (1982) A water-borne outbreak of campylobacter in central Sweden. In: *Campylobacter*, p.278. Ed. Newell D. G., MTP Press, Lancaster.

61 Merrell B. R., Walker R. I. and Coolbaugh J. C. (1982) Experimental morphology and colonisation of the mouse intestine by *Campylobacter jejuni*. In: *Campylobacter*, p.183. Ed. Newell D. G., MTP Press, Lancaster.

62 Neu H.C., Cherubin C. E., Longo E. D. and Winter W. (1975) Antimicrobial resistance of *Shigella* isolated New York City in 1973. *Antimicrob. Agents Chemother.* **7**, 833.

63 Newell D. G. (1982) Ed. *Campylobacter*, MTP Press, Lancaster.

64 Newell D. G. and Pearson A. D. (1982) Pathogenicity of *Campylobacter jejuni* — an *in vitro* model of adhesion and invasion? In: *Campylobacter*, p.196. Ed. Newell D. G., MTP Press, Lancaster.

65 Normore W. M. (1973) Guanine-plus-cytosine (GC) composition of the DNA of bacteria, fungi, algae and protozoa. In: *CRC Handbook of Microbiology, II. Microbial Composition*, p. 585, Eds Laskin A. I., Lechevalier H. A., CRC Press, Cleveland.

66 O.Brien A. D., Thompson M. R., Gemski P., Doctor B. P. and Formal S. B. (1977) Biological properties of *Shigella flexneri* 2A toxin and its serological relationship to *Shigella dysenteriae* 1 toxin. *Infect. Immun.* **15**, 796.

67 Office of Population Censuses and Surveys (1982) Communicable Disease Statistics 1980, HMSO, London.

68 Ogawa H., Nakamura A., Nakaya R., Mise K., Honjo S., Takasaka M., Fujiwara T. and Imaizumi K. (1967) Virulence and epithelial cell invasiveness of dysentery bacilli. *Jpn. J. Med. Sci. Biol.* **20**, 315.

69 Petrovskaya V. G. and Bondarenko V. M (1977) Recommended corrections to the classification of *Shigella flexneri* on a genetic basis. *Int. J. System. Bacteriol.* **27**, 171.

70 Prescott J. F., Manninen K. I. and Baker I. K. (1982) Experimental pathogenesis of *Campylobacter jejuni* enteritis — studies in gnotobiotic dogs, pigs and chickens. In: *Campylobacter*, p.170. Ed. Newell D. G., MTP Press, Lancaster.

71 Public Health Laboratory Service Working Group, Skorgaard N. and Nielsen B.B. (1972). Salmonellas in pigs and animal feeding stuffs in England and Wales and in Denmark. *J. Hyg.* **70**, 127.

72 Rahaman M. M., Huq I., Dey C. R., Kibriya A. K. M. G. and Curlin G. (1974) Ampicillin-resistant Shiga bacillus in Bangladesh. *Lancet* **i**, 406.

73 Report (1978) Persistent excretion of salmonellas. *Br. Med. J.* **5**, 509.

74 Robinson D. A., Edgar W. M., Gibson G. L., Matchett A. A. and Robertson L. (1979) Campylobacter enteritis associated with the consumption of unpasteurised milk. *Br. Med. J.* **1**, 1171.

75 Rosenberg M. L., Hazlet K. K., Schaefer I., Wells J. G. and Pruneda R. C. (1976) Shigellosis from swimming. *J. Am. Med. Assoc.* **16**, 1849.

76 Rout W. R., Formal S. B., Gianella R. A. and Dammin G. J. (1975) The pathophysiology of Shigella diarrhoea in the Rhesus monkey; intestinal transport, morphology and bacteriological studies. *Gastroenterology* **68**, 270.

77 Rowe B., Frost J. A., Threlfall E. J. and Ward L. R. (1980) Spread of a multiresistant clone of *Salmonella typhimurium* phage type 66/122 in South-East Asia and the Middle East. *Lancet* **i**, 1070.

78 Rowe B. and Gross R. J. (1976) Shiga dysentery in England and Wales. *Br. Med. J.* **i**, 532.

79   Rowe B., Gross R. J. and Allen H. A. (1974) *Shigella dysenteriae* and *Shigella boydii* in England and Wales during 1972 and 1973. *Br. Med. J.* **iv**, 641.

80   Rowe B., Gross R. J. and Guiney M. (1976) Antigenic relationships between *Escherichia coli* O antigens O149 to O163 and *Shigella* O antigens. *Int. J. System. Bacteriol.* **26**, 76.

81   Rowe B., Gross R. J. and van Oye E. (1975) An organism differing from *Shigella boydii* 13 only in its ability to produce gas from glucose. *Int. J. System. Bacteriol.* **25**, 301.

82   Rowe B., Hall M. L. M., Ward L. R. and de Sa J. D. H. (1980) Epidemic spread of *Salmonella hadar* in England and Wales. *Br. Med. J.* **280**, 1065.

83   Rowe B. and Threlfall E. J. (1981) Multiple antimicrobial drug resistance in enteric pathogens. *J. Antimicrob. Chemother.* **7**, 1.

84   Sakazaki R., Tamura K., Nakamura A. and Kurata T. (1974) Enteropathogenic and enterotoxigenic activities on ligated gut loops in rabbits of salmonella and some other enterobacteria isolated from human patients with diarrhea. *Jpn. J. Med. Sci. Biol.* **27**, 45.

85   Sakazaki R., Tamura K., Nakamura A., Kurata T., Gohda A. and Takeuchi S. (1974) Enteropathogenicity and enterotoxigenicity of human enteropathogenic *Escherichia coli*. *Jpn. J. Med. Sc. Biol.* **27**, 19.

86   Sandefur P. D. and Peterson J. W. (1976) Isolation of skin permeability factors from culture filtrates of *Salmonella typhimurium*. *Infect. Immun.* **14**, 671.

87   Saphra I. and Winter J. W. (1957) Clinical manifestations of salmonellosis in man. *N. Engl. J. Med.* **256**, 1128.

88   Sebald M. and Veron M. (1963) Teneur en bases de l'ADN et classification des vibrions. *Ann. Inst. Pasteur* **105**, 897.

89   Shaw C. H. (1953) Sonne dysentery in Ipswich. A study of infection in the home. Monthly Bulletin of the Ministry of Health and the Public Health Laboratory Service **12**, 44.

90   Shiga K. (1898) Ueber den Dysenterie bacillus (*Bacillus dysenteriae*). *Zentralbl. Bakteriol.* **24**, 913.

91   Shmilovitz M., Kretzer O. and Levy E. (1974) The anaerogenic serotype 147 as an etiologic agent of dysentery in Israel. *Isr. J. Med. Sci.* **10**, 1425.

92   Skirrow M. B. and Benjamin J. (1982) The classification of 'thermophilic' campylobacters and their distribution in man and domestic animals. In: *Campylobacter*, p.40. Ed. Newell D. G., MTP Press, Lancaster.

93   Smith T. and Taylor M. S. (1919) Some morphological and biological characters of *Spirilla* (*Vibrio fetus* n.sp.) associated with disease of fetal membranes in cattle. *J. Exp. Med.* **30**, 299.

94   Stenzel W. (1978) Problems of *Escherichieae* systematics and the classification of atypical dysentery bacilli. *Int. J. System. Bacteriol.* **28**, 597.

95   Taylor D. J. (1982) Natural and experimental enteric infections with catalase-positive campylobacters in cattle and pigs. In: *Campylobacter*, p.163. Ed. Newell D. G., MTP Press, Lancaster.

96   Thomas M. E. M. and Tillett H. E. (1973) Dysentery in general practice: a study of cases and their contacts in Enfield and an epidemiological comparison with salmonellosis. *J. Hyg.* **71**, 373.

97   Tiehan W. and Vogt R. L. (1978) Waterborne campylobacter gastroenteritis-Vermont. *Morbid. Mortal. Wkly Rept* **27**, 207.

98   Trifonova A., Bratoeva M. and Tekelieva R. (1974) Studies on biochemical variants of *Sh. flexneri*. I. Studies on the lactose positive variants of *Sh. flexneri* 2a. *Zentralbl. Bakteriol. A* **226**, 343.

99   Vernon E. (1977) Food poisoning and salmonella infections in England and Wales, 1973–75. *Public Health* **91**, 225.

100 Weissman J. B., Marton K. I., Lewis J. N., Freidmann C. T. H. and Gangarosa E. J. (1974) Impact in the United States of the Shiga dysentery pandemic in Central America and Mexico. Review of Surveillance Data through 1972. *J. Infect. Dis.* **129**, 218.

101   Weissman J. B., Schmerler A., Weiler P., Filice G., Godbey N. and Hansen I. (1974) The role of pre-school children and day-care centres in the spread of Shigellosis in urban communities. *J. Pediatr.* **84**, 797.

102   World Health Organization (1978) Salmonella surveillance 1975, *Weekly Epidemiological Record* **53**, 53.

103   Young S. E. J. (1982) Human campylobacter infections 1977–80; national data based on routine laboratory reporting. In: *Campylobacter*, p.17. Ed. Newell D. E., MTP Press, Lancaster.

4 *Escherichia coli* diarrhoea

R. J. Gross and B. Rowe

Introduction	79
Infantile enteropathogenic *E. coli* (EPEC)	80
Epidemiology	80
Pathogenesis	82
Laboratory investigations	83
Enterotoxigenic *E. coli* (ETEC)	83
Epidemiology	83
Infantile enteritis in developed countries	83
Diarrhoea in the community in developed countries	84
Traveller's diarrhoea	84
Diarrhoea in developing countries	85
Nature and mode of action of *E. coli* enterotoxins	86
Adhesive factors	87
Laboratory techniques	89
Antisera for the identification of ETEC	90
Enteroinvasive *E. coli* (EIEC)	90
Epidemiology	90
Pathogenesis	91
Laboratory investigation	91
Treatment and control	92
Vaccines	92
Inhibition of enterotoxin activity	93
Antimicrobial prophylaxis	94
References	94

INTRODUCTION

Although *Escherichia coli* was first isolated in 1885[28] from the stools of infants with enteritis, it was soon shown that this organism was also present in the faeces of healthy infants. The problem of recognizing those strains capable of causing diarrhoea was therefore apparent at an early stage. Lesage found in 1897[75] that the serum of infants with enteritis agglutinated *E. coli* isolated from other infants in the same epidemic but not those from healthy subjects. In 1933 Goldschmidt[44] studied epidemics of infantile enteritis in institutions by a slide agglutination method and therefore anticipated the serotyping methods now used routinely in clinical investigations. Bray[5] investigated an outbreak of infantile enteritis in a London hospital in 1945 and showed that the infants were infected with a strain of *E. coli* that belonged to a serogroup which was subsequently recognized as *E. coli* O111. Similar studies in Aberdeen during 1947 and 1948 showed that two serogroups of *E. coli* were the cause of epidemics of infantile enteritis. These strains were first designated as Aberdeen alpha and Aberdeen beta but were later allocated to *E. coli* serogroups O111 and O55 respectively.[43,137] Subsequent studies were facilitated by Kauffmann's description in 1947[64] of a serotyping scheme for *E. coli*, and in 1961 Taylor[139] was able to state that 170 serogroups of *E. coli* had been involved in epidemics of infantile enteritis.

In 1953 the rabbit ileal loop was reported to demonstrate the production of an enterotoxin by *V. cholerae*[11] and the same method was subsequently used to show that certain *E. coli* strains isolated from adults with diarrhoea in Calcutta also produced enterotoxin.[10] Other ileal loop tests proved valuable for the study of *E. coli* diarrhoea in animals. Smith and Gyles in 1970[133] used the pig intestine to show that strains enteropathogenic for swine produced two different enterotoxins. One enterotoxin was antigenic and heat labile (LT) and the other non-antigenic and heat stable (ST). In 1972 a method was developed using intragastric challenge of infant mice to test for ST production by strains of *E. coli* which had previously been shown to be enterotoxigenic in the rabbit ileal loop test.[12] Two years later two different tissue culture methods were described which could detect both the *V. cholerae* enterotoxin and *E. coli* LT.[14,51] Studies using these tests soon showed that strains of *E. coli* could produce ST, LT or both and that the genetic determinants of enterotoxin production were carried by plasmids.

Field studies soon established the importance of enterotoxigenic *E. coli* (ETEC) as a cause of human diarrhoeal disease. It was shown in 1976, however, that strains of *E. coli* that were responsible for epidemics of infantile enteritis in Britain were not enterotoxigenic as judged by the infant mouse test or tissue culture tests.[49] It became clear that *E. coli* could cause diarrhoea by more than one pathogenic mechanism.

Since infantile enteropathogenic *E. coli* (EPEC) were discovered by epidemiological studies using serotyping they belong, by definition, to a restricted range of serotypes. It has now been found that enterotoxigenic *E. coli* (ETEC) also frequently belong to particular serotypes which are different from those associated with EPEC.[88,95] In addition it has been shown that some strains of *E. coli* belonging to another range of serotypes cause dysentery-like symptoms and resemble *Shigella* in their ability to cause experimental keratoconjunctivitis in guinea pigs and to penetrate HeLa cells in tissue culture.[40,85,122] On the basis of these observations Rowe and his colleagues[106,111] have suggested that *E. coli* strains that cause diarrhoea may conveniently be considered as three groups, as follows:

(a) Enteropathogenic *E. coli* (EPEC): common serogroups, O26, O55, O86, O111, O114, O119, O125, O126, O127, O128, O142.

(b) Enterotoxigenic *E. coli* (ETEC): common serogroups, O6, O8, O15, O25, O27, O63, O78, O115, O148, O153, O159.

(c) Enteroinvasive *E. coli* (EIEC): common serogroups, O28ac, O112ac, O124, O136, O143, O144, O152, O164.

INFANTILE ENTEROPATHOGENIC *E. COLI* (EPEC)

Epidemiology

During the first quarter of this century outbreaks of 'summer diarrhoea' occurred each year among infants in Europe and the United States and were associated with a high mortality. The cause was never discovered although it was thought likely that infants were infected by contaminated cows' milk. The incidence of the disease declined during the 1920s and 1930s. This was also difficult to explain although it was suggested that contributing factors might include the introduction of dried and pasteurized milk and general improvements in hygiene and sanitation.[26] Between 1940 and 1950, outbreaks of infantile enteritis occurred in hospitals and nurseries and these outbreaks were seen more frequently during the winter months. At this time neither the aetiological agent nor the manner of spread of infection were recognized. Nevertheless, it was observed that outbreaks could be controlled by the sterilization of feeding bottles, the pasteurization or sterilization of milk feeds shortly before use, and the application of strict measures to control the transmission of the disease from patient to patient. In 1948 Hinden[54,55] reported that while the highest incidence of infantile enteritis in hospitals occurred during the winter months, cases in the community were distributed evenly throughout the year. During the investigations of outbreaks of infantile enteritis in Aberdeen in 1948, Giles and Sangster[43] noticed two peaks in the seasonal incidence of the disease. The highest incidence was in March and April, was mainly due to cases in hospitals and was accompanied by a high mortality. A smaller peak occurred in July and was mainly due to cases in the community. It was concluded that an outbreak in the community had occurred before or at the same time as the hospital outbreaks and that these outbreaks resulted from cross-infection in the hospital following the admission from the community of babies who were excreting the causative organism.

There was great debate concerning the aetiology of infantile enteritis but studies using serotyping showed convincingly that epidemics were caused by strains of *E. coli* belonging to particular O serogroups. Members of these serogroups later became known as enteropathogenic *E. coli* (EPEC). Between 1950 and 1960 outbreaks of infantile enteritis due to EPEC were reported among infants in hospitals and nurseries in Europe and North America, but in late 1967 an epidemic occurred in several hospitals in the Teesside area which was accompanied by a high mortality.[1] Two EPEC strains were involved: *E. coli* O119H6 and O128H2. About a year later an outbreak due to *E. coli* O114H2 occurred in hospitals in the Manchester area.[62] In late 1970 and early 1971 outbreaks due to *E. coli* O142H6 occurred in several hospitals in the Glasgow area[67,80] and later in the same year the same serotype was responsible for an outbreak in a Dublin hospital.[60] In Dublin, it appeared that the outbreak was due to cross-infection in the hospital after the admission of infected infants from the community, thus confirming the observations of Giles and Sangster in 1948.[43]

Since 1971 serious outbreaks of EPEC enteritis have rarely been reported in Britain or the United States but no satisfactory explanation has been put forward for this. In the absence of hospital outbreaks of infantile enteritis the incidence of sporadic infections in Britain is highest in the summer months.

Although EPEC enteritis now appears to be of relatively little importance in temperate areas with good standards of hygiene, surveys have confirmed that EPEC are still a common cause of enteritis in tropical countries[82] and among communities with poor standards of hygiene.[52] However the epidemiology of EPEC enteritis in tropical countries differs in some respects from that in Europe and North America. Although outbreaks in institutions are often reported in the tropics, sporadic cases and outbreaks occur more frequently in the community. Many authors have stressed the protective effect of breast-feeding and it has been shown that the peak incidence of enteritis in several countries occurs in the few months after the beginning of the weaning period.[128] Weaning often occurs later in developing countries and the age distribution of EPEC enteritis consequently differs from that in Europe and North America.

The importance of EPEC as a cause of enteritis in adults is difficult to assess since few laboratories look for EPEC in patients older than 3 years. However, a few outbreaks have been reported. A water-borne outbreak due to E. coli O111 affected adults attending a conference centre in the USA[125] and two food-borne outbreaks have been reported in Britain.[102,146] It has been shown that about 50% of children acquire haemagglutinating antibody to EPEC by the age of 1 year and it is possible that most babies are infected with EPEC early in life and thus acquire some resistance.[92]

Pathogenesis

Oral challenge experiments in infants and adults have confirmed the ability of EPEC strains to cause diarrhoea but their pathogenic mechanism remains obscure.[37,76] Postmortem studies[142] and intubation techniques[71] have shown that colonization of the duodenum and upper ileum occurs, although these regions of the gut are usually free of E. coli in healthy individuals. However, most EPEC strains do not produce ST or LT and are noninvasive, although a few strains of E. coli O114[7] and O128[101] have been shown to be enterotoxigenic by means of the infant mouse and tissue culture tests. Furthermore some strains of E. coli O26 and O126 produce a cytotoxin which can be detected using Vero cells.[70,126] 'Vero toxin' (VT) is distinct from ST and LT and its role in disease is unknown.

A report in the United States described the isolation of E. coli O125 from the duodenal aspirate of a 7 day old infant with protracted diarrhoea.[145] The E. coli strain was found to be nonenterotoxigenic and noninvasive but biopsy showed the organism to adhere closely to the epithelium of the small bowel. The authors proposed that this represented a new mechanism of diarrhoea although E. coli O125 is a well known EPEC serogroup.

Several studies have shown that EPEC strains cause accumulation of fluid in the rabbit ligated ileal loop test and these results suggest the production of an enterotoxin by these strains.[134,140] More recently, Klipstein and his colleagues[68] examined strains of EPEC from outbreaks of infantile enteritis which did not produce ST or LT but had been shown to have retained their virulence by human feeding experiments. Extracts of these strains caused a net efflux of water in experiments using a rat gut perfusion technique. These results suggest that EPEC may produce enterotoxins which affect water transport but which are not detectable in the infant mouse or tissue culture tests.

Laboratory investigations

Stool specimens from children less than 3 years old with diarrhoea are usually investigated for the presence of EPEC. Specimens are plated on nonselective media such as MacConkey or eosinmethylene blue agar and several colonies are examined by slide agglutination using polyvalent antisera for the EPEC serogroups. Colonies giving positive reactions are then tested using monovalent antisera. Identification is finally confirmed by tube agglutinations using heated antigen suspensions.[27] Strains provisionally serogrouped in this way should also be identified as *E. coli* by means of biochemical tests since there is widespread sharing of antigens among the members of the Enterobacteriaceae.

In outbreaks of infantile enteritis when EPEC are not found the assistance of a reference laboratory should be sought. Complete serotyping with more than 160 O antisera and more than 50 H antisera occasionally leads to the recognition of new EPEC serogroups.

ENTEROTOXIGENIC *E. COLI* (ETEC)

Epidemiology

Infections due to ETEC may conveniently be classified into a number of categories. In areas of good hygiene and nutrition ETEC are uncommon but they may occasionally cause outbreaks of diarrhoea both among infants in hospital nurseries and among individuals of all ages in the community. In addition, ETEC are the most common cause of diarrhoea among those travelling from such areas to regions with poor hygiene, especially in the tropics. In the developing countries diarrhoeal disease, together with underlying malnutrition, is a major cause of death in children under 5. Since ETEC are responsible for a high proportion of the acute diarrhoeas of childhood in these areas they contribute significantly to the high level of infant mortality. The most severe illness caused by ETEC is indistinguishable on admission to hospital from that due to *V. cholerae*. This syndrome has been described in western countries but is more commonly reported in areas where cholera is endemic.

These categories are clearly arbitrary and there is overlap between them. Certain populations may exist within a developed country which have a relatively poor standard of hygiene and, particularly if the climate is warm, there may be a high incidence of ETEC infections similar to that found in the tropics. For example, in a study in 1975 of Apache indian children in an Arizona reservation, ETEC were found in 16% of those hospitalized with acute diarrhoea.[121]

Infantile enteritis in developed countries

The first report of an outbreak of infantile enteritis due to ETEC was in 1976.[48] Twenty-five babies in the nursery of a Glasgow hospital were infected. Five babies required intravenous therapy, but there were no fatalities. The causative organism belonged to a previously undescribed serogroup, E. coli O159, and produced ST but not LT. In the same year an outbreak was reported which affected 55 of 205 infants in the special-care nursery of a large hospital in the United States.[116] The epidemic strain belonged to serogroup O78 and again produced ST but not LT. Another outbreak in Britain which affected 10 of 18 babies in the special-care unit of a Gloucester hospital was caused by a strain of E. coli O6 which produced ST and LT.[109] The source and route of transmission of infection in these outbreaks was uncertain. In the Gloucester outbreak the evidence suggested that the index case was a premature baby who developed diarrhoea 4 days after birth and subsequent cases resulted from cross-infection. The outbreak in the United States continued for 9 months and investigations of the hospital environment revealed heavy contamination with E. coli O78. The epidemic strain was also isolated from milk feeds.

Diarrhoea in the community in developed countries

Several surveys have shown that ETEC are probably not an important cause of sporadic diarrhoea in developed countries with good standards of hygiene. A study of Boston children in 1975[20] suggested that ETEC were unimportant and studies in Canada in 1977 reached the same conclusion.[52] In Europe a Swedish study in 1977[2] and a small survey in Britain in 1979[50] found that ETEC were uncommon as a cause of indigenous sporadic diarrhoea in those countries. However, two studies in the USA found a high incidence of ETEC in infants and children with enteritis. Gorbach and Khurana in 1972[46] found ETEC in 80% of faecal specimens from children under 4 years old in Chicago, and Rudoy and Nelson reported similar findings in infants and children in Texas in 1975.[113] These reports did not gain wide acceptance since the first group used an infant rabbit test, which has not been used by other workers; the well known tissue culture tests and the infant mouse test being preferred. The second group adopted unusual criteria for the interpretation of the infant mouse test and have been criticized for failing to share their strains with other laboratories for confirmation.[42]

In the summer of 1975 more than 2000 staff and visitors at a national park in the United States developed diarrhoea caused by a strain of E. coli O6 which produced ST and LT.[105] The source of the infection was found to be drinking water which had been contaminated with sewage. In Japan seven outbreaks of adult enteritis were studied in Tokyo between 1969 and 1974.[72] Six were caused by

E. coli O159 and one by *E. coli* O11. In all the outbreaks the *E. coli* produced ST but not LT. Two outbreaks were caused by contaminated water supplies and two others were thought to be due to food-borne infection.

Traveller's diarrhoea

Traveller's diarrhoea is a worldwide illness, usually of brief duration, often beginning with the rapid onset of loose stools and sometimes accompanied by other symptoms including nausea, vomiting and abdominal cramps. It occurs most frequently among those travelling from areas of good hygiene and temperate climate to areas with lower standards, particularly in the tropics.

Rowe and his colleagues first demonstrated a relationship between *E. coli* and traveller's diarrhoea in a study of British troops in South Arabia in 1970.[112] In this study serotyping provided evidence to suggest that about 50% of diarrhoea among new arrivals might be due to *E. coli* O148, a previously undescribed serogroup. Only later was it discovered that this strain produced ST.[108] Enterotoxigenic *E. coli* O148 was also a cause of diarrhoea among United States soldiers in Vietnam.[17] ETEC belonging to a number of serotypes were the most common pathogens found among US military personnel in the Philippines in a 1979 study.[22] In contrast, in the same year a study of US troops in South Korea, an area with a relatively temperate climate, showed that ETEC infections were uncommon even though 55% of the soldiers developed diarrhoea.[24]

There have been several studies of traveller's diarrhoea in Mexico where 'Turista' has an attack rate of 29–48%. In one study ETEC was the most common cause and accounted for 45% of the diarrhoea cases,[87] while in another survey 72% of those with diarrhoea were excreting ETEC.[45]

Civilian travellers from Europe to tropical or even Mediterranean countries may develop diarrhoea due to ETEC. In a study in Sweden in 1977[2] ETEC were found in 11% of those developing diarrhoea while abroad or shortly after returning from abroad, and in a similar study in Great Britain in 1979[50] the figure was also 11%.

The sea cruise is a form of travel which has often been plagued by outbreaks of diarrhoea. *Salmonella* or *Shigella* are often the cause but some outbreaks have been associated with ETEC. Hobbs and her colleagues[56] reported that a strain of *E. coli* O27 that produced ST was isolated from 55%, 61% and 20% of travellers with diarrhoea on three successive cruises by the same ship. On this ship the infections were probably food-borne. In another ship it was reported that an *E. coli* O25 strain that produced ST was isolated from 83% of diarrhoea cases in outbreaks occurring during two successive cruises.[103] Studies on board the ship revealed many deficiencies in the handling of food and drinks. When these procedures were improved no further outbreaks of diarrhoea occurred.

Diarrhoea in developing countries

There is no doubt that ETEC are an important cause of diarrhoea in all age groups in areas of poor hygiene, particularly in the tropics. In a study of 354 Ethiopian children and infants with diarrhoea ETEC were isolated from 14% of the patients.[147] In black South African infants with acute summer gastroenteritis ETEC were found in 9 of 34 infants,[124] while in a survey in Taiwan ETEC were found in 9 of 57 children (16%).[23] In Mexico, Donta and his colleagues[15] found ETEC in 16% of 50 children admitted to hospital with diarrhoea while Evans and her colleagues[30] isolated ETEC from 40% of 71 children in a retrospective study. In a separate study of 62 children with diarrhoea at a Mexico City hospital outpatient clinic, Evans and her group found ETEC in 29 patients (47%).[32] In the Philippines Echeverria and his colleagues[21] found ETEC in 11% of 82 children hospitalized with diarrhoea.

Although clinical cholera characterized by profuse 'rice-water' stools is traditionally associated with *V. cholerae*, there was, prior to the discovery of ETEC, a significant proportion of patients from whom no aetiological agent could be isolated. In 1971 Sack and his colleagues[120] used the rabbit ileal loop test to demonstrate LT production by ETEC isolated from jejunal aspirates of four adult patients with cholera-like diarrhoea in Calcutta. A subsequent survey in Bangladesh showed that LT-producing ETEC could be isolated from 19.2% of all patients with diarrhoea, from 55% of hospital inpatients with diarrhoea and from 70% of those severely ill with non-vibrio cholera.[91] In a further study in rural Bangladesh, ETEC were not found in 22 patients less than 2 years old, but were isolated from 11 of 18 patients (56%) who were more than 10 years old.[115] Sack and his colleagues[118] studied patients with acute cholera-like disease in Dacca, Bangladesh, and isolated ETEC from 23 of 65 patients (35%). Diarrhoea caused by ETEC affected individuals of all ages and could not be distinguished from cholera on clinical grounds.

The sources and methods of transmission of ETEC infection in developing countries are poorly understood. In one Bangladesh study ETEC were found in only one of 39 drinking water sources,[115] while in a study in the Philippines ETEC were not found in foods or surface waters, although they were isolated from a small number of pigs and water buffalo.[25] In a more recent Bangladesh study[3] it was shown that in 9% of dwellings where patients with ETEC diarrhoea lived, the drinking water was contaminated with ETEC belonging to the same serotype as that causing the illness. The incidence of infection was highest in the dwellings with contaminated water. It seems likely that water contaminated by human or animal sewage is an important cause of ETEC infection but further studies are needed to confirm this.

Nature and mode of action of *E. coli* enterotoxins

HEAT-LABILE ENTEROTOXIN (LT)

LT consists of two polypeptide subunits. Subunit A has a molecular weight of about 25 000 and has the ability to stimulate adenylate cyclase activity. Subunit B has a molecular weight of about 11 500 and has the ability to form aggregates of

4 or 5 monomers which are able to adsorb to Y1 adrenal cells used in LT tests. Immunological and biological neutralization tests show that there is a close similarity between *E. coli* LT and the *V. cholerae* enterotoxin. Furthermore there is significant homology between the amino acid sequences of the B subunits of LT and *V. cholerae* enterotoxin. In both toxins the B subunit is responsible for binding to the Gm1 ganglioside of the epithelial cells of the small intestine, while subunit A stimulates adenylate cyclase activity thereby increasing the concentration of cyclic AMP in the cells. The increased level of cAMP appears to act in two ways to cause fluid and electrolyte loss into the gut lumen. In the villus cells cAMP inhibits the absorption of Na^+ and hence of Cl^- and water. In the crypt cells cAMP exerts a direct secretory effect by increasing Na^+ secretion and consequently causing loss of Cl^- and water.[38]

HEAT-STABLE ENTEROTOXIN (ST)

Estimates of the molecular weight of the ST polypeptide have varied. However, the situation was clarified to some extent when it was shown that more than one form of ST exists: STa is methanol soluble and active in the infant mouse test and in neonatal piglets while STb is methanol insoluble, inactive in infant mice and active in ligated intestinal loops of older piglets and rabbits.[6] *E. coli* strains may produce STa, STb or both. Furthermore, ST produced by strains isolated from different host species may differ both in molecular weight and in amino-acid sequence.[100] For example, a strain of porcine origin has been shown to produce ST of molecular weight 3580 with 33 amino acid residues while ST from a strain of human origin had a molecular weight of 1972 with 18 residues.

ST does not affect the concentration of cAMP but instead stimulates the activity of guanylate cyclase and therefore causes an increase in cGMP levels. This occurs only in intestinal epithelial cells and not in a variety of other tissues and cell lines suggesting that a unique toxin receptor is present in intestinal cells. The mechanism by which increased cGMP leads to a net secretion of water and electrolytes is not well understood but the action of ST appears to be mainly antiabsorptive and lacks the secretory activity of LT and cholera toxin.[39,93]

Adhesive factors

Studies of piglet enteritis first showed that the ability to produce enterotoxin is not sufficient to enable an *E. coli* strain to cause diarrhoea.[136] The organism must also be able to colonize the mucosal surface of the epithelial cells of the small intestine. This colonization depends on adhesion mediated by pilus-like filamentous protein structures which bind to specific receptors in the cell membrane. Adhesive factors are antigenic and can be recognized by means of agglutination or immunodiffusion tests using specific antisera. Their presence can also be demonstrated by haemagglutination, by experimental colonization of animal intestines or by tissue or organ culture methods. In contrast to the haemagglutination due to type 1 pili of *E. coli*, that due to adhesive factors associated with diarrhoeal disease is not inhibited by the presence of mannose. The genetic determinants controlling the production of *E. coli* adhesive factors are carried on plasmids which may be transferable. Plasmids exist which simultaneously carry genes for both an adhesive factor and enterotoxin production.[132]

The first adhesive factor found to be important in *E. coli* diarrhoea was an antigen (K88) which was shown to be controlled by a transferable plasmid.[96] K88 could also be detected by its ability to cause mannose-resistant haemagglutination (MRHA) of guinea pig red blood cells.[63] Its importance in piglet enteritis was demonstrated by Smith and Linggood in 1971.[136] In an elegant series of experiments they showed that the loss of the K88 plasmid from a strain of *E. coli* O141 resulted in the loss of its ability to cause diarrhoea when given orally to piglets. This ability was restored by introducing a K88 plasmid from another strain of *E. coli*. It was later shown that there is a gene in pigs themselves that is inherited in a simple Mendelian manner and which determines the presence of receptors for K88 in the cells of the pig intestinal epithelium. Pigs lacking this receptor are resistant to small intestine colonization by *E. coli* possessing the K88 antigen.[114]

Another antigen designated as 987P is important in infections of pigs,[61] while the K99 antigen causes MRHA of sheep red blood cells and has been shown to be important in diarrhoea of sheep and cattle.[97]

In 1975[33] an enterotoxigenic strain of *E. coli* O78 isolated from a human patient with cholera-like diarrhoea was found to possess an adhesive factor now known as colonization factor antigen 1 (CFA/I). Small numbers of this organism injected into the duodenum of infant rabbits grew to large numbers and caused diarrhoea. A laboratory-passaged derivative did not increase in population and did not cause diarrhoea. Antiserum prepared using the original strain as the vaccine and absorbed with the laboratory derivative agglutinated the original strain only. The agglutination depended on the presence of a pilus-like surface structure, the loss of which correlated with the loss of a particular plasmid. Strains of *E. coli* which possess CFA/I cause MRHA of human group A erythrocytes[31] but this is of little value as a test for CFA/I since strains from extraintestinal sources frequently cause group A MRHA but are not enterotoxigenic and do not possess CFA/I.[9] The presence of CFA/I appears to be restricted mainly to a few serogroups of ETEC including O25, O63, O78 and O153.[47] The frequency with which CFA/I strains are found in surveys therefore depends on the serotypes of ETEC found in the area studied. It has been confirmed by oral challenge experiments in human volunteers that the original CFA/I strain causes diarrhoea while its laboratory derivative without CFA/I does not.[123] Nevertheless, strains of ETEC belonging to other serotypes and lacking CFA/I have also been shown to cause diarrhoea in volunteers.[77]

A second colonization factor (CFA/II) has also been found and differs from CFA/I antigenically and also in its ability to cause MRHA of bovine but not human red blood cells. CFA/II was found in ETEC belonging to serogroups O6 and O8 and was found to be common in strains of these serogroups isolated from patients with traveller's diarrhoea in Mexico.[29] Another antigenically distinct colonization factor known as E8775 has also been found in ETEC of other serogroups including O25, O115 and O167.[141] It seems likely that further colonization factors are yet to be recognized.

Laboratory techniques

DETECTION OF LT

Tissue culture methods using Y1 mouse adrenal cells[14] and Chinese hamster ovary (CHO) cells[51] are widely used for the detection of LT, although other cell lines, including Vero monkey kidney cells, are also sensitive.[138] In these tests the cells are exposed to culture supernatants and if LT or cholera toxin are present an increase in the intracellular concentration of cAMP results and leads to a morphological response which can be seen microscopically. CHO cells respond by elongation while Y1 cells become rounded. The response is distinct from the cytotoxic effect of supernatants of some *E. coli* O26 and O126 cultures in Vero cells.[69,126]

Injection of LT or cholera toxin intradermally in rabbits causes a local increase in vascular permeability which can be detected as an area of induration and blue colouration following intravenous injection of Evans Blue dye. This reaction forms the basis of the permeability factor (PF) test which has not been widely used for the detection of LT but has proved more valuable as an assay for antitoxin directed against LT or cholera toxin.[35]

Antisera to LT can be prepared in animals and immunological techniques may therefore be used for the detection of LT. A passive immune haemolysis method has been described in which sheep erythrocytes sensitized with LT were lysed by exposure to antitoxin and complement.[34] An enzyme-linked immunosorbent assay (ELISA) has also been described which used cholera antitoxin prepared in guinea pigs and a goat anti-guinea pig serum conjugated with alkaline phosphatase. The ELISA method was used in a study of diarrhoea in adults in Bangladesh and Kenya.[148]

A solid phase radio-immunoassay (RIA) for *E. coli* LT has also been described.[8] In this method an LT antitoxin prepared in goats was bound to polystyrene tubes and LT was assayed by competitive inhibition of the binding of radioiodinated LT. A development of the passive immune haemolysis method enabled tests to be performed in media solidified with agar.[4] In this way large numbers of individual colonies of *E. coli* or *V. cholerae* could be tested for LT production and mutants could be selected for genetic studies. The discovery that the Gm1 ganglioside binds LT and cholera toxin led to the development of a ganglioside ELISA test for the detection of these toxins.[117] Microtiter wells were coated with Gm1 ganglioside and the test samples were then added. Bound toxin was detected by the addition of guinea pig cholera antitoxin followed by enzyme-labelled goat anti-guinea pig serum. Finally, a precipitin test (the 'Biken test') performed directly on cultures growing on special agar media has recently been described and promises to be a valuable, simple technique.[59]

DETECTION OF ST

Surveys suggest that almost half of all enterotoxigenic *E. coli* isolates produce only ST while only a small number produce LT alone.[86] For this reason it is important to include tests for ST production in any survey. Unfortunately the usual tests are cumbersome, time consuming and extravagant in their use of experimental animals.

Injection of enterotoxin preparations into ligated ileal loops of rabbits,[10] pigs, calves[135] and dogs[90] causes accumulation of fluid. In these tests the action of ST can be distinguished from that of LT by its relative stability to heat and by its rapidity of action. Nevertheless, these tests have not been widely used in investigations of human disease. So far it has proved impossible to develop tissue culture tests for ST and the most widely used method is the infant mouse test described by Dean and his colleagues in 1972.[12] In this test infant mice are challenged by injection of culture supernatants through the abdominal wall into the milk filled stomach. After 4 hours the mice are killed and the intestines examined for dilation due to accumulated fluid. The intestines are then removed and the ratio of gut weight to remaining body weight determined as an objective measure of fluid accumulation. The test works well for *E. coli* of human and bovine origin but some strains of porcine origin produce ST which can be detected using a ligated intestinal loop test in pigs but not by the infant mouse test.[53]

The non-antigenic nature of ST prevented the development of more convenient immunological test methods until recently but antiserum to purified ST has now been prepared by coupling the toxin to a bovine serum albumin carrier.[41] The antiserum has been used to develop a radioimmunoassay and other studies should lead to the development of further convenient test methods, including ELISA, in the near future.

Antisera for the identification of ETEC

Many ETEC belong to a restricted range of serogroups and it has been suggested that serogrouping might provide a simple test for the preliminary recognition of ETEC in clinical laboratories. In a study in Bangladesh,[86] 12 antisera were used for the examination of *E. coli* from 618 patients with acute diarrhoea. The survey yielded 798 *E. coli* isolates, of which 130 produced ST and LT, 115 produced ST and 9 produced LT. Using the 12 antisera the local laboratory identified 110 of the 130 ST/LT strains (85%) but only 46 of the 115 ST strains (40%). Similar studies are needed in other parts of the world to evaluate this method and to determine whether any changes to the constituent serogroups might improve its sensitivity.

ENTEROINVASIVE *E. COLI* (EIEC)

Epidemiology

In contrast to the attention given to ETEC during the last 10 years, there have been few studies of EIEC and our understanding of their epidemiology is limited. The first description of EIEC diarrhoea was in American troops in the Mediterranean region in 1947.[36] An organism regarded at the time as a 'paracolon bacillus' was isolated from diarrhoeal stools and from food handlers and was later identified as *E. coli* O124. Strains of this serogroup have caused outbreaks in hospitals in Britain[57,107] and water-borne outbreaks in the community in Hungary.[74] A large outbreak in the USA in 1971 resulted from the importation of contaminated French cheese.[83] Enteroinvasive *E. coli* O164 have also been the subject of several reports. The organism was first isolated in 1946 from the faeces of a British prison inmate who developed dysentery. Outbreaks and sporadic cases were subsequently reported in Australia,[104] Britain[110] and Israel.[130]

In most reports adults and children have been affected and the age distribution therefore contrasts with that seen in EPEC. Patients often develop the symptoms of bacillary dysentery including fever and diarrhoea with blood and mucus in the stools.

Pathogenesis

The ability of EIEC to cause the symptoms of bacillary dysentery has been confirmed in human volunteers by means of feeding experiments using strains of *E. coli* O124, O136 and O143.[17] Sigmoidoscopy of infected volunteers showed changes similar to those seen in mild *Shigella* dysentery. Sigmoidoscopy of patients in the cheese-borne outbreak in the United States showed ulceration of the colon.[83] Laboratory tests using rabbits and guinea pigs have shown the importance of epithelial cell invasion and thus confirm that the pathogenesis of EIEC diarrhoea resembles that of *Shigella* dysentery and depends on epithelial invasion in the large bowel leading to inflammation and ulceration of the mucosa.

Laboratory investigation

The identification of EIEC is difficult for several reasons. They are frequently atypical in their biochemical reactions and may ferment lactose late or not at all, and may be anaerogenic and non-motile. In addition, most of the serogroups to which EIEC most commonly belong are antigenically related to various *Shigella* serogroups.[27] For these reasons clinical laboratories may mistakenly identify these strains as *Shigella*. Such a misidentification is of little consequence clinically since EIEC diarrhoea is indistiguishable from *Shigella* dysentery but, for epidemiological purposes, accurate identification is important.

The correlation between serogroup and pathogenicity in the EIEC is far from perfect and serogrouping is therefore of limited value in distinguishing EIEC from non-pathogenic *E. coli* strains. It has recently been reported that most EIEC strains fail to decarboxylate lysine and differ in this respect from most other *E. coli* strains.[131] It is possible that serogrouping and biochemical testing combined might be valuable in the recognition of EIEC but more studies are needed.

Laboratory tests are available for the detection of 'invasiveness' in EIEC and *Shigella* but these are not widely used in clinical laboratories. In the Sereny test a suspension of live organisms is instilled into the guinea pig eye; EIEC and virulent *Shigella* strains cause an ulcerative keratoconjunctivitis.[129] Tissue culture tests have also been described using either HeLa[17] or HEp-2 cells.[85]

TREATMENT AND CONTROL

For detailed consideration of the treatment of diarrhoea the reader is referred to the recent texts edited by Lambert[73] and by DuPont and Pickering.[18] Most otherwise healthy and well-nourished patients with diarrhoea recover uneventfully. It must be emphasized, however, that in severe cases the early correction of fluid and electrolytes balance is the most important single factor in preventing the death of the patient. Infants and the elderly are particularly susceptible to the effects of dehydration.

The value of antimicrobial therapy in *E. coli* diarrhoea has not been definitively established and it should certainly not be used routinely. Nevertheless, infants with severe EPEC infections have sometimes been reported to respond dramatically to antibiotic treatment and such treatment should be considered for prolonged or severe illness. Studies to establish the value of antimicrobial treatment of ETEC diarrhoea are still required. It is, however, reasonable to assume that such treatment would decrease the total fluid loss in view of the similarity of the disease to cholera.

There are a number of different approaches to the prevention of *E. coli* diarrhoea and these are best considered separately. First of all it should be remembered that the most important aspect in the prevention of illness is the prevention of exposure to the infecting agent. The transmission of ETEC in tropical countries is probably by means of contaminated food and water and the prevention of diarrhoeal disease in the indigenous population depends on the establishment of adequate standards of hygiene and nutrition. The traveller in such areas is advised to take advice from those with local experience before selecting eating places, and to depend on hot food and drinks or bottled water. While peeled fruits are likely to be safe, leafy vegetables are likely to be contaminated. Milk should be considered unsafe unless pasteurized. The spread of infantile enteritis in hospitals and nurseries depends on the transmission of the infecting organism from patient to patient by way of the environment or the hands of hospital staff. Outbreaks can usually be contained by the isolation of infected patients and the institution of strict barrier nursing techniques. In some cases only the closure of the ward or nursery and its complete disinfection before reopening will be effective.

Vaccines

Veterinary investigations of *E. coli* enteritis have often preceded similar studies in human medicine. It was shown in 1976[13] that LT preparations administered to pregnant sows could protect newborn piglets against challenge with LT or ST and a 1977 study showed that immunization of rats with cholera toxoid protected against challenge with LT.[98] A report in 1978 described the use of heated antigens derived from a number of enteropathogenic serotypes of *E. coli* as an additive to the diet of pigs at weaning.[78] Although such preparations would not be expected to contain exterotoxin in an immunogenic form, it was found that pigs became insensitive to ST and LT. In the same year it was shown that vaccination of pregnant sows with purified K99 or 987 pili could protect suckling pigs against subsequent challenge with ETEC strains possessing these adhesive factors.[89] The development of human vaccines based either on toxoid antigens or on colonization factor antigens is an important area of research and considerable progress may be expected during the next few years.

Inhibition of enterotoxin activity

Several substances have been shown to inhibit or reverse the secretory effects of enterotoxins in experimental animals and may be of value in the prevention of diarrhoea. Phenylbutazone administered subcutaneously to the infant mouse 30 minutes before intragastric injection of ST significantly reduces the resulting fluid accumulation.[94] Activated attapulgite or charcoal given prior to, or simultaneously with, LT or cholera toxin prevents fluid accumulation in the rabbit ileal loop.[16] Nicotinic acid is known to lower tissue levels of cAMP and it has been shown that subcutaneous or intraluminal injection of rabbits with nicotinic acid blocks the rise in cAMP and fluid secretion caused by cholera toxin in the rabbit ileal loop.[143] Chlorpromazine inhibits adenylate cyclase in several tissues and has been investigated as a possible antisecretory drug for the treatment of dehydrating diarrhoea. Experiments in mice[58] showed it to be effective in inhibiting the effects of LT and cholera toxin and studies of natural ETEC diarrhoea in pigs confirmed its antisecretory effects.[79] Clinical trials using chlorpromazine in the treatment of patients with severe cholera showed that a significant reduction in fluid loss was achieved.[99] The effect of indomethacin on the secretion of fluid caused by ST in the infant mouse has been studied and a significant decrease reported.[81] Bismuth subsalicylate has been shown to inhibit the effect of crude *V. cholerae* and *E. coli* enterotoxins in the rabbit intestinal loop and a controlled trial has been undertaken in the prophylaxis of traveller's diarrhoea in young adults visiting Mexico from the USA.[19] Treated individuals experienced fewer intestinal complaints and were less likely to pass loose stools than control subjects. Once diarrhoea developed, enteropathogens were found less commonly in the stools of those receiving bismuth subsalicylate than in those receiving placebo.

Further clinical trials of such agents appear to be warranted, especially in view of the problems associated with the use of antimicrobial drugs for prophylaxis.

Antimicrobial prophylaxis

There is little doubt that a number of antimicrobial drugs reduce the incidence of diarrhoea in travellers to tropical areas. Reports in 1962,[66] 1963,[65] and 1967[144] indicated that phthalylsulphathiazole, neomycin and streptotriad might be effective while more recent studies have demonstrated the value of doxycycline.[119] Nevertheless, the widespread use of antibiotic prophylaxis has been criticized both on the grounds of drug toxicity and because of the possibility that the development and spread of drug resistance might be encouraged among a variety of enteropathogenic organisms. Plasmids have been discovered which carry the genetic determinants of both drug resistance and enterotoxin production and these plasmids can be transferred from one strain of *E. coli* to another.[84,127] Antibiotics might therefore encourage the spread of enterotoxigenicity as well as drug resistance and thus increase the incidence of drug-resistant, enterotoxigenic strains of *E. coli*.

REFERENCES

1 Annotations (1968) Gastroenteritis due to *Escherichia coli. Lancet* **i**, 32.
2 Back E., Blomberg S. and Wadstrom T. (1977) Enterotoxigenic *Escherichia coli* in Sweden. *Infection* **5**, 2.
3 Black R. E., Merson M. H., Rowe B., Taylor P. R., Abdul Alim A. R. M., Gross R. J. and Sack D. A. (1981) Enterotoxigenic *Escherichia coli* diarrhoea: acquired immunity and transmission in an endemic area. *Bull. WHO* **59**, 263.
4 Bramucci M. G. and Holmes R. K. (1978) Radial passive immune hemolysis assay for detection of heat-labile enterotoxin produced by individual colonies of *Escherichia coli* or *Vibrio cholerae. J. Clin. Microbiol.* **8**, 252.
5 Bray J. (1945) Isolation of antigenically homogeneous strains of *Bact. coli neapolitanum* from summer diarrhoea of infants. *J. Pathol.* **57**, 239.
6 Burgess M. N., Bywater R. J., Cowley C. M., Mullan N. A. and Newsome P. M. (1978) Biological evaluation of a methanol-soluble heat-stable *Escherichia coli* enterotoxin in infant mice, pigs, rabbits and calves. *Infect. Immun.* **21**, 526.
7 Burnham G. M., Scotland S. M., Gross R. J. and Rowe B. (1976) New enterotoxigenic bacteria isolated. *Br. Med. J.* **2**, 1256.
8 Ceska M., Grossmuller F. and Effenberger F. (1978) Solid-phase radioimmunoassay method for determination of *Escherichia coli* enterotoxin. *Infect. Immun.* **19**, 347.
9 Cravioto A., Gross R. J., Scotland S. M. and Rowe B. (1979) Mannose-resistant haemagglutination of human erythrocytes by strains of *Escherichia coli* from extraintestinal sources: lack of correlation with colonization factor antigen (CFA/I). *FEMS Microbiol. Lett.* **6**, 41.
10 De S. N., Bhattacharya K. and Sarkar J. K. (1956) A study of pathogenicity of strains of *Bacterium coli* from acute and chronic enteritis. *J. Pathol. Bacteriol.* **71**, 201.
11 De S. N. and Chatterje D. N. (1953) An experimental study of the mechanism of action of *Vibrio cholerae* on the intestinal mucous membrane. *J. Pathol. Bacteriol.* **66**, 559–62.
12 Dean A. G., Ching Y., Williams R. G. and Harden L. B. (1972) Test for *Escherichia coli* enterotoxin using infant mice: application in a study of diarrhea in children in Honolulu. *J. Infect. Dis.* **125**, 407.
13 Dobrescu L. and Huygelen C. (1976) Protection of piglets against neonatal *E.coli* enteritis by immunization of the sow with a vaccine containing heat-labile enterotoxin (LT). *Zentralbl. Veterinarmed.* **B23**, 79.

14 Donta S. T., Moon H. W. and Whipp S. C. (1974) Detection of heat-labile *Escherichia coli* enterotoxin with the use of adrenal cells in tissue culture. *Science* **183**, 334.

15 Donta S. T., Wallace R. B., Whipp S. C. and Olarte J. (1977) Enterotoxigenic *E.coli* and diarrheal disease in Mexican children. *J. Infect. Dis.* **135**, 482.

16 Drucker M. M., Goldhar J., Ogra P. L. and Neter E. (1977) The effect of attapulgite and charcoal on enterotoxicity of *Vibrio cholerae* and *Escherichia coli* enterotoxins in rabbits. *Infection* **5**, 211.

17 DuPont H. L., Formal S. B., Hornick R. B., Snyder M. J., Libonati J. P., Sheahan D. G., Labrec E. H. and Kalas J. P. (1971) Pathogenesis of *Escherichia coli* diarrhea. *N. Eng. J. Med.* **285**, 1.

18 DuPont H. L. and Pickering L. K. (Eds) (1980) *Infections of the Gastrointestinal Tract*, Plenum, New York.

19 DuPont H. L., Sullivan P., Evans D. G., Pickering L. K., Evans D. J., Vollet J. L., Ericsson C. D., Ackerman P. B. and Tjoa W. S. (1980) Prevention of travelers' diarrhea (emporiatric enteritis). Prophylactic adminstration of subsalicylate bismuth. *J. Am. Med. Assoc.* **243**, 237.

20 Echeverria P., Blacklow N. R. and Smith D. H. (1975) Role of heat-labile toxigenic *Escherichia coli* and reovirus-like agent in diarrhoea in Boston children. *Lancet* **ii**, 1113.

21 Echeverria P., Blacklow N. R., Vollet J. L., Ulyangco C. V., Cukor G., Soriano V. B., DuPont H. L., Cross J. H., Ørskov F. and Ørskov I. (1978) Reovirus-like agent and enterotoxigenic *Escherichia coli* infections in pediatric diarrhea in the Philippines. *J. Infect. Dis.* **138**, 326.

22 Echeverria P., Blacklow N. R., Zipkin C., Vollet J. L., Olson J. A., DuPont H. L. and Cross J. H. (1979) Etiology of gastroenteritis among Americans living in the Philippines. *Am. J. Epidemiol.* **109**, 493.

23 Echeverria P., Ho M. T., Blacklow N. R., Quinnan G., Portnoy B., Olson J. G., Conklin R., DuPont H. L. and Cross J. H. (1977) Relative importance of viruses and bacteria in the etiology of pediatric diarrhea in Taiwan. *J. Infect. Dis.* **136**, 383.

24 Echeverria P., Ramirez G., Blacklow N. R., Ksiazek T., Cukor G. and Cross J. H. (1979) Travelers' diarrhea among U.S. Army troops in South Korea. *J. Infect. Dis.* **139**, 215.

25 Echeverria P., Verhaert L., Basaca-Sevilla V., Banson T., Cross J., Ørskov F. and Ørskov I. (1978) Search for heat-labile enterotoxigenic *Escherichia coli* in humans, livestock, food, and water in a community in the Philippines. *J. Infect. Dis.* **138**, 87.

26 Editorial (1936) Infantile diarrhoea in hospital. *Lancet* **ii**, 85.

27 Edwards P. R. and Ewing W. H. (1972) *Identification of Enterobacteriaceae.* Burgess Publishing Co., Minneapolis.

28 Escherich T. (1885) Die Darmbakterien des Neugeborenen und Säuglings. *Fortsch. Med.* **3**, 515.

29 Evans D. G. and Evans D. J. (1978) New surface-associated heat-labile colonization factor antigen (CFA/II) Produced by enterotoxigenic *Escherichia coli* of serogroups 06 and 08. *Infect. Immun.* **21**, 638.

30 Evans D. G., Evans D. J. and DuPont H. L. (1977) Virulence factors of enterotoxigenic *Escherichia coli*. *J. Infect. Dis.* **136**, S118.

31 Evans D. G., Evans D. J. and Tjoa W. (1977) Hemagglutination of human group A erythrocytes by enterotoxigenic *Escherichia coli* isolated from adults with diarrhea: correlation with colonization factor. *Infect. Immun.* **18**, 330.

32 Evans D. G., Olarte J., DuPont H. L., Evans D. J., Galindo E., Portnoy B. L. and Conklin R. H. (1977) Enteropathogens associated with pediatric diarrhea in Mexico City. *J. Pediat.* **91**, 65.

33 Evans D. G., Silver R. P., Evans D. J., Chase D. G. and Gorbach S. L. (1975) Plasmid controlled colonization factor associated with virulence in *Escherichia coli* enterotoxigenic for humans. *Infect. Immun.* **12**, 656.

34 Evans D. J. and Evans D. G. (1977) Direct serological assay for the heat-labile enterotoxin of *Escherichia coli*, using passive immune hemolysis. *Infect. Immun.* **16**, 604.

35 Evans D. J., Evans D. G. and Gorbach S. L. (1973) Production of vascular permeability factor by enterotoxigenic *Escherichia coli* isolated from man. *Infect. Immun.* **8**, 725.

36 Ewing W. H. and Gravatti J. L. (1947) *Shigella* types encountered in the Mediterranean area. *J. Bacteriol.* **53**, 191.

37 Ferguson W. W. and June R. C. (1952) Experiments on feeding adult volunteers with *Escherichia coli* 111, B₄, a coliform organism associated with infant diarrhea. *Am. J. Hyg.* **55**, 155.

38 Field M. (1979) Modes of action of enterotoxins from *Vibrio cholerae* and *Escherichia coli*. *Rev. Infect. Dis.* **1**, 918.

39 Field M., Graf L. H., Laird W. J. and Smith P. L. (1978) Heat-stable enterotoxin of *Escherichia coli*: in vitro effects on guanylate cyclase activity, cyclic GMP concentration, and ion transport in small intestine. *Proc. Natl. Acad. Sci. U.S.A.* **75**, 2800.

40 Formal S. B. and Hornick R. B. (1978) Invasive *Escherichia coli*. *J. Infect. Dis.* **17**, 641.

41 Frantz J. C. and Robertson D. C. (1981) Immunological properties of *Escherichia coli* heat-stable enterotoxins: development of a radioimmunoassay specific for heat-stable enterotoxins with suckling mouse activity. *Infect. Immun.* **33**, 193.

42 Gangarosa E. J. (1978) Epidemiology of *Escherichia coli* in the United States. *J. Infect. Dis.* **137**, 634.

43 Giles C. and Sangster G. (1948) An outbreak of infantile gastroenteritis in Aberdeen. The association of a special type of *Bact. coli* with the infection. *J. Hyg.* **46**, 1.

44 Goldschmidt T. (1933) Untersuchungen zur Atiologie der Durchfallserkrankungen des Säuglings. *Jahrb. Kinderheilkunde* **89**, 318.

45 Gorbach S. L., Kean B. H., Evans D. G., Evans D. J. and Bessudo D. (1975) Travelers' diarrhea and toxigenic *Escherichia coli*. *N. Eng. J. Med.* **292**, 933.

46 Gorbach S. L. and Khurana C. M. (1972) Toxigenic *Escherichia coli*. *N. Eng. J. Med.* **287**, 791.

47 Gross R. J., Cravioto A., Scotland S. M., Cheasty T. and Rowe B. (1978) The occurrence of colonization factor (CF) in enterotoxigenic *Escherichia coli*. *FEMS Microbiol. Lett.* **3**, 231.

48 Gross R. J., Rowe B., Henderson A., Byatt M. E. and Maclaurin J. C. (1976) A new *E. coli* O group, O159, associated with outbreaks of enteritis in infants. *Scand. J. Infect. Dis.* **8**, 195.

49 Gross R. J., Scotland S. M. and Rowe B. (1976) Enterotoxin testing of *Escherichia coli* causing epidemic enteritis in the United Kingdom. *Lancet* **i**, 629.

50 Gross R. J., Scotland S. M. and Rowe B. (1979) Enterotoxigenic *Escherichia coli* causing diarrhoea in travellers returning to the United Kingdom. *Br. Med. J.* **i**, 1463.

51 Guerrant R. L., Brunton L. L., Schnaitman T. C., Rebhun L. I. and Gilman A. G. (1974) Cyclic adenosine monophosphate and alteration of Chinese hamster ovary cell morphology; a rapid sensitive *in vitro* assay for the enterotoxins of *Vibrio cholerae* and *Escherichia coli*. *Infect. Immun.* **10**, 320.

52 Gurwith M. J. and Williams T. W. (1977) Gastroenteritis in children: a two year review in Manitoba. I. Etiology. *J. Infect. Dis.* **136**, 239.

53 Gyles C. L., (1979) Limitations of the infant mouse test for *Escherichia coli* heat stable enterotoxin. *Can. J. Comp. Med.* **43**, 371.

54 Hinden E. (1948) Etiological aspects of gastro-enteritis. I. *Arch. Dis. Childh.* **23**, 27.

55 Hinden E. (1948) Etiological aspects of gastro-enteritis. II. *Arch. Dis. Childh.* **23**, 33.

56 Hobbs B. C., Rowe B., Kendall M., Turnbull P. C. B. and Ghosh A. C. (1976) *Escherichia coli* O27 in adult diarrhoea. *J. Hyg.* **77**, 393.

57 Hobbs B. C., Thomas E. M. and Taylor J. (1949) School outbreak of gastro-enteritis associated with a pathogenic paracolon bacillus. *Lancet* **ii**, 530.

58 Holmgren J., Lange S. and Lonnroth I. (1978) Reversal of cyclic AMP-mediated intestinal secretion in mice by chlorpromazine. *Gastroenterology* **75**, 1103.

59 Honda T., Taga S., Takeda Y. and Miwatani T. (1981) Modified Elek test for detection of heat-labile enterotoxin of enterotoxigenic *Escherichia coli*. *J. Clin. Microbiol.* **13**, 1.

60 Hone R., Fitzpatrick S., Keane C., Gross R. J. and Rowe B. (1973) Infantile enteritis in Dublin caused by *Escherichia coli* O142. *J. Med. Microbiol.* **6**, 505.

61 Isaacson R. E., Nagy B. and Moon H. W. (1977) Colonization of porcine small intestine by *Escherichia coli*: colonization and adhesion factors of pig enteric pathogens that lack K88. *J. Infect. Dis.* **22**, 771.

62 Jacobs S. I., Holzel A., Wolman B., Keen J. H., Miller V., Taylor J. and Gross R. J. (1970) Outbreak of infantile gastro-enteritis due to *Escherichia coli* O114. *Arch. Dis. Childh.* **45**, 656.

63 Jones G. W. and Rutter J. M. (1974) The association of K88 antigen with haemagglutinating activity in porcine strains of *E.coli*. *J. Gen. Microbiol.* **84**, 135.

64 Kauffmann F. (1947) The serology of the coli group. *J. Immunol.* **57**, 71.

65 Kean B. H. (1963) The diarrhea of travelers to Mexico: survey of five year study. *Ann. Intern. Med.* **59**, 605.

66 Kean B. H., Schaffner W., Brennan R. W. and Waters S. R. (1962) The diarrhea of travelers: V. Prophylaxis with phthalylsulfathiazole and neomycin sulfate. *J. Am. Med. Assoc.* **162**, 367.

67 Kennedy D. H., Walker G. H., Fallon R. J., Boyd J. F., Gross R. J., and Rowe B. (1973) An outbreak of infantile gastro-enteritis due to *E.coli* O142. *J. Clin. Pathol.* **26**, 731.

68 Klipstein F. A., Rowe B., Engert R. F., Short H. B. and Gross R. J. (1978) Enterotoxigenicity of enteropathogenic serotypes of *Escherichia coli* isolated from infants with epidemic diarrhea. *Infect. Immun.* **21**, 171.

69 Konowalchuk J., Dickie N., Stavric S. and Speirs J. I. (1978) Properties of an *Escherichia coli* cytotoxin. *Infect. Immun.* **20**, 575.

70 Konowalchuk J., Speirs J. I. and Stavric S. (1977) Vero response to a cytotoxin of *Escherichia coli*. *Infect. Immun.* **18**, 775.

71 Koya G., Kosakai N., Kono M., Mori M. and Fukasawa Y. (1954) Observations on the multiplication of *Escherichia coli* O111 B4 in the intestinal tract of adult volunteers in feeding experiments. The intubation study with Miller-Abbots double lumen tube. *Jpn. J. Med. Sci. Biol.* **7**, 197.

72 Kudoh Y., Zen-Yoji H., Matsushita S., Sakai S. and Maruyama T. (1977) Outbreaks of acute enteritis due to heat-stable enterotoxin-producing strains of *Escherichia coli*. *Microbiol. Immunol.* **21**, 175.

73 Lambert H. P. (Ed.) (1979) 'Infections of the G.I. tract', *Clinics in Gastroenterology 8*, No. 3, W. B. Saunders Co., London.

74 Lanyi B., Szita J., Ringelham B. and Lovach K. (1959) A water-borne outbreak of enteritis associated with *Escherichia coli* serotype 124:72:32. *Acta Microbiol. Acad. Sci. Hung.* **6**, 77.

75 Lesage A. A. (1897) Contribution à l'étude des enterites infantiles serodiagnostique des races de *Bacterium coli*. *Comptes Rendus Soc. Bio.* **49**, 900.

76 Levine M. M., Berquist E. J., Nalin D. .R., Waterman D. H., Hornick R. B., Young C. R., Sotman S. and Rowe B. (1978) *Escherichia coli* strains that cause diarrhoea but do not produce heat-labile or heat-stable enterotoxins and are non-invasive. *Lancet* **i**, 119.

77 Levine M. M., Rennels M. B., Daya V. and Hughes T. P. (1980) Hemagglutination and colonization factors in enterotoxigenic and enteropathogenic *Escherichia coli* that cause diarrhea. *J. Infect. Dis.* **141**, 733.

78 Linggood M. A. and Ingram P. L. (1978) The effect of oral immunization with heat-stable *E.coli* antigens on the sensitivity of pigs to enterotoxins. *Res. Vet. Sci.* **25**, 113.

79 Lonnroth I., Andren B., Lange S., Martinsson K. and Holmgren J. (1979) Chlorpromazine reverses *Escherichia coli* diarrhea in piglets. *Infect. Immun.* **24**, 900.

80 Love W. C., Gordon A. M., Gross R. J. and Rowe B (1972) Infantile gastro-enteritis due to *Escherichia coli* O142. *Lancet* **ii**, 355.

81 Madsen G. L. and Knoop F. C. (1978) Inhibition of the secretory activity of *Escherichia coli* heat-stable enterotoxin by indomethacin. *Infect. Immun.* **22**, 143.

82 Maiya P. P., Pereira S. M., Mathan M., Bhat P., Albert M. J. and Baker S. J. (1977)

Aetiology of acute gastroenteritis in infancy and early childhood in southern India. *Arch. Dis. Childh.* **52**, 482.

83   Marier R., Wells T. G., Swanson R. C., Callahan W. and Mehlman I. J. (1973) An outbreak of enteropathogenic *Escherichia coli* food-borne disease traced to imported French cheese. *Lancet* **ii**, 1376.

84   McConnell M. M., Willshaw G. A., Smith H. R., Scotland S. M. and Rowe B. (1979) Transposition of ampicillin resistance to an enterotoxin plasmid in an *Escherichia coli* strain of human origin. *J. Bacteriol.* **139**, 346.

85   Mehlman I. J., Eide E. L., Sanders A. C., Fishbein M. and Aulisio C. C. G. (1977) Methodology for recognition of invasive potential of *Escherichia coli*. *J. Assoc. Analyt. Chem.* **60**, 546.

86   Merson M. H., Black R. E., Gross R. J., Rowe B., Huq I. and Eusof A. (1980) Use of antisera for identification of enterotoxigenic *Escherichia coli*. *Lancet* **ii**, 222.

87   Merson M. H., Morris G. K., Sack D. A., Wells J. G., Feeley J. C., Sack R. B., Creech W. B., Kapikian A. Z. and Gangarosa E. J. (1976) Travelers' diarrhea in Mexico. *N. Engl. J. Med.* **294**, 1299.

88   Merson M. H., Ørskov F., Ørskov I., Sack R. B., Huq I. and Koster F. T. (1979) Relationship between enterotoxin production and serotype in enterotoxigenic *Escherichia coli*. *Infect. Immun.* **23**, 325.

89   Morgan R. L., Isaacson R. E., Moon H. W., Brinton C. C. and To C. C. (1978) Immunization of suckling pigs against enterotoxigenic *Escherichia coli*-induced diarrheal disease by vaccinating dams with purified 987 or K99 pili: protection correlates with pilus homology of vaccine and challenge. *Infect. Immun.* **22**, 771.

90   Nalin D. R., Levine M. M., Young C. R., Bergquist E. J. and McLaughlin J. C. (1978) Increased *Escherichia coli* enterotoxin detection after concentrating culture supernatants: possible new enterotoxin detectable in dogs but not in infant mice. *J. Clin. Microbiol.* **8**, 700.

91   Nalin D. R., Rahaman M., McLaughlin J. C., Yunus M. and Curlin G. (1975) Enterotoxigenic *Escherichia coli* and idiopathic diarrhoea in Bangladesh. *Lancet* **ii**, 1116.

92   Neter E., Westphal O., Luderitz O., Gino R. M. and Gorzynski E. A. (1955) Demonstration of antibodies against enteropathogenic *Escherichia coli* in sera of children of various ages. *Paediatr. (Springfield)* **16**, 801.

93   Newsome P. M., Burgess M. N. and Mullan N. A. (1978) Effect of *Escherichia coli* heat-stable enterotoxin on cyclic GMP levels in mouse intestine. *Infect. Immun.* **22**, 290.

94   Ohgke H. and Wagner D. (1977) Heat-stable *Escherichia coli* enterotoxin: reduced action after administration of phenylbutazone in infant mice. *Zentralbl. Bakteriol.* **A238**, 350.

95   Ørskov F., Ørskov I., Evans D. J., Sack R. B., Sack D. A. and Wadstrom I. (1976) Special *Escherichia coli* serotypes among enterotoxigenic strains from diarrhoea in adults and children. *Med. Microbiol. Immunol.* **162**, 73.

96   Ørskov I. and Ørskov F. (1966) Episome-carried surface antigen K88 of *Escherichia coli*. *J. Bacteriol.* **91**, 69.

97   Ørskov I., Ørskov F., Smith H. W. and Sojka W. J. (1975) The establishment of K99, a thermolabile, transmissible, *Escherichia coli* K antigen, previously called 'Kco', possessed by calf and lamb enterotoxigenic strains. *Acta Patholog. Microbiolog. Scand.* **83B**, 31.

98   Pierce N. (1977) Protection against challenge with *Escherichia coli* heat-labile enterotoxin by immunization of rats with cholera toxin/toxoid. *Infect. Immun.* **18**, 338.

99   Rabbani G. H., Holmgren J., Greenough W. B. and Lonnroth I. (1979) Chlorpromazine reduces fluid-loss in cholera. *Lancet* **i**, 410.

100 Rao M. C., Orellana S. A., Field M., Robertson D. C. and Gianella R. A. (1981) Comparison of the biological actions of three purified heat-stable enterotoxins: effects on ion transport and guanylate cyclase activity in rabbit ileum *in vitro*. *Infect. Immun.* **33**, 165.

101 Reis M. H. L., Castro A. F. P., Toledo M. R. F. and Trabulsi L. R. (1979) Production of heat-stable enterotoxin by the O128 serogroup of *Escherichia coli*. *Infect. Immun.* **24** 289.

102 Report (1974) Chief Medical Officer of the Department of Health and Social Security. Annual Report for 1973. London, HMSO.

103 Report (1976) Diarrheal illness on a cruise ship caused by enterotoxigenic *Escherichia coli*. *Morbid. Mortal. Wkly Rept* **25**, 229.

104 Riley W. B (1968) An outbreak of diarrhoea in an infants' home due to a Shigella-like organism. *Med. J. Aust.* **2**, 1175.

105 Rosenberg M. L., Koplan J. P., Wachsmuth I. K., Wells J. G., Gangarosa E. J., Guerrant R. L. and Sack D. A. (1977) Epidemic diarrhea at Crater Lake from enterotoxigenic *Escherichia coli*. *Ann. Intern. Med.* **86**, 714.

106 Rowe B. (1979) The role of *Escherichia coli* in gastroenteritis. *Clin. Gastroenterol.* **8**, 625.

107 Rowe B., Gross R. J. and Allen H. A. (1974) Enteropathogenic *E. coli* O124 in the United Kingdom. *Lancet* **i**, 224.

108 Rowe B., Gross R. J. and Scotland S. M. (1976) Serotyping of *E. coli*. *Lancet* **ii**, 37.

109 Rowe B., Gross R. J., Scotland S. M., Wright A. E., Shillom G. N. and Hunter N. J. (1978) An outbreak of infantile enteritis caused by enterotoxigenic *Escherichia coli* O6H16. *J. Clin. Pathol.* **31**, 217.

110 Rowe B., Gross R. J. and Woodroof D. P. (1977) Proposal to recognise Serovar 145/46 (Synonyms: 147, *Shigella* 13, *Shigella sofia*, and *Shigella manolovii*) as a new *Escherichia coli* O group, O164. *Int. J. System. Bacteriol.* **27**, 15.

111 Rowe B., Scotland S. M. and Gross R. J. (1977) Enterotoxigenic *Escherichia coli* causing infantile enteritis in Britain. *Lancet* **i**, 90.

112 Rowe B., Taylor J. and Bettelheim K. A. (1970) An investigation of travellers' diarrhoea. *Lancet* **i**, 1.

113 Rudoy R. C. and Nelson J. D. (1975) Enteroinvasive and enterotoxigenic *Escherichia coli*. *Am. J. Dis. Child.* **129**, 668.

114 Rutter J. M., Burrows M. R., Selwood R. and Gibbons R. A. (1975) A genetic basis for resistance to enteric disease caused by *E. coli*. *Nature* **257**, 135.

115 Ryder R. W., Sack D. A., Kapikian A. Z., McLaughlin J. C., Chakraborty J., Rahman A. S. M. M., Merson M. H. and Wells J. G. (1976) Enterotoxigenic *Escherichia coli* and reovirus-like agent in rural Bangladesh. *Lancet* **i**, 659.

116 Ryder R. W., Wachsmuth I. K., Buxton A. E., Evans D. G., DuPont H. L., Mason E. and Barrett F. F. (1976) Infantile diarrhea produced by heat-stable enterotoxigenic *Escherichia coli*. *N. Engl. J. Med.* **295**, 849.

117 Sack D. A., Huda S., Neogi P. K. B., Daniel R. R. and Spira W. M. (1980) Microtiter ganglioside enzyme-linked immunosorbent assay for Vibrio and *Escherichia coli* heat-labile enterotoxins and antitoxin. *J. Clin. Microbiol.* **11**, 35.

118 Sack D. A., McLaughlin J. C., Sack R. B., Ørskov F. and Ørskov I. (1977) Enterotoxigenic *Escherichia coli* isolated from patients at a hospital in Dacca. *J. Infect. Dis.* **135**, 275.

119 Sack R. B., Froehlich J. L., Zulich A. W., Sidi Hidi D., Kapikian, A. Z., Ørskov F., Ørskov I. and Greenberg H. B. (1979) Prophylactic doxycycline for travelers' diarrhea. *Gastroenterol.* **76**, 1368.

120 Sack R. B., Gorbach S. L., Banwell J. G., Jacobs B., Chatterjee B. D. and Mitra R. C. (1971) Enterotoxigenic *Escherichia coli* isolated from patients with severe cholera-like disease. *J. Infect. Dis.* **123**, 378.

121 Sack R. B., Hirschhorn N., Brownlee I., Cash R. A., Woodward W. E. and Sack D. A (1975) Enterotoxigenic *Escherichia coli*-associated diarrheal disease in Apache children. *N. Engl. J. Med.* **292**, 1041.

122 Sakazaki R., Tamura K. and Saito M. (1968) Enteropathogenic *Escherichia coli* associated with diarrhoea in children and adults. *Jpn. J. Med. Sci. Biol.* **20**, 387.

123   Satterwhite T. K., DuPont H. L., Evans D. G. and Evans D. J. (1978) Role of *Escherichia coli* colonization factor antigen in acute diarrhoea. *Lancet* **ii**, 181.

124   Schoub B. D., Greeff A. S., Lecatsas G., Prozesky O. W., Hay I. T., Prinsloo J. G. and Ballard R. C. (1977) A microbiological investigation of acute gastroenteritis in Black South African infants. *J. Hyg.* **78**, 377.

125   Schroeder S., Caldwell J. R., Vernon T. M., White P. C., Grainger S. I. and Bennett J. V. (1968) A water-borne outbreak of gastroenteritis in adults associated with *Escherichia coli*. *Lancet* **i**, 737.

126   Scotland S. M., Day N. P. and Rowe B. (1980) Production of a cytotoxin affecting Vero cells by strains of *Escherichia coli* belonging to traditional enteropathogenic serogroups. *FEMS Microbiol. Lett.* **7**, 15.

127   Scotland S. M., Gross R. J., Cheasty T. and Rowe B. (1979) The occurrence of plasmids carrying genes for both enterotoxin production and drug resistance in *Escherichia coli* of human origin. *J. Hyg.* **83**, 531.

128   Scrimshaw N. S., Taylor C. E. and Gordon S. E. (1968) *Interactions of Nutrition and Infection*, WHO Geneva.

129   Serény B. (1957) Experimental keratoconjunctivitis shigellosa. *Acta Microbiologica Academiae Scientiarum Hungaricae* **4**, 367.

130   Shmilovitz M., Kretzer B. and Levy E. (1974) The anaerogenic serotype 147 as an etiologic agent of dysentery in Israel. *Isr. J. Med. Sci.* **10**, 1425.

131   Silva R. M., Toledo M. R. F. and Trabulsi L. R. (1980) Biochemical and cultural characteristics of invasive *Escherichia coli*. *J. Clin. Microbiol.* **11**, 441.

132   Smith H. R., Willshaw G. A., McConnell M. M., Scotland S. M., Gross R. J. and Rowe B. (1979) A plasmid coding for the production of colonisation factor antigen I and heat-stable enterotoxin in strains in *Escherichia coli* of serogroup O78. *FEMS Microbiol. Lett.* **6**, 255.

133   Smith H. W. and Gyles C. L. (1970) The relationship between two apparently different enterotoxins produced by enteropathogenic strains of *Escherichia coli* of porcine origin. *J. Med. Microbiol.* **3**, 387.

134   Smith H. W. and Gyles C. L. (1970) The effect of cell-free fluids prepared from cultures of human and animal enteropathogenic strains of *Escherichia coli* on ligated intestinal segments of rabbits and pigs. *J. Med. Microbiol.* **3**, 403.

135   Smith H. W. and Halls S. (1967) Observations by the ligated intestinal segment and oral inoculation methods on *Escherichia coli* infections in pigs, calves, lambs and rabbits. *J. Pathol. Bacteriol.* **93**, 499.

136   Smith H. W. and Linggood M. A. (1971) Observations on the pathogenic properties of the K88, Hly and Ent plasmids of *Escherichia coli* with particular reference to porcine diarrhoea. *J. Med. Microbiol.* **4**, 467.

137   Smith J. (1949) The association of certain types (α and β) of *Bact. coli* with infantile gastro-enteritis. *J. Hyg.* **47**, 221.

138   Speirs J. I., Stavric S. and Konowalchuk J. (1977) Assay of heat-labile enterotoxin with Vero cells. *Infect. Immun.* **16**, 617.

139   Taylor J. (1961) Host-specificity and enteropathogenicity of *Escherichia coli*. *J. Appl. Bacteriol.* **24**, 316.

140   Taylor J., Maltby M. P. and Payne J. M. (1958) Factors influencing the response of ligated rabbit gut segments to injected *Escherichia coli*. *J. Pathol. Bacteriol.* **76**, 491.

141   Thomas L. V., Cravioto A., Scotland S. M. and Rowe B. (1982) New fimbrial antigenic type (E8775) that may represent a colonization factor in enterotoxigenic *Escherichia coli* in humans. *Infect. Immun.* **35**, 1119.

142   Thomson S. (1955) The role of certain varieties of *Bacterium coli* in gastro-enteritis of babies. *J. Hyg. (Camb.)* **53**, 357.

143   Turjman N., Gotterer G. S. and Hendrix T. R. (1978) Prevention and reversal of cholera enterotoxin effects in rabbit jejunum by nicotinic acid. *J. Clin. Invest.* **61**, 1155.

144   Turner A. C. (1967) Travellers' diarrhoea; a survey of symptoms, occurrence and possible prophylaxis. *Br. Med. J.* **4**, 653.

145 Ulshen M. H. and Rollo J. L. (1980) Pathogenesis of *Escherichia coli* gastro-enteritis in man — another mechanism. *N. Engl. J. Med.* **302**, 99.
146 Vernon E. (1969) Food-poisoning and Salmonella infections in England and Wales 1967. *Public Health (London)* **83**, 205.
147 Wadstrom T., Aust-Kettis A., Habte D., Holmgren J., Meeuwisse G., Mollby R. and Soderlind O. (1976) Enterotoxin-producing bacteria and parasites in stools of Ethiopian children with diarrhoeal disease. *Arch. Dis. Childh.* **51**, 865.
148 Yolken R. H., Greenberg H. B., Merson M. H., Sack R. B. and Kapikian A. Z. (1977) Enzyme-linked immunosorbent assay for detection of *Escherichia coli* heat-labile enterotoxin. *J. Clin. Microbiol.* **6**, 439.

5 Cholera and other vibrios, *Aeromonas* and *Plesiomonas*

C. S. Goodwin

Cholera	104
Clinical features	104
Causative organisms	105
Pathogenesis	105
Cholera toxins	106
Epidemiology	108
Laboratory diagnosis	109
Treatment of cholera	110
Control	111
Non-cholera vibrios	113
Causative organisms and laboratory diagnosis	113
Clincial features	113
Epidemiology	114
Pathogenesis	114
Antibacterial treatment	114
Halophilic vibrios particularly *Vibrio parahaemolyticus*	114
Epidemiology and clinical features	115
Pathogenesis and causative organisms	115
Laboratory diagnosis	116
Treatment and control	116
Aeromonas species	117
Causative organisms and clinical features	117
Epidemiology	118
Pathogenesis	118
Laboratory diagnosis	119
Antibacterial treatment and control	119
Plesiomonas shigelloides	120
Causative organisms and clinical features	120
Pathogenesis	121
Laboratory diagnosis	121
Epidemiology	121
References	122

In this chapter the vibrios that cause gut infection in man will be considered. *Vibrio fetus* is now placed in the genus *Campylobacter*, this organism is discussed in Chapter 3. The cause of cholera, *Vibrio cholerae* can be cultured in the absence of salt and thus is a non-halophilic vibrio. A distinction is made between cholera vibrios that agglutinate with O–1 antiserum and other non-halophilic vibrios that agglutinate with antisera against antigens O2 or others, up to at least O70;[43] the latter are called non-cholera vibrios. *V. parahaemolyticus* and *V. alginolyticus* are halophilic vibrios, which, for growth in culture media, require salt. *Aeromonas hydrophila* and *Plesiomonas shigelloides* are discussed at the end of this chapter.

CHOLERA

During the 19th century classical cholera due to *Vibrio cholerae* repeatedly spread from Bengal to Europe, but it was brought under control and virtually eliminated in Britain by the provision of uncontaminated water supplies. During the 20th century classical cholera has been largely confined to the Indian subcontinent and to China, but in 1958 an epidemic due to the El Tor variant of *Vibrio cholerae* occurred in the Philippines. This variant produced in adults more cases of mild disease than the classical cholera vibrio, with many asymptomatic carriers which allowed widespread dissemination of the organism. El Tor cholera spread to Hong Kong in 1962, to Afghanistan and Iran in 1965, and then to the Mediterranean and South Europe, to East Africa and to South Africa. The current epidemic strain,[43] and isolates from the USA[64] have characteristics intermediate between the original El Tor biotype and the classical biotype. If and when it reaches South America it will cause pandemics in the insanitary suburbs of the great cities there.

Clinical features

In adults classical cholera may have a gradual onset[22] or a sudden onset with diarrhoea with profuse watery stools, vomiting, rapid dehydration, acidosis, muscular cramps and circulatory collapse. The stools rapidly lose their faecal character and become like rice-water, with flecks of mucus. Enormous volumes may be passed; it is not unusual for 20 litres a day to be passed per rectum. Vomitus also becomes like rice-water. The body surface temperature can fall to 34° C, while the rectal temperature may be 39° C. Anuria may supervene; or a typhoid-like state may develop.[84] In a very few cases called 'cholera sicca' collapse and death may occur after only a short period of diarrhoea and vomiting. In patients who recover there is a gradual cessation of vomiting and diarrhoea with the reappearance of the pulse at the wrist and a rise in body surface temperature. Secretion of urine returns and in a few days the patient may be practically well again. Recovery from anuria is marked by the passage of a small amount of turbid urine, which may be followed by a 'critical diuresis'. If hyperpyrexia occurs this is almost invariably fatal. All the clinical symptoms can be reversed by rehydration with appropriate fluid and electrolytes. Death may occur from dehydration or collapse during a few hours after onset, and in untreated cases the case fatality rate may be 70%. El Tor cholera in untreated adults has a lower mortality rate of 10–20%, but especially in children it is a fearsome disease; in 1963 in Jakarta in Indonesia the mortality rate in children was 46% even when intravenous glucose-saline was available.[52] In adults with El Tor cholera the diarrhoea may be short lived, and many infected patients do not show disease but become carriers of the organism. For classical cholera the incubation period may be only a few hours but 3 to 6 days is common.[84] In El Tor cholera the incubation period is 1 to 3 days. Patients with cholera in the early stages may be differentiated clinically from patients with other forms of bacterial gastroenteritis, because in cholera nausea is absent, vomiting causes little distress, headache is absent, abdominal pain is mild, tenesmus is absent, while muscular cramps may be constant and severe. An attack of cholera confers short-lived immunity. Vibriocidal IgM antibody persists for about 3 months although antitoxin persists longer.[22,25,126] Thus in endemic areas repeated infections are common, with or without clinical symptoms.[140]

Causative organisms

Classical cholera is caused by *Vibrio cholerae*, a Gram-negative, comma-shaped, highly motile organism with a single terminal flagellum. *V. cholerae* biotype El Tor was originally isolated from pilgrims at El Tor in the Sinai peninsula, and was thought to be a non-pathogenic variant. It was originally characterized as haemolytic, but some strains are non-haemolytic.[34] Both cholera vibrios possess the somatic O1 antigen which has three polysaccharide fractions A, B and C. There are two common serotypes Ogawa (AB) and Inaba (AC), a rarer Hikojima (ABC) serotype, and a very rare serotype A.[25] Isolates from chronic carriers of *V. cholerae* may lack the O antigen, but may be detected by an antiserum prepared from an O-antigen deficient strain. The H antigen is shared with non-cholera vibrios. *V. cholerae* biotype El Tor is now distinguished from *V. cholerae* by its ability to agglutinate chick erythrocytes, by its resistance to classical choleraphage IV, its resistance to polymyxin B and by haemagglutination tests,[114] and by its sensitivity to El Tor phage 5.[43] There are five classical *V. cholerae* bacteriophage types, and six El Tor phage types, but some El Tor strains are resistant to all the El Tor phages.[43] When *V. cholerae* is grown in nitrate-peptone broth nitroso-indole is produced and this is detected by the addition of sulphuric acid when a 'cholera-red' colour is seen. However, this reaction is not confined to *V. cholerae* although it was thought to be specific for this organism. *V. cholerae* produces a powerful exotoxin, choleragen, a protein which is responsible for the catastrophic diarrhoea. The organism also produces at least one haemagglutinin which is probably important in the attachment of *V. cholerae* to the intestinal villi.[24] Some *V. cholerae* O1 strains isolated from the environment may be non-enterotoxigenic.[133]

Pathogenesis

After oral ingestion of cholera vibrios and their multiplication in the intestine, disease may not follow.[22] In volunteers a dose of 10^4 organisms of classical *V. cholerae* with sodium bicarbonate caused disease, but without bicarbonate the disease occurred only if the dose was 10^8 organisms.[22] Some volunteers had formed stools from which *V. cholerae* could be isolated, while others had catastrophic diarrhoea. In 45% of volunteers *V. cholerae* could be cultured from the stools before the onset of diarrhoea.

Stomach acid is capable of destroying *V. cholerae* but a few organisms may survive passage through the stomach. People with hypochlorhydria are more prone to develop cholera.[74] In the volunteer study mentioned above[22] the bicarbonate could have neutralized the effect of stomach acid, and allowed infectivity with a lower dose of bacteria. The infrequency with which the El Tor vibrio may produce disease was shown during an El Tor outbreak in Hong Kong; of 46 employees in one restaurant 18 were found to be carriers of *V. cholerae* El Tor but only one of them had mild diarrhoea.[35] Seventeen cases of cholera were traced to this restaurant with four deaths. It was calculated that the case : infection ratio was 1 : 100,[35] but in classical cholera the case: infection ratio is considered to be about 1:7.[95]

Cholera toxins

V. cholerae produces a powerful protein exotoxin called choleragen, and a haemagglutinin;[24] and most strains of the El Tor variant produce a haemolysin. It has been possible to duplicate cholera diarrhoea in the isolated small intestine of mammals, but there are variations in different models such as pigs,[37] rabbits[120] and rodents.[24] However a consistent picture emerges of the effect of the major toxin choleragen,[47] which is very similar to the heat-labile toxin of entero-toxigenic *Escherichia coli*.[109,145] Choleragen is a protein of 84 000 daltons consisting of three peptide chains, A_1, A_2 and B[80] which weigh about 22 000, 5000 and 11 600 daltons respectively. Each toxin molecule contains one each of the A chains and five B chains. A_1 A_2 are connected by a single disulphide bond. The activity of choleragen resides in the A_1 peptide, as described below. The B chains can be isolated as a single subunit which is known as choleragenoid. Subunit B is probably responsible for binding choleragen to gangliosides on the mucosal cell membrane. Binding is complete within 2 minutes of contact but there is then a lag of up to 3 hours before biological effects are observed. This lag may be due to the time taken for the subunits A_1 and A_2 to become detached from the B subunit and traverse the membrane of the villus cell. Subunits A_1 and A_2 are probably synthesized as a single polypeptide which is nicked, apparently extracellularly,[78] forming A_1 and A_2 which remain coupled by the disulphide bond.[48,89] The mode of transport of the complex choleragen molecule across the inner and outer membranes of *V. cholerae* is of interest. Two peptides in the outer and inner membranes of *V. cholerae* have been found,[32] which may be the form in which the toxin subunits are transported across the membranes. When *V. cholerae* was grown aerobically at 37° C most of the synthesized choleragen was membrane-bound but under anaerobic conditions at 37° C choleragen was released into the growth medium. Sodium deoxycholate, which releases membrane-bound toxin, released several peptides from *V. cholerae* including two with molecular weights of 22 000 and 66 000. Trypsin also released these two peptides. These two membrane peptides may be the precursors of the subunits A_1 and A_2 of choleragen.[32] In humans with cholera the bulk of the fluid secretion occurs in the duodenum and jejunum.[81] The small intestinal mucosa is intact and retains its capacity to absorb glucose and other nutrients.[124] Glucose-coupled sodium and chloride transport into the villus cell permits successful oral rehydration. There is neither epithelial invasion by bacteria nor evidence of damage to epithelial cells, even at the ultrastructural level.[123] The importance of adherence as well as exotoxin production was demonstrated in the ileal loops of adult rabbits.[127] Non-adherent and adherent strains multiplied to the same extent in the intestine. A good correlation was found between adherence and pathogenesis. Adhesive strains were pathogenic, but poorly adhesive strains proved to be poor pathogens. There was no toxicity in the ileal loops which were inoculated with poorly adhesive strains. It is generally agreed that adherence occurs before release of toxin and thus plays an important role in the pathogenesis of cholera. Adherence may be mediated by the haemagglutinin[24] or the B subunit of choleragen;[33] an L-fucose-containing receptor has been described.[72] However pathogenic *V. cholerae* must also possess the ability to initially penetrate the mucus gel on the intestinal villi, adhere to receptors in the gel, and penetrate deep into the intervillous spaces.[38] In human milk and colostrum a nonimmunoglobulin fraction inhibits adhesion of *V. cholerae*.[61]

The diarrhoeal process can be reproduced in animals by inoculating the small intestine with either cholera organisms, or a bacteria-free culture filtrate, or the purified toxin.[33] In animal preparations choleragen but not choleragenoid stimulates the activity of mucosal adenylate cyclase which converts ATP to cyclic AMP, and this leads to increased tissue levels of cyclic AMP.[124] Two ion transport processes are controlled by cyclic AMP (see p.86); firstly coupled *absorption* of sodium chloride is *inhibited* in intestinal villus cells, and secondly in crypt cells active *secretion* of chloride and bicarbonate into the gut lumen is *stimulated* by cyclic AMP. In the healthy gut guanosine triphosphatase regulates the activity of adenylate cyclase. The A_1 subunit of choleragen catalyses the transfer of adenosine diphosphate ribose from NAD to the membrane-bound guanosine triophosphatase (GTP) thereby inhibiting this enzyme. Thus choleragen releases adenylate cyclase from its repression by GTP.[23,47] The released adenylate cyclase promotes the formation of cyclic AMP; sodium chloride absorption from the gut lumen is stopped, and active secretion from the crypt cells results in an outpouring of fluid into the gut lumen.

Prostaglandins, especially PGE1 and PGE2, increase the activity of adenyl cyclase in the tissue and levels of cyclic AMP in animal intestinal mucosa. In rat ileal loops exposed to cholera toxin fluid accumulation is reduced by salicylates and indomethacin. The prostaglandin inhibitor acetylsalicylic acid has been used successfully to reduce intestinal fluid loss in acute diarrhoea in children, some of whom had cholera.[18]

Gm1-ganglioside is probably the membrane receptor to which choleragen must bind before it can produce intestinal secretion and diarrhoea.[60] In ligated rabbit intestinal loops, experimentally induced cholera can be completely prevented by the presence of free Gm1-ganglioside.[59] Gm1-ganglioside can be attached to finely divided charcoal and a trial of this combination was undertaken in Bangladesh. Gm1-charcoal was made up as a slurry containing 1 g charcoal per 10 ml. Cholera patients were given 20 ml of fluid, either Gm1-charcoal, charcoal alone, or water every 2 hours beginning 4 hours after admission and continuing for 48 hours. Patients treated with Gm1-ganglioside tended to have a greater reduction in purging than patients treated with either charcoal alone or water. This difference was statistically significant soon after beginning medication, and up to 15 hours, and the reduction in fluid loss was especially pronounced in patients with very severe initial purging who had been ill for a short time before admission.[128] The results suggest that toxin produced in the gut lumen increases fluid-loss early, but later in the course of the disease toxin which is inaccessible to luminal binding agents, is the major stimulus of purging.

The haemolysin produced by *V. cholerae* El Tor has been clarified and characterized.[62] Although it was found to be cytotoxic to cultured Y-1 adrenal cells and cardiotoxic and rapidly lethal to mice, identical diseases are produced by both haemolytic and non-haemolytic cholera vibrios. Thus the El Tor haemolysin may be presumed to be pathogenetically irrelevant.[62]

Epidemiology

Cholera is primarily a disease of poor people living in areas with unchlorinated water supplies and inadequate or absent sewage disposal. In 1855 in London John Snow[125] made a careful study of the epidemiology of cholera. He showed that the disease could be spread directly from person to person, that it could be water-borne by water contaminated with human faeces, and flies might carry the 'poison'; storage, or heating of water led to the water becoming safe. He laid down rational preventive measures, and stopped one famous outbreak when he removed the handle of the Broad Street pump in Golden Square.

Cholera is endemic in the river deltas of the Ganges and Brahmaputra. In 1892 the Elbe was contaminated, and in Hamburg 18 000 cases of cholera occurred with 8200 deaths.[73] Altona was downstream from Hamburg but its efficient sand-filtration plant made the water safe. In water the vibrio remains alive depending on the pH, and the degree of contamination by other organisms; in Nile water it was found to survive 4 days.[51] *V. cholerae* El Tor may survive longer than *V. cholerae*.[11] A study of a Queensland river indicated that *V. cholerae* may survive a very long time, and may multiply in the water.[106] Both organisms are killed by chlorine. Anything made with raw water such as ice or soft drinks, or contaminated by raw water such as utensils, food and vegetables, can be a vehicle for the vibrio.[12] Vibrios were not found *inside* fruit and vegetables with intact skins.[100] Cooked crab,[126] and pelecypods[113] have transmitted cholera, but some isolates from shell fish such as oysters may be non-enterotoxigenic.[133] Mussels and other seafood were vehicles of infection in Italy in 1973,[8] and a history of gastric surgery was more common among patients than asymptomatic contacts. Spread can occur by food, and from case to case.[43] The vibrio may be deposited by faeces or vomit onto linen, and if this is kept moist the vibrio can survive for days or weeks. Survival times on different articles have been documented.[51] Asymptomatic carriers of *V. cholerae* do not remain so for a long time; in one series only 2% were carriers for longer than 3 weeks.[49] However one carrier of *V. cholerae* El Tor was documented as being a carrier for 23 weeks.[137] The carrier state may not be preceded by illness. During an epidemic in Hong Kong of *V. cholerae* El Tor a carrier rate of 5%–16% was found.[36] Geographically cholera can be transferred not only to contiguous areas but also to far away places by carriers; an outbreak in Nigeria was attributed to the return of pilgrims from Mecca.[118] In this latter outbreak the University Campus and Hospital staff in Zaria were immunized with two doses of cholera vaccine; none developed cholera. The area in which Government staff lived had a piped water supply and good sanitation and no cholera occurred there. However, in the surrounding area there were 500 cases which were concentrated in certain areas suggesting that the water supply in each case had become contaminated. Among 200 patients with reliable histories only 15 had definitely received immunization, and these all with only one dose. There was no recurrence of the epidemic the following year.[118]

The rapid spread of *V. cholerae* El Tor from the Philippines in 1958 to Africa has been mentioned at the beginning of the chapter. In 1971 there were reports of 100 000 cases in Africa and 72 000 in Asia.[139] The use of tetracycline as chemoprophylaxis for close contacts of cholera patients has led in Tanzania in 1972 to the rapid emergence of an Ogawa strain resistant to tetracycline in 76% of isolates and resistant in a lower percentage to chloramphenicol, nitrofurantoin, neomycin, ampicillin and sulphadimidine.[92]

Laboratory diagnosis

Only patients who have passed through a cholera-endemic area need be examined for *V. cholerae*, but other vibrios may occur in any temperate or tropical sea, and laboratory diagnosis of these will be considered later in this chapter. During an epidemic, cholera vibrios may be identified rapidly by microscopy; either a fleck of mucus is stained with dilute carbol-fuchsin, or in a 'hanging-drop' preparation motile 'darting' vibrios may be seen, and this motility can be inhibited by specific antiserum. A fluorescent antibody technique, and dark ground microscopy[14] have been described. Other authors deny the value of microscopy.[43] Stool specimens for culture of vibrios can be preserved in a borate saline mixture[135] or Cary-Blair medium.[21] For rectal swabs and small quantities of faeces the tranport medium of Barua[13] is probably more efficient. Stool specimens from carriers, with fewer organisms should be inoculated into a liquid medium usually alkaline peptone water,[43] but sodium-gelatin-phosphate broth is very efficient.[103] From the liquid media, subculture is made onto the solid medium. Probably all stools suspected of containing vibrios should be inoculated into a liquid medium and onto a solid medium. Vibrios grow faster in alkaline peptone water than other bacteria, and accumulate on the surface; a loopful from the surface can be subcultured onto a solid medium after 3–6 hours, although overnight culture in sodium-gelatin-phosphate broth should be used for carriers.[103] Many solid media suitable for vibrios have been described,[43,139] but the thiosulphate-citrate-bile-salts-sucrose (TCBS) medium is probably the best, but some brands are too inhibitory.[43] Sucrose-fermenting yellow colonies are easily seen, but some vibrios from carriers do not ferment sucrose.[94] *V. cholerae* is oxidase positive, is agglutinated by O group 1 antiserum, and has a characteristic biochemical profile.[25,43] Agglutination by O1 antiserum may be unsuccessful until a suspension of the organism has been heated at 100° C for 2 hours. Agglutination with antisera to the Inaba and Ogawa subtypes should be attempted. The major distinguishing characteristics of the El Tor biotype[25,43,139] have been delineated in the section on causative organisms. Some carriers of *V. cholerae* may only be detected after the use of a purgative or aspiration of duodenal juice.[98] Vibrios from such people may not agglutinate with O antiserum but can be agglutinated by antiserum against an O-deficient strain, and other characteristics may indicate the organism as *V. cholerae*.[25,43,139] A serum specimen collected intially, and another serum 6 days after the onset of symptoms may show a fourfold rise in agglutinins and vibriocidal antibodies.[139] To isolate *V. cholerae* from environmental sources salt-free alkaline peptone-water is best, and the pH must be kept in the range 8.5–9.0.[43] Techniques required to process seafood and sea water, and enumeration methods have been described by Furniss *et al.*[43]

Treatment of cholera

Nothing should take priority over the urgent replacement of lost fluid and electrolytes, but the value of chemotherapy is still equivocal. The elucidation of the pathogenesis of cholera has indicated that glucose absorption in the intestine remains intact, and is even enhanced by the low intracellular sodium, and with glucose, sodium and chloride are transported into the villus cells. However the mucosal cells may still lose sodium, until the disease process is overcome by the body. Oral rehydration therapy with glucose and salts as recommended by the World Health Organization is described on p.209, and is adequate unless dehydration is severe, or the rate of purging exceeds 100 ml/kg/24 hours.[54] Oral fluids should be warmed to body temperature so that they do not stimulate vomiting. Solid food and milk should not be given during the period of severe diarrhoea. Antidiarrhoeal agents such as diphenoxylate (Lomotil) are not recommended. Simultaneous oral and intravenous rehydration was used successfully in children in Indonesia;[52] children could be discharged after 8 hours treatment. Intravenous lactated Ringer's solution plus oral glucose solution was adequate in 85% of children in Nigeria,[83] but 15% of children under 6 required intravenous glucose-saline solution. Other intravenous fluids have been described including one containing 4 g NaCl, 4 g $NaHCO_3$ and 0.5 g KCl, or a saline-bicarbonate solution or saline-lactate solution.[139] The intravenous fluids must not be sterilized by boiling. Under medical supervision the management of intravenous therapy should be monitored by the blood pressure, which should rise, replacement of rapid deep breathing by normal respiration, and the patient becoming less confused as the acidosis is corrected. If excessive intravenous therapy is given pulmonary oedema may ensue.

In severely affected children, but not in babies, the first litre of fluid can be given during 20 minutes. After the first litre of saline, lactated bicarbonate or acetate should be given, and potassium chloride 1 g per litre can be added to the fluid. As soon as the patient can tolerate oral therapy this should replace intravenous therapy. Other details of intravenous therapy are given by Maegraith.[82]

Intramuscular or oral chlorpromazine 1 mg/kg has been shown in Bangladesh to significantly reduce stool output[101] and to decrease nausea; the use of soluble aspirin 25 mg/kg, which significantly reduced daily stool volume in Indonesian children with diarrhoea due to a variety of organisms[18] is discussed in Chapter 9.

Tetracycline, chloramphenicol, and cotrimoxazole all hasten the eradication of *V. cholerae* from the stools of patients with cholera.[43] Tetracycline 250 mg 6-hourly for 48 hours should be given, after vomiting has stopped, to patients and to carriers to reduce environmental contamination.

In view of the rapid emergence of El Tor vibrios resistant to antimicrobial agents after the widespread use of tetracycline for prophylaxis this drug should be reconsidered and possibly replaced with cotrimoxazole or furazolidone.[92]

Control

Public health measures which control any disease spread by faeces will control cholera, but it may be helpful to itemize these measures:

(a) Sanitary disposal of human faeces.

(b) Protection and purification of water supplies. Chlorination is obviously necessary, but individuals whose only water supply is raw contaminated water, should boil the water.

(c) Raw milk and other dairy products which may be contaminated should be pasteurized or boiled.

(d) If foods are eaten raw these must be prepared only under sanitary conditions, and not be allowed to be contaminated by flies. However, in most developing countries, to avoid faecal borne disease, it is probably necessary to eat only cooked food, and peeled or disinfected fruit. The public should be informed that fish and especially shellfish collected from waters that could be contaminated with sewage, and vegetables irrigated or freshened with sewage-contaminated water must be cooked very thoroughly.

(e) Destruction of flies, and control of fly breeding, and especially screening of food to prevent fly contamination.

(f) Education of the public in personal hygiene, especially washing hands before eating and after defaecation. The public should be informed that infection can be acquired not only by drinking water, but by bathing or washing articles in sewage-contaminated water. They should realize that eating and drinking in the homes of sick people can be a hazard.

In the event of an outbreak of cholera the following procedures should be adopted:

(a) Active case finding with the help of community leaders, and notification of the cases to the local health authority.

(b) Isolation of the patients under conditions which prevent transfer of infection from faeces or vomit to the environment or to those who care for the patient. A gown and gloves or meticulous handwashing will be adequate for most situations. Health personnel should have been vaccinated, see (h) below.

(c) Sanitary disposal of faeces and vomit and of articles used by the patient. If clothing is not discarded then it should be thoroughly disinfected, as should the utensils and environs of cholera patients — by boiling utensils or the use of phenolic disinfectants. Dead bodies of cholera victims should be disposed of with the minimum of transportation and rites, which can spread the disease.

(d) Provision of early and proper treatment of cases. This may include the establishment of temporary treatment centres, so that infected people travel as little as possible.

(e) Monitoring of faeces for the presence of cholera vibrios so that isolation is maintained until after three daily stools have yielded no vibrios.

(f) Contacts of cases should be monitored by stool examination. If a contact is found to be excreting the vibrio the contact must also be put in some form of isolation such as hostel accommodation until their stools no longer yield cholera vibrios. This is one of the most effective measures of controlling an epidemic, and was probably the reason why the epidemic in Hong Kong in 1962 was brought under control so efficiently. Chemoprophylaxis of family contacts with tetracycline is probably less satisfactory, although those found to be excreting organisms should be given tetracycline.

(g) When a case of cholera occurs the vehicle of infection should be determined and if this is polluted water or contaminated food the source should be adequately treated or isolated so that further cases do not occur.

(h) Active immunization with cholera vaccine for any person at risk of infection. Two doses of killed whole organism vaccine given at an interval of 1 week provide the best protection, but this is probably only in the region of 60%. The usual strength of cholera vaccine is 8×10^9 vibrios per ml with a dose of 0.25–1.0 ml according to the age of the subject.

The principles of immunization against cholera are discussed in Chapter 12. Much work has been done with animals to compare different vaccines. The different subunits of choleragen have been compared with toxoid, and the latter has been shown to be more effective in rabbits.[97] Although some authorities indicate that in an endemic area one dose is sufficient, it was found in one outbreak in Nigeria that cholera could occur after one dose.[118] In general, immunization with cholera vaccine is inferior in its protective value to the practice of ingesting only chlorinated or boiled water and food either cooked or peeled. Breast-fed infants ingest antibodies against intestinal pathogens to which their mothers are immune. Antibodies against *Vibrio cholerae* have been found in breast milk.[138] Vaccination of lactating women with killed cholera vaccine produced a booster effect of specific milk SIgA antibody levels.[129] After a cholera toxoid vaccine or whole-cell vaccine was given to volunteers in Bangladesh a significant increase was found in anticholera toxin IgA titres in the milk of five of six lactating mothers; three of the five mothers also had a significant increase in anticholera-toxin IgG titres in the milk.[91] Purified cholera toxoid although antigenic when given parenterally and orally failed to provide protection against experimental challenge.[77] It is suggested that the predominant immune mechanisms are antibacterial rather than antitoxic, and probably the antibacterial effect occurs during the adherence stage of the pathogenesis.

NON-CHOLERA VIBRIOS

Causative organisms and laboratory diagnosis

Non-cholera vibrios are distinguishable from halophilic vibrios by the fact that they grow in the absence of added salt, although growth is enhanced by the addition of salt to the medium. These non-cholera vibrios (NCVs) are biochemically indistinguishable from the cholera vibrios but they fail to be agglutinated by O1 antiserum. Methods of isolation of NCVs are essentially the same as for cholera vibrios.[43] In order to isolate NCVs from a marine environment, enrichment techniques need to be designed to suppress halophilic vibrios.

On TCBS medium (p.109) NCVs are indistinguishable from cholera vibrios, although some do not ferment sucrose and therefore will appear as green colonies. As with other vibrios they are sensitive to the vibriostatic compound 0129 (2,4-diamino-6,7-diisopropyl-pteridine phosphate). Discs containing 10 μg and 150 μg of compound 0129 are placed on a plate of nutrient agar; some organisms will be sensitive only around the stronger disc.

The heat-labile flagellar H antigen of vibrios may be of value in the study of NCVs. However agglutination with antiserum against the O1 antigen has become the essential test for the identification of an organism as a cholera vibrio.

Heiberg[57] subdivided vibrios into six groups on the basis of their fermentation reactions. Group I were the cholera vibrios. By agglutination the remaining Groups II–VI were confirmed as non-cholera vibrios.[44] In 1970 Sakazaki[111] described 57 O-serotypes of non-halophilic vibrios. At least 70 serotypes are now recognized.[43] The original group II is Sakazaki serotype 7, group III is Sakazaki serotype 2, group V is serotype 3, and VI is serotype 4. However, some strains agglutinate with more than one specific antiserum. Cholera vibrios are still Sakazaki serotype 1. Another somatic antigen R has been described,[121] but some R strains also agglutinate with O-antiserum. More usually a strain exhibits either an R antigen or an O antigen. Furniss[42] only recognizes three fermentation groups of NCVs: those in group I ferment sucrose and mannose, in group II sucrose only and those in group V of Heiberg ferment mannose only. Vibrios that ferment arabinose are halophilic. Cholera vibrios are in Group I, and NCVs from human sources are usually in Groups I or II. A phage-typing system for NCVs has been proposed.[122]

Clinical features

If a non-cholera vibrio (NCV) is the only intestinal pathogen isolated from a patient with diarrhoea it may be considered as aetiologically significant. Most patients have only mild diarrhoea but a very few have symptoms almost resembling cholera. Vibrios are excreted for only a few days. A very severe case of gastroenteritis due to a non-cholera vibrio was reported from Western Australia in 1977.[56] In the USA from 1972–75 there were 13 cases of acute diarrhoea due to NCVs, and NCV was isolated from four people without diarrhoea, and in nine patients an NCV was isolated from tissues outside the gut and four of them died.[67]

Severe diarrhoea and vomiting followed by systemic invasion and death due to an NCV serotype 27 was reported in a woman of 64 years in Australia;[55] the organism was isolated from a large multi-lobular liver abscess at postmortem, and was highly enterotoxigenic by the mouse adrenal tumour cell-assay.

Epidemiology

Non-cholera vibrios have caused cholera-like epidemics during cholera outbreaks,[29,87] a food-borne outbreak in Czechoslovakia,[1] a water-borne outbreak in the Sudan,[104] and traveller's diarrhoea in Saudi Arabia[141] and in India.[105] In the 13 people with acute diarrhoea in the United States[67] most had a history of recent shell-fish ingestion, and another nine cases have been due to oysters.[94] This indicates that non-cholera vibrios may be sometimes present in seawater. Acquisition of NCV infection through direct contact with salt water has been reported.[7]

Pathogenesis

A toxin very similar to the choleragen of *V. cholerae* has been isolated from some NCVs,[43,145] and some serotypes can invade the body.[55]

Antibacterial treatment

Mild cases of gastroenteritis may need no treatment. For severe diarrhoea the same treatment is indicated as for cholera (p.110). Tetracycline will shorten the period of excretion of vibrios. For severe systemic invasion an aminoglycoside such as gentamicin, or chloramphenicol, is warranted.

HALOPHILIC VIBRIOS PARTICULARLY *VIBRIO PARAHAEMOLYTICUS*

These vibrios will not grow in the laboratory on media lacking salt. Five species are recognized of which two cause disease in humans, *Vibrio parahaemolyticus* and *V. alginolyticus*.[42] *V. alginolyticus* rarely causes gastroenteritis, and so will not be considered separately in this chapter. In addition to these two species a halophilic 'lactose-positive' vibrio has been described, which has caused two forms of infection, one being gastroenteritis.[15] This latter organism appeared to be ingested with raw oysters, and has caused fatalities. It will also not be considered in a separate section in this chapter. These organisms will not grow on CLED (cysteine-lactose-electrolyte deficient) medium; although non-halophilic vibrios will grow readily on CLED.

Epidemiology and clinical features

V. parahaemolyticus was first isolated in 1950 from postmortem specimens of patients who died during a food-borne outbreak of gastroenteritis traced to semi-dried sardines in Japan.[39,40] The organism is one of the commonest causes of gastroenteritis in Japan[41] and in Singapore.[50] It has been reported as a cause of gastrointestinal illness usually associated with seafood in India,[26] Thailand,[5] Malaysia,[71] Great Britain,[65] United States[10] and Panama.[67]

In view of the confused nomenclature of vibrios it is not surprising that some outbreaks of gastroenteritis have been attributed to 'non-agglutinating vibrios' — organisms that did not agglutinate with *V. cholerae* O1–antiserum — when in fact the causative organism was a halophilic vibrio, probably *V. parahaemolyticus*. Unless an organism is tested for its ability to grow on media without salt no conclusion can be reached as to its true identity; the organism may be a halophilic vibrio or a non-cholera vibrio. Between 1969 and 1979 in the USA there were only 16 reported gastroenteritis outbreaks caused by *V. parahaemolyticus*, but in some outbreaks large numbers of people were infected.[76] *V. parahaemolyticus* is seldom involved in traveller's diarrhoea.[90] The organism is widely distributed in British coastal waters, in sediments and shellfish, especially in the southern and western areas, although it is present in relatively small numbers.[6] Symptoms include abdominal pain, nausea, vomiting and diarrhoea usually without blood in the stools.[76]

Illness follows the ingestion of infected shellfish, including shrimps and prawns. *V. parahaemolyticus* can cause explosive diarrhoea, and in a confined space such as an aircraft can produce an unpleasant situation. The clinical symptoms are usually limited to 3 days.[76]

V. parahaemolyticus has been reported in Bangladesh as a cause of gastro-enteritis only 2½ hours after fish was eaten in a restaurant.[67] In outbreaks in the United States the incubation period was usually 12–24 hours.

Pathogenesis and causative organisms

Most strains of *V. parahaemolyticus* that are isolated from stools of gastro-enteritis patients are Kanagawa-positive, which indicates that the strain hae-molyses human red cells in a special medium.[136] The haemolytic reaction is known as the Kanagawa phenomenon and the haemolysin responsible has been isolated and purified; it is a thermostable cytotoxic protein of 45 000 daltons and is cardiotoxic in rats.[63] Kanagawa-positive strains also cause dilatation of the isolated rabbit ileal loop.[16] Strains isolated from epidemiologically-incriminated seafoods from estuarine environments rarely are Kanagawa-positive, and do not show toxicity in the rabbit ileal loop. However if sufficient colonies are tested, Kanagawa-positive strains can usually be detected.[43] Volunteers have ingested 10^{10} cells of Kanagawa-negative *V. parahaemolyticus* with no ill-effects.[110] In contrast the number of Kanagawa-positive organisms required to produce clinical symptoms in volunteers has ranged from 2×10^5 to 3×10^7.[115] For an effective response in the rabbit ileal loop model — 50% of loops dilated — more than 10^5 organisms must be injected.[132] Kanagawa-positive strains adhere rapidly to human fetal intestinal cells, while Kanagawa-negative strains do not.[20] A heat-labile factor has been isolated from a culture filtrate of a Kanagawa-positive strain of *V. parahaemolyticus* and separated from a heat-stable haemolysin. This heat-labile factor caused morphological changes in Chinese hamster-ovary cells similar to those caused by choleragen and the heat-labile enterotoxin of *E. coli*.[63] In an outbreak in Bangladesh bloody diarrhoea occurred suggesting that tissue invasion can occur with this organism in contrast to the infection without invasion which occurs with *V. cholerae*.

V. parahaemolyticus also produces a haemolysin that is active against goat erythrocytes; and it grows at 42° C, which none of the non-halophilic vibrios do. An antigenic scheme consisting of at least 11 O-antigens, and of up to 58 K-antigens[70] has been established for *V. parahaemolyticus*. *Vibrio alginolyticus* is a halophilic vibrio which requires salt to grow, but it ferments sucrose which differentiates it from *V. parahaemolyticus*. *V. alginolyticus* occurs in retail fish in Australia;[96] in this study the gills of 56 fish were swabbed and 39 yielded *V. alginolyticus*. An organism, 'lactose-positive halophilic vibrio' has been reported to show toxicity in the ligated ileal loop of rats and rabbits.[99]

Laboratory diagnosis

It has been suggested that to add a special medium to the range used for routine faeces culture would be rather expensive, but the addition of 1.5% sodium chloride to existing media would allow the detection of *V. parahaemolyticus*.[107] However when a clear history has been obtained of seafood ingestion prior to gastroenteritis, the same media as for *Vibrio cholerae* should be used to isolate halophilic vibrios. Salt-colistin broth is particularly suitable for *V. para-haemolyticus*.[43]

Treatment and control

Patients suffering only from gastroenteritis merely require fluid replacement. Seafood should be kept in a refrigerator until eaten to avoid any dangerous rise in temperature which could allow *V. parahaemolyticus* to multiply. On a cruise ship coastal sea water had contaminated purified seafood, and when this contamination was stopped, further outbreaks of gastroenteritis due to this organism stopped.[76]

AEROMONAS SPECIES

As with other newly-recognized occasional causes of diarrhoea it is only when a microbiology laboratory is alerted to look for *Aeromonas* sp. that these organisms may be considered significant when isolated from a patient with gastro-enteritis.[9,102] In such a patient *Aeromonas* sp. especially *A. hydrophila* may be present in large numbers; and treatment that eliminates this organism may be accompanied by clinical cure.[9] Many strains of *A. hydrophila*[19] and some of *A. punctata* produce enterotoxin.[146] Thus *A. hydrophila* and possibly *A. punctata* should be considered as possible enterotoxigenic causes of gastroenteritis. However, the significance of these organisms as enteric pathogens has not yet been generally accepted, and further epidemiological studies are needed to assess their significance as a cause of diarrhoea. Children may be more frequently affected than adults.[144]

Causative organisms and clinical features

A. hydrophila and *A. punctata* are Gram-negative rods which are facultatively anaerobic. Other species of the genus *Aeromonas* can be found in water, and in fish, frogs and salamanders; experimental animals such as mice, guinea pigs and rabbits can be infected.[119] Previously the organism *Plesiomonas shigelloides* was included in the genus *Aeromonas*.

    A. hydrophila was first isolated from human faeces in 1937 by Miles and Halnan,[93] who termed it *Proteus melanovogenes*; the organism was recovered from a patient with 'chronic colitis'. *A. hydrophila* was first suggested to be a cause of severe gastroenteritis in 1961 in Colombia;[85] the organism was found to be the predominant bacterium in the aerobic stool flora of several patients with diarrhoea, and was isolated in pure culture from a few neonates with gastroenteritis. Since then diarrhoea due to *A. hydrophila* has been reported from Europe, Africa, India, Asia and North America.[58,108,130] Severe gastroenteritis has been associated with the organism especially in the elderly; from an 82 year old female with foul smelling liquid stools a pure culture of *A. hydrophila* was obtained.[9]

    In India, among 206 infants and children with diarrhoea, there were seven isolates of *A. hydrophila* and one isolate from 138 children without diarrhoea.[117] In a study of 188 patients without diarrhoea, 3.2% had *Aeromonas* species in their stools.[53] However in neither of these studies were the isolates of *Aeromonas* tested for enterotoxin production. To establish whether *A. hydrophila* and possibly *A. punctata* are causes of diarrhoea isolates must be tested for enterotoxin production, for example by the suckling-mouse test.[19] A study of 1156 children in

Perth, Western Australia, with gastroenteritis and 1156 matched controls has shown that 10.2% of children with gastroenteritis, but only 0.6% of those without diarrhoea, excreted enterotoxigenic *Aeromonas* species.[144] From adult patients in Western Australia during a period of 9 months, among 600 faecal specimens enterotoxigenic *A. hydrophila* was isolated without any other bacterial pathogen in 32 adults with diarrhoea, but five of these only had a brief period of diarrhoea.[143] In some of the patients severe diarrhoea had persisted for many weeks. Two patients had carcinoma of the large bowel; all but two of the patients were over the age of 60. A few patients had experienced vomiting but the predominant symptom was the passage of numerous fluid stools, usually without blood or mucus.

A. hydrophila can frequently be isolated from sites outside the gut. In one series of 30 patients from whom *A. hydrophila* was isolated, only two patients had diarrhoea;[53] the organism was isolated from bile, blood, and pus from a head wound. *A. hydrophila* has been implicated as the cause of meningitis, peritonitis, septicaemia and wound infection, particularly in the immunologically compromised.[130] A biotype variant of *A. hydrophila* has been called *A. sobria.*[147]

Epidemiology

A. hydrophila can be isolated from water, particularly surface waters, and from fish.[17] *A. hydrophila* has been cultured from tap water in the USA, during the summer.[88]

Pathogenesis

Some strains of *A. hydrophila* have been reported to produce a toxin cytopathic for mouse Y1 adrenal cells, and some strains produced a toxin that caused fluid accumulation in the ligated rabbit ileal loop.[116] However strains that produce a cytotoxin may not produce an enterotoxin as shown by the suckling-mouse test. Toxins produced by *A. hydrophila* have been reported not to be neutralized by anticholera toxin or anti-*E. coli* toxin,[79] but toxin detected by jejunal perfusion has been neutralized by anti-*V. cholerae* toxin.[142] Of 103 strains of *Aeromonas* species, including 95 from faeces, which were obtained from patients in Australia, India and Bangladesh, 79 were found to produce heat-stable enterotoxins as shown by the suckling-mouse test[19] and by rat jejunal perfusion. In the suckling-mouse test the effect of the enterotoxin is to produce diarrhoea of varying amounts and accumulation of fluid in the intestine as shown by the ratio of intestinal weight to remaining body weight. The cultural conditions required to produce the enterotoxin by *A. hydrophila* were shown to be important, and involved growth in Trypticase-Soy-Broth with yeast extract and shaking in an environmental incubation shaker at 100 rpm. The mice in the assay were not more than 6 days old and the inoculum mixed with blue dye was introduced intragastrically via a fine polyethylene tube. After incubation of the mice for 3 hours at 28° C the intestinal weight : body weight ratio and grade of diarrhoea were recorded. Other aspects of the work are discussed on p.197. In addition to enterotoxin production[148] *A. hydrophila* strains have also been shown to have the ability to attach to buccal epithelial cells, and adherence is a well-known virulence factor of gut pathogens.[147] Some strains of *A. hydrophila* elaborate at least two different lectins that are capable of recognizing L-fucose or D-mannose.[4]

Laboratory diagnosis

Culture of faeces on selective bile-salt-containing media such as deoxycholate citrate agar (DCA) and MacConkey medium can yield *A. hydrophila* either as a lactose fermenting organism, a non-lactose fermenter or one that is a late lactose fermenter. However a few strains of enterotoxigenic *Aeromonas* sp. fail to grow on such media but can be detected by aerobic culture on blood agar containing ampicillin 10 mg/l. The minimum inhibitory concentration of ampicillin for a few strains of *A. hydrophila* is occasionally as low as 12.5 mg/l,[150] and such strains will not grow on blood agar containing ampicillin 30 mg/l. Some workers merely put an ampicillin disc on a blood agar plate, rather than incorporating the ampicillin in the medium. On ampicillin-blood agar *Aeromonas* sp. typically appear as large, flat, grey colonies surrounded by a zone of beta-haemolysis. Enterotoxigenic strains of *Aeromonas* sp. are usually haemolytic,[19] but all oxidase-positive colonies should be studied and identified. Ampicillin-blood agar also has the advantage of being reliable for oxidase testing, which may be unreliable on selective medium.[86] However if the pH of MacConkey medium is greater than 5.2, all strains of *A. hydrophila* are found to be oxidase positive.[68] A 3-hour oxidase test has been described.[69]

A selective medium for *A. hydrophila* without blood or bile salts but containing ampicillin 20 mg/l and xylose was described in 1979,[151] with a minor modification by Moulsdale in 1983.[149] *Aeromonas* sp. appear as pink, non-xylose fermenting colonies. Moulsdale in England found that the hottest months of the year were associated with the highest rates of isolation of *Aeromonas* sp. from faeces, as did Gracey *et al.*,[144] and Goodwin (unpublished), in adults in Perth.

Aeromonas sp. are oxidase-positive but are distinguished from vibrios by their ability to grow in the presence of vibriostatic compound 0129, although a few strains are sensitive to 0129 (Burke, Valerie, personal communication). *A. hydrophila* produces deoxyribonuclease but does not decarboxylate ornithine, both of which distinguish it from *Plesiomonas*. The full biochemical identification of *Aeromonas* has been reported by Furniss *et al.*[43]

Antibacterial treatment and control

If diarrhoea is selflimited antibacterial treatment is not warranted. However, if diarrhoea persists the appropriate active antibiotic will be revealed by antibiotic sensitivity tests. The organism is usually sensitive to tetracycline, co-trimoxazole and chloramphenicol, but is resistant to ampicillin.[150] The organism is also sensitive to cefamandole and cefoxitin, and especially to the third generation cephalosporins, such as latamoxef and cefotaxime.[30] Not until appropriate selective media such as ampicillin-blood agar are used to reveal the full picture of the incidence of *Aeromonas* in patients with gastroenteritis and in those without, and not until the isolates are tested for enterotoxin production will it be possible to ascertain the importance of this organism as a cause of gastroenteritis. If *Aeromonas* is present in tap water this may be due to low levels of chlorine, and high levels should eliminate the organism. *A. hydrophila* seems to be more common among immuno-suppressed patients and in those with carcinoma.

PLESIOMONAS SHIGELLOIDES

Causative organism and clinical features

Plesiomonas shigelloides is a motile, oxidase-positive Gram-negative rod which may agglutinate with shigella antisera. The organism was first isolated in 1947,[31] and it used to be called *Aeromonas shigelloides*. The reported incidence of the organism in patients, and particularly children with gastroenteritis[45] is obviously related to the significance attached to the organism by different laboratories. In Adelaide, South Australia, from 1963 to 1967 the organism was cultured from 36 children and two adults; 12 of the children were less than 3 months old. One of the adults had an illness lasting 1 day with diarrhoea and some vomiting, and the other adult had moderately severe diarrhoea and vomiting for 3 days. Of the 13 children the organism was isolated at the beginning of an episode of gastroenteritis and there was no other organism isolated, although at that time rotavirus would not have been considered. From eight children the organism was isolated without any evidence of intestinal disease. In another nine children the organism was isolated in addition to either *Salmonella* or *Shigella* or enteropathogenic *E. coli*.[27] In Calcutta, during 1970, of 3433 diarrhoeal stool specimens *Plesiomonas shigelloides* was isolated as the only pathogen from 24 specimens;[112] it was isolated with *Vibrio cholerae* in 15 specimens, with *V. parahaemolyticus* in 8 specimens, with both vibrios in another 6 specimens, and with *Shigella* sp. in 1 specimen. A total of 56 strains of *P. shigelloides* were isolated.[112]

Two epidemics of water-borne diarrhoeal disease involving a total of 1000 people have been reported from Japan, and in both epidemics the only organism isolated was *P. shigelloides*.[131] The main clinical symptoms were diarrhoea in 88% of patients, abdominal pain in 82% and fever in 22%. Most patients recovered within 2 or 3 days. Tap water was the only common factor noted. In one epidemic 124 stool specimens were cultured for all known bacterial pathogens and 21 specimens yielded *P. shigelloides*. One of eight samples of tap water yielded

P. shigelloides of the same serotype O17:H2 as the predominant type isolated from the patients. In addition *P. shigelloides* were isolated from 4 of 12 water samples obtained from a water treatment plant in the area. In the second outbreak which only involved 35 people, of eight faecal specimens three yielded *P. shigelloides* in pure culture. The organism has been isolated from patients with diarrhoea in Australia,[27] India[112] and Africa[134] and from Cuba[2] and other countries.[131] The biochemical features of *P. shigelloides* have been described.[27,43]

Pathogenesis

In ileal loops of adult rabbits some isolates of *P. shigelloides* did produce fluid accumulation.[116] Multiplication of *P. shigelloides* was observed, although the multiplication rate was much lower than that of *A. hydrophila*; the strains of *P. shigelloides* had been isolated from four children with diarrhoea, and two other strains were tested. An enterotoxin, detected by the suckling-mouse test,[19] has been obtained from *P. shigelloides* (Burke, Valerie, personal communication.)

Laboratory diagnosis

Culture of faeces on deoxycholate citrate agar yields *P. shigelloides* as colourless colonies. The colonies are oxidase positive, with characteristic biochemical features.[27,43] *P. shigelloides* differ from *Aeromonas* in that the former produce acid from inositol and are non-haemolytic; they are sensitive to 0129.[43] Faeces may be enriched in GN broth,[28] and this is a good method of detecting small numbers of organisms. Some strains agglutinate with shigella antisera,[66] but of 35 isolates of *P. shigelloides* in Africa none agglutinated with anti-*Shigella sonnei* serum.[134] In South Australia 4 of 38 isolates agglutinated either with *Shigella sonnei* or *Shigella flexneri* antisera.[27]

Epidemiology

In Japan, of 342 samples of water and mud from ponds, rivers and shallow streams, *P. shigelloides* was isolated from 38% of the samples.[3] The rate of isolation was higher in the warmer rather than the cold seasons. Fish, shellfish and newts have been found to harbour the organism; and as mentioned above in the two Japanese outbreaks *P. shigelloides* was isolated from tap water.[131] Other authorities have also suggested that *P. shigelloides* may be water-borne.[2]

Treatment and control are similar to those for *A. hydrophila*, although *P. shigelloides* strains are frequently sensitive to ampicillin. Most strains appear to be sensitive to tetracycline and chloramphenicol and aminoglycosides, with many strains sensitive to sulphonamides.[27]

REFERENCES

1 Aldova E., Laznickova K., Stepankova E. and Lietava J. (1968) Isolation of non-agglutinable vibrios from an enteritis outbreak in Czechoslovakia. *J. Infect. Dis.* **118**, 23.

2 Aldova E, Rakovsky J. and Chovancova A. (1966) The microbiological diagnostics of strains of *Aeromonas shigelloides* isolated in Cuba. *J. Hyg. Epidemiol. Microbiol. Immunol.* **10**, 470.

3 Arai T., Ikejima N., Itoh T., Sakai S., Shimada T. and Sakazaki R. (1980) A survey of *Plesiomonas shigelloides* from aquatic environments, domestic animals, pets and humans. *J Hyg. (Camb.)* **84**, 203.

4 Atkinson H. M. and Trust T. J. (1980) Hemagglutination properties and adherence ability of *Aeromonas hydrophila. Infect. Immun.* **27**, 938.

5 Attasampunna P. (1974) *Vibrio parahaemolyticus* food poisoning in Thailand. In: International Symposium on Vibrio parahaemolyticus, p. 21, Eds Fugino T, Sakaguchi G., Sakazaki R. and Takeda Y. Saikon Publishing, Tokyo.

6 Ayres P. A. and Barrow G. I. (1978) The distribution of *Vibrio parahaemolyticus* in British coastal waters: report of a collaborative study 1975-6. *J. Hyg. (Camb.)* **80**, 281.

7 Back E., Ljunggren A. and Smith H. (1974) Non-cholera vibrios in Sweden. *Lancet* **i**, 723.

8 Baine W.B., Zampieri A., Mazzotti M., *et al.* (1974) Epidemiology of cholera in Italy in 1973. *Lancet* **ii**, 1370.

9 Baman S. I. (1980) *Aeromonas hydrophila* as the etiologic agent in severe gastroenteritis: Report of a case. *Am. J. Med. Technol.* **46**, 179.

10 Barker W. H. Jr (1974) *Vibrio parahaemolyticus* outbreaks in the United States. *Lancet* **i**, 551.

11 Bart K. J., Huq Z., Khan M. and Mosley W. H. (1970) Seroepidemiologic studies during a simultaneous epidemic of infection with El Tor Ogawa and Classical Inaba *Vibrio cholerae. J. Infect. Dis.* **121** Suppl. S17.

12 Barua D. (1970) In: Principles and practice of cholera control. Publ. Hlth Papers, WHO, No. 40, p. 29.

13 Barua D. and Mukherjee A. C. (1964) Observations on the El Tor vibrios isolated from cases of cholera in Calcutta. *Bull. Cal. Sch. Trop. Med.* **12**, 147.

14 Benenson A. S., Islam M. R. and Greenough W. B. (1964) Rapid identification of *Vibrio cholerae* by dark-field microscopy. *Bull. WHO* **30**, 827.

15 Blake P. A., Merson M. H., Weaver R. E., Hollis D. G. and Heublein P. C. (1979) Disease caused by a marine vibrio. Clinical characteristics and epidemiology. *N. Engl. J. Med.* **300**, 1.

16 Brown D. F., Spaulding P. L. and Twedt R. M. (1977) Enteropathogenicity of *Vibrio parahaemolyticus* in the ligated rabbit ileum. *Appl. Environ. Microbiol.* **33**, 10.

17 Boulanger Y., Lallier R. and Cousineau G. (1977) Isolation of enterotoxigenic *Aeromonas* from fish. *Can. J. Microbiol.* **23**, 1161.

18 Burke V., Gracey M., Suharyono and Sunoto (1980) Reduction by aspirin of intestinal fluid loss in acute childhood gastroenteritis. *Lancet* **i**, 1329.

19 Burke V., Robinson J., Berry R. J. and Gracey M. (1981) Detection of enterotoxins of *Aeromonas hydrophila* by a suckling mouse test. *J. Med. Microbiol.* **14**, 401.

20 Carruthers M. M. (1977) In vitro adherence of Kanagawa-positive *Vibrio parahaemolyticus* to epithelial cells. *J. Infect. Dis.* **136**, 588.

21 Cary S. G. and Blair E. B. (1964) New transport medium for shipment of clinical specimens. I. Fecal specimens. *J. Bact.* **88**, 96.

22 Cash R. A., Music S. I., Libonati M. J., Wenzel R. P. and Hornick R. B. (1974) Response of man to infection with *Vibrio cholerae*. I. Clinical, serologic, and bacteriologic responses to a known inoculum. *J. Infect. Dis.* **129**, 45.

23 Cassel D. and Selinger Z. (1977) Mechanisms of adenylate cyclase activation by cholera toxin: inhibition of GTP hydrolysis at the regulatory site. *Proc. Natl Acad. Sci. USA* **74**, 3307.

24 Chaicumpa W. and Atthasisiha N. (1977) Study of intestinal immunity against *V. cholerae*: Role of antibody to *V. cholerae* haemagglutinin in intestinal immunity. *Southeast Asian J. Trop. Med. Public Health* **8**, 13.

25 Chatterjee B. D. (1981) Vibrios. In: *Medical Microbiology and Infectious Diseases*, Vol. II, p. 353, Ed. Braude A. I., Saunders, Philadelphia.

26 Chatterjee B. D., Neogy K. N. and Gorbach S. L. (1970) Study of *Vibrio parahaemolyticus* from cases of diarrhoea in Calcutta. *Ind. J. Med. Res.* **58**, 234.

27 Cooper R. G. and Brown G. W. (1968) *Plesiomonas shigelloides* in South Australia. *J. Clin. Pathol.* **21**, 715.

28 Edwards P. R. and Ewing W. H. (1962) *Identification of Enterobacteriacae*, p. 236, 2nd edn, Burgess, Minneapolis.

29 El-Shawi N. and Thewaini A. J. (1969) Non-agglutinable vibrios isolated in the 1966 epidemic of cholera in Iraq. *Bull. WHO* **40**, 163.

30 Fass R. J. and Barnishan J. (1981) In vitro susceptibilities of Aeromonas hydrophila to 32 antimicrobial agents. *Antimicrob. Agents Chemother.* **19**, 357.

31 Ferguson W. W. and Henderson N. D. (1947) Description of strains C27: a motile organism with the major antigen of *Shigella sonnei* phase 1. *J. Bact.* **54**, 179.

32 Fernandes P. B. and Bayer M. E. (1977) Membrane-bound enterotoxin of *Vibrio cholerae*. *J. Gen Microbiol.* **103**, 381.

33 Field M. (1979) Mechanisms of action of cholera and *Escherichia coli* enterotoxins. *Am. J. Clin. Nutr.* **32**, 189.

34 Finkelstein R. A. (1966) Pre-selection of hemolytic variants of El Tor vibrios. *J. Bacteriol.* **92**, 513.

35 Forbes G. I. (1966) An outbreak of cholera El Tor in Hong Kong: the Temple Street Well. *Public Health* **8**, 188.

36 Forbes G. I., Lockhart J. D. F., Robertson M. J. and Allan W. G. L. (1968) Cholera case investigation and the detection and treatment of cholera carriers in Hong Kong. *Bull. WHO* **39**, 381.

37 Forsyth G. W., Hamilton D. L., Goertz K. E. and Johnson M. R. (1978) Cholera toxin effects on fluid secretion, adenylate cyclase, and cyclic AMP in porcine small intestine. *Infect. Immun.* **21**, 373.

38 Freter R. (1980) Prospects of preventing the association of harmful bacteria with host mucosal surfaces. In: *Bacterial Adherence*, p. 439, Ed. Beachey E. H., Chapman and Hall, London.

39 Fujino T. (1974) Discovery of *Vibrio parahaemolyticus*. In: International symposium on *Vibrio parahaemolyticus*, p. 1, Eds Fujino T., Sakaguchi G., Sakazaki R. and Takeda Y., Saikon Publishing, Tokyo.

40 Fujino T., Okemo Y., Nakada D., Aoyama A., Fukai K., Mukai T. and Ueho T. (1953) On the bacteriological examination of Shirasu-food poisoning. *Med. J. Osaka Univ.* **4**, 299.

41 Fujino T., Sakaguchi G., Sakazaki R. and Takeda Y. (1974) International symposium on *Vibrio parahaemolyticus*, Tokyo, Japan, 1973, Saikon Publishing, Tokyo.

42 Furniss A. L. (1978) Non-Cholera Vibrios. In: *Modern Topics in Infection*, p. 126. Ed. Williams J. D., Heinemann, London.

43 Furniss A. L., Lee J. V. and Donovan T. J. (1978) The Vibrios. Public Health Lab. Service Monograph Series No. 11.

44 Gardner A. D. and Venkatraman K. V. (1935) The antigens of the cholera group of vibrios. *J. Hyg.* **35**, 262.

45 Geizer E., Kopecky K. and Aldova E. (1966) Isolation of *Aeromonas shigelloides* in a child. *J. Hyg. Epidemiol. Microb. Immunol.* **10**, 190.

46 Gharagozloo R. A., Naficy K., Mouin M., Nassirzadeh M. H. and Yalda R. (1970) Comparative trial of tetracycline, chloramphenicol and trimethoprim/sulphamethoxazole in eradication of *Vibrio cholerae* El Tor. *Br. Med. J.* **4**, 281.

47 Gill D. M. and Enomoto D. M. (1980) Intracellular, enzymic action of enterotoxins: the biochemical basis of cholera. In: Cholera and related diarrhoeas, 43rd Nobel Symposium, Stockholm 1978, p. 104, Eds Ouchterlony O. and Holmgren J., Karger, Basel.

48 Gill D. M. and Rappaport R. S. (1979) Origin of the enzymatically active A_1 fragment of cholera toxin. *J. Infect. Dis.* **139**, 674.

49 Gilmour C. C. B. (1952) Period of excretion of *Vibrio cholerae* in convalescents. *Bull. WHO* **7**, 343.

50 Goh K. T. and Lam S. (1981) Vibrio infections in Singapore. *Ann. Acad. Med. Sing.* **10**, 2.

51 Gohar M. A. and Makkawi M. (1948) Cholera in Egypt. Laboratory diagnosis and protective inoculation. *J. Trop. Med. Hyg.* **51**, 95.

52 Gracey M. (1977) ROSE system of treatment of cholera dehydration. *Br. Med. J.* **1**, 839.

53 Graevenitz A. von and Mensch A. H. (1968) The genus Aeromonas in Human Bacteriology. *N. Engl. J. Med.* **278**, 245.

54 Greenough W. B. (1980) Principles and prospects in the treatment of cholera and related dehydratory diarrhoeas. In: Cholera and related diarrhoeas, 43rd Nobel Symposium, Stockholm 1978, p. 211, Eds Ouchterlony O and Holmgren J., Karger, Basel.

55 Guard R. W., Brigden M. and Desmarchelier P. (1980) Fulminating systemic infection caused by *Vibrio cholerae* species which does not agglutinate with O–1 *V. cholerae* antiserum. *Med. J. Aust.* **1**, 659.

56 Harris A. R. (1977) A case of non-agglutinable vibrio gastroenteritis with anuria. *Med. J. Aust.* **1**, 405.

57 Heiberg B. (1934) Des réactions de fermentation chez les vibrions. *Comptes rendus Soc. Biol.* **115**, 984.

58 Helm E. B. and Stille W. (1970) Akute enteritis durch *Aeromonas hydrophila. Dtsch Med. Wochensch.* **95**, 18.

59 Holmgren J., Lonnroth I. and Svennerholm L. (1973) Tissue receptor for cholera exotoxin: postulated structure from studies with GMI ganglioside and related glycolipids. *Infect. Immun.* **8**, 208.

60 Holmgren J. and Lonnroth I. (1980) Structure and function of enterotoxins and their receptors. In: Cholera and related diarrhoeas, 43rd Nobel Symposium, Stockholm 1978, p. 88, Eds Ouchterlony O. and Holmgren J., Karger, Basel.

61 Holmgren J., Svennerholm A. and Ahren C. (1981) Nonimmunoglobulin fraction of human milk inhibits bacterial adhesion (hemagglutination) and enterotoxin binding of *Escherichia coli* and *Vibrio cholerae. Infect. Immun.* **33**, 136.

62 Honda T. and Finkelstein R. A. (1979) Purification and characterization of a hemolysin produced by *Vibrio cholerae* biotype El Tor: Another toxic substance produced by cholera vibrios. *Infect. Immun.* **26**, 1020.

63 Honda T., Taga S., Takeda T., Hasibuan M. A., Takeda Y. and Miwatani T. (1976) Identification of lethal toxin with the thermostable direct hemolysin produced by *Vibrio parahaemolyticus* and some physiochemical properties of the purified toxin. *Infect. Immun.* **13**, 133.

64 Hood M. A., Ness G. E. and Roderick G. E. (1981) Isolation of *Vibrio cholerae* Serotype O1 from the Eastern Oyster, *Crassostrea virginica. Appl. Environ. Microbiol.* **41**, 559.

65 Hooper W. L., Barrow G. I. and McNab D. J. N. (1974) *Vibrio parahaemolyticus* food poisoning in Britain. *Lancet* **i**, 1100.

66 Hori M., Hayashi K., Maeshima K., Kigawa M., Miyasato T., Yoneda Y. and Hagihara Y. (1966) Food poisoning caused by *Aeromonas shigelloides* with an antigen common to *Shigella dysenteriae* 7. *J. Jpn. Assoc. Infect. Dis.* **39**, 433.

67 Hughes J. M., Hollis D. G., Gangarosa E. J. and Weaver R. E. (1978) Non-cholera vibrio infections in the United States. Clinical, epidemiologic, and laboratory features. *Ann. Int. Med.* **88**, 602.

68 Hunt L. K., Overman T. L. and Otero R. B. (1981*a*) Role of pH in oxidase variability of *Aeromonas hydrophila. J. Clin. Microbiol.* **13**, 1054.

69 Hunt L. K., Overman T. L. and Otero R. B. (1981*b*). Rapid oxidase method for testing oxidase-variable *Aeromonas hydrophila* strains. *J. Clin. Microbiol.* **13**, 1117.

70 Ishibashi M., Kinoshita Y., Yanai Y., Abe H., Takeda Y. and Miwatani T. (1980) Analysis of antigens of *Vibrio parahaemolyticus* strains possessing new O-and K-antigens. *Jpn. J. Bacteriol.* **35**, 701.

71 Jegathesan M. and Paramasivam T. (1976) Emergence of *Vibrio parahaemolyticus* as an important cause of diarrhoea in Malaysia. *Am. J. Trop. Med. Hyg.* **25**, 201.

72 Jones G. W. and Freter R. (1976) Adhesive properties of *Vibrio cholerae:* Nature of the interaction with isolated rabbit brush border membranes and human erythrocytes. *Infect. Immun.* **14**, 240.

73 Koch R. (1894) *The Bacteriological Diagnosis of Cholera,* Translation by Duncan, Edinburgh.

74 Lancet (1976) Cholera Research: What next? *Lancet* **ii**, 1283.

75 Lancet (1977) Bacterial adhesiveness and the gut. *Lancet* **i**, 1293.

76 Lawrence D. N., Blake P. A., Yashuk J. C., Wells J. G., Creech W. B. and Hughes J. H. (1979) *Vibrio parahaemolyticus* gastroenteritis outbreaks aboard two cruise ships. *Am. J. Epidemiol.* **109**, 71.

77 Levine M. M., Nalin D. R., Craig J. P., Hoover D., Bergquist E. J., Waterman D., Holley H. P., Hornick R. B., Pierce N. P. and Libonati J. P. (1979) Immunity of cholera in man: Relative role of antibacterial versus antitoxic immunity. *Trans. R. Soc. Trop. Med. Hyg.* **73**, 3.

78 Levner M., Urbano C. and Rubin B. A. (1980) Polymyxin B release of unnicked cholera toxin subunit A. *J. Bacteriol.* **144**, 1203.

79 Ljungh A., Wretlind B. and Wadstrom T. (1978) Evidence for enterotoxin and two cytolytic toxins in human isolates of *Aeromonas hydrophila.* In: *Toxins: Animal, Plant and Microbiol,* Ed. Rosenberg P., p. 947, Pergamon, Oxford.

80 Lonnroth I., Holmgren J. (1973) Subunit structure of cholera toxin. *J. Gen. Microbiol.* **76**, 417.

81 Love A. H. G., Phillips R. A., Rhode J. E. and Veall N. (1972) Sodium-ion movement across intestinal mucosa in cholera patients. *Lancet* **ii**, 151.

82 Maegraith B. (1980) Cholera. In: *Adams and Maegraith: Clincial Tropical Diseases,* p. 50, 7th edn, Blackwell Scientific Publications, Oxford.

83 Mahalanabis D., Brayton J. B., Mondal A. and Pierce N. F. (1972) The use of Ringer's lactate in the treatment of children with cholera and acute noncholera diarrhoea. *Bull. WHO* **46**, 311.

84 Manson-Bahr P. (1966) *Manson's Tropical Diseases,* 16th edn, p. 398, Bailliere, Tindall, London.

85 Martinez-Silva R., Guzmann-Urrego M. and Caselitz F. H. (1961) On the problem of the significance of *Aeromonas* strains in enteritis in infants. *Z. Tropenmed. Parasitol.* **12**, 445.

86 McGrath V. A., Overman S. B. and Overman T. L. (1977) Media-dependent oxidase reaction in a strain of *Aeromonas hydrophila. J. Clin. Microbiol.* **5**, 112.

87 McIntyre O. R., Feeley J. C. Greenhough W. B. III, Benenson A. S., Hassan S. I. and Saad A. (1965) Diarrhoea caused by non-cholera vibrios. *Am. J. Trop. Med. Hyg.* **14**, 412.

88 Meeks M. V. (1963) The genus Aeromonas: methods for identification. *Am. J. Med. Technol.* **29**, 361.

89 Mekalanos J., Collier R. and Romig W. (1979) Enzymic activity of cholera toxin. II. Relationships to proteolytic processing, disulfide bond reduction and subunit composition. *J. Biol. Chem.* **254**; 5855.

90 Merson M. H., Morris G. K., Sack D. A. *et al.* (1976) Traveller's diarrhoea in Mexico: a prospective study of physicians and family members attending a Congress. *New Engl. J. Med.* **294**, 1299.

91 Merson M. H., Black R. E., Sack D. A., Svennerholm A. M. and Holmgren J. (1980) Maternal cholera immunisation and secretory IgA in breast milk. *Lancet* **i**, 931.

92 Mhalu F. S., Mmari P. W. and Ijumba J. (1979) Rapid emergence of El Tor *Vibrio cholerae* resistant to antimicrobial agents during first six months of fourth cholera epidemic in Tanzania. *Lancet* **i**, 345.

93 Miles A. A. and Halnan E. T. (1937) New species of micro-organism (*Proteus melanovogenes*) causing black rot in eggs. *J. Hyg. (Camb.)* **37**, 79.

94 Morris J. G., Wilson R., Davis B. R., Wachsmuth I. K., Riddle C. F., Wathen H. G., Pollard R. A. and Blake P. A. (1981) Non-O Group 1 *Vibrio cholerae* gastroenteritis in the United States. Clinical, epidemiologic and laboratory characteristics of sporadic cases. *Ann. Int. Med.* **94**, 656.

95 Mosley W. H. (1970) In: Principles and practice of cholera control. *Pub. Hlth Papers, WHO* **40**, 23.

96 O'Connor R. F. (1979) *Vibrio alginolyticus* in retail fish. *Med. J. Aust.* **1**, 396.

97 Peterson J. W. (1979) Protection against experimental cholera by oral or parenteral immunization. *Infect. Immun.* **26**, 594.

98 Pierce N. F., Banwell J. G., Gorbach S. L., Mitra R. C., Mondal A. and Manji P. M. (1969) Bacteriological studies of convalescent carriers of cholera vibrios. *Ind. J. Med. Res.* **57**, 706.

99 Poole M. D. and Oliver J. D. (1978) Experimental pathogenicity and mortality in ligated ileal loop studies of the newly reported halophilic lactose-positive *Vibrio* sp. *Infect. Immun.* **20**, 126.

100 Prescott L. M. and Bhattacharjee N. K. (1969) Viability of El Tor Vibrios in common foodstuffs found in an endemic cholera area. *Bull. WHO* **40**, 980.

101 Rabbani G. H. *et al.* (1979) Chlorpromazine reduces fluid-loss in cholera. *Lancet* **i**, 410.

102 Rahman A. F. M. S. and Willoughby J. M. T. (1980) Dysentery-like syndrome associated with *Aeromonas hydrophila*. *Br. Med. J.* **281**, 976.

103 Rennels M. B., Levine M. M., Daya V., Angle P. and Young C. (1980) Selective vs. nonselective media and direct plating vs. enrichment technique in isolation of *Vibrio cholerae*: Recommendations for clinical laboratories. *J. Infect. Dis.* **142**, 328.

104 Report (1969) Outbreak of gastroenteritis by non-agglutinable (NAG) vibrios. *WHO, Weekly Epidemiol. Record* **44**, 10.

105 Report (1975) Non-cholera vibrio importation. *Can. Dis. Weekly Rep.* **1**, 65.

106 Rogers R. C., Cuffe R. G. C. J, Cossins Y. M., Murphy D. M. and Bourke A. I. C. (1980) The Queensland cholera incident of 1977. 2. The epidemiological investigation. *Bull. WHO* **58**, 665.

107 Roland F. P (1979) Isolated causes of *Vibrio parahaemolyticus* gastroenteritis. *J. Am. Med. Assoc.* **241**, 2504.

108 Rosner R. (1964) *Aeromonas hydrophila* as etiologic agent in case of severe gastroenteritis. *Am. J. Clin. Path.* **42**, 402.

109 Sack B. (1980) Pathogenesis and pathophysiology of diarrhoeal diseases caused by *Vibrio cholerae* and enterotoxigenic *Escherichia coli*. In: Cholera and related diarrhoeas, 43rd Nobel Symposium, Stockholm 1978, p. 53, Eds Ouchterlony O. and Holmgren J., Karger, Basel.

110 Sakazaki R., Tamura K., Kato T., Obara Y., Yamai S. and Hobo K. (1968) Studies on the enteropathogenic facultatively halophilic bacteria, *Vibrio parahaemolyticus*. III Enteropathogenicity. *Jpn. J. Med. Sci. Biol.* **21**, 325.

111 Sakazaki R., Tamura K., Gomez C. Z. and Sen R. (1979) Serological studies on the cholera group of vibrios. *Jpn. J. Med. Sci. Biol.* **23**, 13.

112 Sakazaki R., Tamura K., Prescott L. M. and Bencic Z. (1971) Bacteriological examination of diarrhoeal stools in Calcutta. *Ind. J. Med. Res.* **59**, 1025.

113 Salmaso S., Greco D., Bonfiglio B. *et al.* (1980) Recurrence of pelecypod-associated cholera in Sardinia. *Lancet* **ii**, 1124.

114 Sanyal S. C., Sakazaki R., Murase M. and Prescott L. M. (1972) Characterization of *V. cholerae* strains isolated in Calcutta during 1969–70. *Ind. J. Med. Res.* **60**, 844.

115 Sanyal S. C. and Sen P. C. (1974) Human volunteer study on the pathogenicity of *Vibrio*

parahaemolyticus. In: International Symposium on *Vibrio parahaemolyticus*, p. 227, Eds Fujino T., Sakaguchi G., Sakazaki R. and Takeda Y., Saikon Publishing, Tokyo.
116   Sanyal S. C., Singh S. J. and Sen P. C. (1975) Enteropathogenicity of *Aeromonas hydrophila* and *Plesiomonas shigelloides. J. Med. Microbiol.* **8**, 195.
117   Sanyal S. C., Sen P. C., Tiwari I. C., Bhattia B. D. and Singh S. J. (1977) Microbial agents in stools of infants and young children with and without acute diarrhoeal disease. *J. Trop. Med. Hyg.* **80**, 2.
118   Schram R. (1972) The 1971 cholera epidemic in Zaria, Nigeria. *Lancet* i, 213.
119   Schubert R. H. (1967) Die Pathogenität der Aeromonaden für Mensch und Tier. *Arch. Hyg. Bakteriol.* **150**, 709.
120.   Sherr H. P., Stifel F. B. and Herman R. H. (1978) Effect of cholera toxin on rabbit jejunal carbohydrate-metabolizing enzymes. *Gastroenterology* **75**, 711.
121   Shimada T. and Sakazaki R. (1973) R antigen of *Vibrio cholerae. Jpn. J. Med. Sci. Biol.* **26**, 155.
122   Sil J., Dutta N. M., Sanyal S. C. and Mukerjee S. (1974) Bacteriophage typing of *Vibrio cholerae* other than O serotype 1. *Ind. J. Med. Res.* **62**, 15.
123   Sladen G. E. and Dawson A. M. (1969) Cholera — a clue to functional diarrhoea? *Gut* **10**, 82.
124   Sladen G. E. (1975) Lessons from cholera. In: *Topics in Gastroenterology*, p. 169, Vol. 2, Eds Truelove S. C. and Trowell J., Blackwell Scientific Publications, Oxford.
125   Snow J. (1855) *On the Mode of Communication of Cholera*, 2nd edn, John Churchill, London.
126   Snyder J. D., Allegra D. T., Levine M. M. *et al.* (1981) Serologic studies of naturally acquired infection with *Vibrio cholerae* serogroup O1 in the United States. *J. Infect. Dis.* **143**, 182.
127   Srivastava R. *et al.* (1980) Events in pathogenesis of experimental cholera: Role of bacterial adherence and multiplication. *J. Med. Microbiol.* **13**, 1.
128   Stoll B. J., Bardhan P. K., Greenough W. B., Holmgren J., Huq I., Fredman P. and Svennerholm L. (1980) Binding of intraluminal toxin in cholera: Trial of GM1 Ganglioside charcoal. *Lancet* ii, 888.
129   Svennerholm A. M., Hanson L. A., Holmgren J., Lindblad B. S. Nilsson B. and Quereshi F. (1980) Different secretory immunoglobulin A antibody responses to cholera vaccination in Swedish and Pakistani women. *Infect. Immun.* **30**, 427.
130   Trust T. J. and Chipman D. C. (1979) Clinical involvement of *Aeromonas hydrophila. C.M.A. Journal* **120**, 942.
131   Tsukamoto T., Kinoshita Y., Shimada T. and Sakazaki R. (1978) Two epidemics of diarrhoeal disease possibly caused by *Plesiomonas shigelloides. J. Hyg. (Camb.)* **80**, 275.
132   Twedt R. M., Peeler J. T. and Spaulding P. L. (1980) Effective Ileal Loop Dose of Kanagawa-Positive *Vibrio parahaemolyticus. Appl. Environ. Microbiol.* **40**, 1012.
133   Twedt R. M., Madden J. M., Hunt J. M. *et al.* (1981) Characterization of *Vibrio cholerae* Isolated from Oysters. *Appl. Environ. Microbiol.* **41**, 1475.
134   Van Damme L. R. and Vandepitte J. (1980) Frequent isolation of *Edwardsiella tarda* and *Plesiomonas shigelloides* from healthy Zairese freshwater fish: A possible source of sporadic diarrhoea in the tropics. *Appl. Environ. Microbiol.* **39**, 475.
135   Venkatraman K. V. and Ramakrishnan C. S. (1941) A preserving medium for the transmission of specimens for the isolation of *Vibrio cholerae. Ind. J. Med. Res.* **29**, 681.
136   Wagatsuma S. (1968) A medium for the test of hemolytic reaction of *Vibrio parahaemolyticus. Media Circle* **13**, 159.
137   Wallace C. K., Pierce N. F., Anderson P. N. *et al.* (1967) Probable gallbladder infection in convalescent cholera patients. *Lancet* i, 865.
138   Weisz-Carrington P., Roux M. E., McWilliams M., Phillips-Quagliata J. M. and Lamm M. E. (1978) Hormonal induction of the secretory immune system in the mammary gland. *Proc. Natl Acad. Sci. USA* **75**, 2928.

139 Wilson G. S. and Miles A. A. (1975) *Topley and Wilson's Principles of Bacteriology, Virology and Immunity*, p. 1864, 6th edn, Arnold, London.

140 Woodward W. E. (1971) Cholera reinfection in man. *J. Infect. Dis.* **123**, 61.

141 Zafari Y., Zafari A. Z., Rahmanzaden S. and Fakhar N. (1973) Diarrhoea caused by non-agglutinable *Vibrio cholerae* (non-cholera vibrio), *Lancet* **ii**, 429.

142 James C., Dibley M., Burke V., Robinson J. and Gracey M. (1982) Immunological cross-reactivity of enterotoxins of *Aeromonas hydrophila* and cholera toxins. *J. Clin. Exp. Immunol.* **47**, 34.

143 Goodwin C. S., Harper W. E. S., Stewart J. K., Gracey M., Burke V. and Robinson J. (1983) Enterotoxigenic *Aeromonas hydrophila* and diarrhoea in adults. *Med. J. Aust.* **1**, 25.

144 Gracey M., Burke V., and Robinson J. (1982) *Aeromonas*—associated gastroenteritis. *Lancet* **ii**, 1304.

145 Lahiri A., Agarwal R. K. and Sanyal S. C. (1982) Biological similarity of *Vibrio cholerae* serotypes other than type 1 to cholera toxin and *Esherichia coli* heat-labile enterotoxin. *J. Med. Microbiol.* **15**, 429.

146 Burke V., Robinson J., Atkinson M., and Gracey M. (1982) Biochemical characteristics of enterotoxigenic *Aeromonas* spp. *J. Clin. Microbiol.* **15**, 48.

147 Daily O. P., Joseph S. W., Coolbaugh J. C., Walker R. I., Merrell B. R., Rollins D. M., Seidler R. J., Colwell R. R. and Lissner C. R. (1981) Association of *Aeromonas sobria* with human infection. *J. Clin. Microbiol.* **13**, 769.

148 Pitarangsi C., Echeverria P., Whitmire R., Tirapat C., Formal S., Dammin G. J. and Tingtalapong M. (1982) Enteropathogenicity of *Aeromonas hydrophila* and *Plesiomonas shigelloides:* Prevalence among individuals with and without diarrhea in Thailand. *Infect. Immun.* **35**, 666.

149 Moulsdale M. T. (1983) Isolation of *Aeromonas* from faeces. *Lancet* **i**, 351.

150 Richardson C. J. L., Robinson J. O., Wagener L. B. *et al.* (1982) *In-vitro* susceptibility of *Aeromonas* spp. to antimicrobial agents. *J. Antimicrob. Chem.* **9**, 267.

151 Rogol M., Sechter I., Grinberg L., Gerichter C. B. (1979) Pril-xylose-ampicillin agar, a new selective medium for the isolation of *Aeromonas hydrophila*. *J. Med. Microbiol.* **12**, 229.

6 Enteric fever — due to *Salmonella typhi* and *S. paratyphi*

J. Schneider

Typhoid fever	130
Epidemiology	130
Pathogenesis	131
Pathology	131
Clinical features	132
Typhoid fever in children	134
Paratyphoid fever	135
Laboratory diagnosis	135
Blood culture and clot culture	136
Serological diagnosis	136
Complications	137
Perforation	137
Haemorrhage	138
Typhoid carriers	139
Vi-antibody tests	140
Gelatin capsule string test for detection of chronic faecal carriers	140
Antimicrobial therapy	141
Chloramphenicol	141
Amoxycillin	142
Cotrimoxazole	143
Trimethoprim	143
Mecillinam	143
Pivmecillinam	144
Treatment of chronic enteric carriers	144
Prevention of typhoid	144
Typhoid vaccine	145
References	145

The term 'enteric fever' should not be viewed as old-fashioned, including as it does typhoid and paratyphoid fevers. The causative organism of typhoid is *Salmonella typhi*, and of the paratyphoid fevers *Salmonella paratyphi* A, B and C are the main organisms. Previously *S. paratyphi* B was also known as *S. schottmulleri*, and *S. paratyphi* C as *S. hirschfeldii*.

Salmonella organisms continue to be responsible for a significant number of gastrointestinal infections. No country is exempt. Even in the USA in 1978 there were 28 748 isolations of Salmonella from human sources, including 604 isolates of *Salmonella typhi*.[48]

TYPHOID FEVER

Epidemiology

The developed countries are virtually free from the danger of endemic typhoid fever. This must be attributed to improved hygienic practices, the provision of chlorinated, piped water supplies, and proper sewage disposal which isolate the sources from which infection might occur. Contamination of water supplies is a major factor in the spread of typhoid fever. The very important role played by contaminated water in the spread of typhoid was strikingly illustrated by an epidemic in 1901 in Germany, when there were more than 3000 typhoid patients, of whom 8% died.[35] It was established that the water company had adulterated filtered drinking water with untreated Ruhr river water. In Mexico in 1972 there was an epidemic of typhoid caused by water-borne transmission of a chloramphenicol-resistant strain of *S. typhi*.[27] Typhoid fever is encountered frequently in Africa, India, the Far East and South America.[70] South Africa, which is probably the most highly developed area of Africa, continues to report comparatively large numbers of cases of typhoid fever. For example 2519 cases were reported in 1977 and for the period January to November 1979 there were 3310 cases.[20] Travellers overseas from developed countries may acquire typhoid from an endemic area. In the USA of 1418 clinical cases of typhoid reported in 1947–72, 470 (33%) had acquired their infection outside the country. Infections that were contracted in Mexico, Italy and India accounted for 72% of these travel-associated cases.[66] In a developing country, Indonesia, invasive *S. typhi* or *S. enteritidis* infections accounted for 42% of patients admitted to hospital with febrile illness in Jakarta.[1]

Central to the understanding of *S. typhi* and *S. paratyphi* infections is that there is usually a human source.[24] Very uncommonly outbreaks of some magnitude occur in developed countries, such as the epidemic that occurred in Aberdeen, Scotland in 1964. Imported corned beef was found to be the agent responsible.[71] Cans in Argentina had been cooled by contaminated water.

In microbiological laboratories technologists are at risk and may acquire typhoid fever; aerosols are believed to contribute to 80% of such infections.[47] In Massachusetts, USA, four technologists became ill with typhoid after processing 'unknown simulated clinical specimens' during a laboratory improvement programme![33]

THE INFECTIOUS DOSE OF *SALMONELLA TYPHI* REQUIRED TO PRODUCE DISEASE

A study in volunteers demonstrated that a dose of 10^3 viable organisms did not produce disease but a dose of 10^7 organisms resulted in disease in 50% of volunteers, and 10^9 organisms in disease in 95% of volunteers.[34]

Pathogenesis

Salmonella organisms penetrate the mucosa of both small and large bowel, coming to lie intracellularly where they proliferate. There is not the same tendency to mucosal damage as occurs with Shigella infections but ulceration of lymphoid follicles may occur.[21] The evolution of typhoid is fascinating. Initially *S.typhi* proliferates in the second part of the duodenum. After increase in their numbers they enter and multiply in the Peyer's patches of the lower small intestine from where systemic dissemination occurs, to the liver, spleen and reticuloendothelial system. For a period varying from 1 to 3 weeks the organism multiplies within these organs. Rupture of infected cells occurs, liberating organisms into the blood stream, which signals the onset of illness. The bacilli then enter the bile and for a second time cause infection of the lymphoid tissue of the small intestine particularly in the ileum. It is this phase of heavy infection that brings the classical bowel pathology of typhoid in its train.

Pathology

Huckstep[36] refers to pathology in the Peyer's patches assuming four phases. These phases correspond approximately to the weeks of disease if treatment has not been given.
Phase 1 — Hyperplasia of lymphoid follicles.
Phase 2 — Necrosis of lymphoid follicles during the second week involving both mucosa and submucosa.
Phase 3 — Ulceration in the long axis of the bowel with the possibility of perforation and haemorrhage.
Phase 4 — Healing takes place from the fourth week onward, and unlike tuberculosis of the bowel with its encircling ulcers, does not produce strictures.
Although the ileum is the classical seat of typhoid pathology, lymphoid follicles may be affected in other parts of the gastrointestinal tract, such as the jejunum and ascending colon. The ileum usually contains larger and more numerous Peyer's patches than the jejunum, but this is not an invariable finding.[15] It is not generally appreciated that such lymphoid follicles are also found in the large intestine.[16] The number of solitary follicles in the large intestine decreases with age. Ulceration during paratyphoid B infection may involve stomach and large intestine as well.[17]

TYPHOID PERFORATION

Eggleston *et al.*[18] refer to typhoid perforations as usually being simple and involving the antimesenteric border of the bowel where they appear as punched-out holes. In contrast to other types of perforation omental migration to the affected area does not occur.

RETICULOENDOTHELIAL SYSTEM

Enlargement and congestion of the spleen and mesenteric glands are characteristic findings.

TYPHOID HEPATITIS

So-called 'typhoid hepatitis' has been described[63] when a liver biopsy may show non-specific reactive hepatitis. The salient features on liver biopsy are focal liver cell necrosis with associated infiltration of mononuclears — 'typhoid nodules' — sinusoidal congestion and dilation, and mononuclear cell infiltration of the portal area. Hepatitis should not be forgotten as one of the complications of typhoid and paratyphoid fever.[63]

OTHER SYSTEMIC INVASION

Other organs that may be affected by *Salmonella typhi* include the central nervous system, with meningitis as an infrequent complication, the skeletal system with occasional osteomyelitis, and typhoid abscesses in other areas such as the buttocks.

INCUBATION PERIOD OF TYPHOID FEVER

This is on average 10–14 days but may be a little less than a week or as long as 3 weeks.

Clinical features

No discussion on the clinical features would be complete without paying tribute to the remarkable clinical investigation carried out by Huckstep[36] on 975 cases of typhoid in Kenya.

FEVER

Fever is the most common manifestation of typhoid. In a series of 104 cases of enteric fever reported from the Lebanon, fever was the most constant clinical sign and was present in all patients.[55] In the classical case, there is a step-like rise in temperature during the first week. The temperature stays above normal for the first 3 weeks of the typical untreated case and falls to the normal range during the fourth week. Apart from this typical pattern of pyrexia variations may be encountered. In the pre-antibiotic era in 1946 it was observed that after the temperature reached its maximum by the so-called step-ladder ascent, it was found to maintain its height for approximately 11 days.[80] The clinical picture of typhoid may have undergone considerable change since the introduction of chloramphenicol; Gulati *et al*.[29] reported that 23 out of 57 patients had intermittent fever during the first week of illness. Change in the pattern of fever warrants consideration of other possibilities. Thus if the temperature rises suddenly early in the course of this disease, this could be due to a complication such as lobar pneumonia. A dramatic fall in temperature could be due to bowel haemorrhage or perforation. Temperature maintained at a low level can be seen in mild cases and is an occasional finding in the aged.[36] It should be remembered that pyrexia, although common, is not an invariable accompaniment of typhoid, and in up to 7% of cases infection may be asymptomatic.[62]

TOXAEMIA

In the early stages the typhoid patient may have a dull heavy 'toxic' appearance.[36]

RELATIVE BRADYCARDIA

This is encountered in somewhat less than half of all cases. This sign has also been referred to as 'a low pulse-temperature ratio' and is particularly relevant in the first week of the disease. This is not invariable and a rapid pulse rate can be encountered during the first week of illness in children and in other cases termed 'severe'.[36] In the uncommon instance of typhoid myocarditis the pulse is weak and rapid and the heart sounds are muffled; T-wave changes are seen in the electrocardiogram and the blood pressure is low.

SPLENOMEGALY

This can be detected in a little less than half of all patients with typhoid fever, the spleen becoming palpable during the second week of illness. In one study 64% of patients had enlarged spleens,[80] but in another series of 106 patients the spleen was palpable in only 16% of the patients.[12]

LEUKOPENIA

Leukopenia has been considered to be a common feature of typhoid fever, which will help to make the diagnosis. A transient leukocytosis may occur during the first week and a half of illness, but leukopenia, mainly neutropenia, tends to be most marked during the third week.[23]

ROSE SPOTS

These are mentioned in many reports. They were present in 33% in one series, but were observed more frequently in whites (45%) than in blacks (14.5%).[80] Rose spots were not observed in any of 57 Indian cases.[29] Rose-coloured macules are obviously more difficult to see in patients with deeply pigmented skins. Typically the spots are 2–4 mm in size, are present on the trunk and tend to appear at the end of the first week of illness. Their number does not as a rule exceed twelve.[37]

OTHER SYMPTOMS

Other symptoms occur very commonly in typhoid fever and constitute part of a composite picture. In a series of 360 cases cough occurred in 86%, headache in 90% and constipation in 78%, with diarrhoea in 43%, but as a prodromal complaint in about 10% only.[80] In a large series of 975 typhoid patients in Kenya, the main symptom on admission was headache (74.9%), with abdominal discomfort in 60.7%, and joint pains in 54%.[36]

Typhoid fever in children

The clinical picture of typhoid fever in young children may be atypical. Common presenting features in children under the age of 5 years are meningism, convulsions and diarrhoea, while the relative bradycardia and leukopenia of older patients is less common.[12] Among proven cases of typhoid fever under the age of 15 years, 55% presented with diarrhoea, 10% with constipation and 35% had neither of these symptoms.[62]

TYPHOID AND THE SICKLE CELL TRAIT

Patients with the sickle cell trait are thought to react more severely to typhoid fever[17] and salmonella osteomyelitis is more commonly seen in these patients.

SEPTICAEMIC SALMONELLOSIS AND SCHISTOSOMIASIS

Among 35 cases of septicaemic salmonellosis of long duration *Schistosoma mansoni* infection was present in all patients. *S.typhi* was isolated from seven of these cases by blood culture and in five other instances the disease was identified by serology. *S. paratyphi* A and C were identified in two other cases by serology. Also a number of other Salmonella types were found in the patients. The prolonged septicaemia was stated to have the clinical characteristics of a reticulo-endotheliosis very closely related to that of kala-azar.[56] In two cases that had failed to respond to chloramphenicol the intercurrent schistosomiasis was treated with niridazole and the response was excellent.[57]

PARATYPHOID FEVER

In general, these infections are milder than typhoid fever. Paratyphoid infection often occurs in developed countries such as eastern Europe and the United States. *S. paratyphi* A tends to produce an illness clinically akin to that produced by *S. typhi* with prolonged fever and a tendency to relapse.[37]

SALMONELLA PARATYPHI B

Outbreaks of disease due to this organism are more frequently food-borne than water-borne. Moreover, carrier states are more common. A comprehensive report on 62 cases of paratyphoid fever occurring in American military personnel and their dependants living in southern Turkey has been given by Meals.[52] Fifty-four had *S. paratyphi* B, six had *S. paratyphi* A, and both organisms were isolated from the remaining two patients. According to Huckstep[36] *S. paratyphi* B is milder than typhoid but is more prone to cause jaundice, suppurative lesions and carrier state. Ulceration can occur in the stomach and large intestine as well.[17]

SALMONELLA PARATYPHI C (*Salmonella hirschfeldii*)

Infection with this organism has been reported in Eastern Europe, India, Guyana, and in Central and East Africa. Many isolates from the latter areas differed from the classic strain in that they did not ferment arabinose and were thus labelled as var. *east africa*. *Salmonella paratyphi* C has been encountered in South and South-west Africa (Namibia). Jacobs *et al.*[38] documented 53 such cases, 47 of whom where diagnosed in the Eastern Transvaal. In three of the South-west African patients, the organism was isolated from the urinary tract, *a feature often associated with this organism.*[38] Isolates from a further two cases from South-west Africa were *S. paratyphi* C var. *east africa* — one being obtained from a foot abscess and the other from an area of peripheral gangrene. There is also a description of peripheral gangrene having occurred in two cases of *Salmonella paratyphi* C septicaemia in Nigeria.[61] However, of the 47 patients from the Eastern Transvaal reported by Jacobs *et al.*[38] 46 were stated to have features in keeping with a diagnosis of enteric fever. A history of fever was obtained in 35.

LABORATORY DIAGNOSIS

The presence of *Salmonella typhi* or *S. paratyphi* is detected either by culture of the organism or by the demonstration of specific antibodies or antigen in the serum. The organism may be cultured from blood, bone marrow, stool or urine.

Blood culture and clot culture

In addition to the usual two bottles inoculated with blood, a third bottle containing streptokinase bile-salt broth can significantly increase the isolation rate of *S. typhi*. In 210 cases of enteric fever whole blood conventional bile salt broth yielded the organism in 64% of cases but streptokinase bile salt broth inoculated with blood clot which was minced with scissors yielded a positive result in 92% of eight cases.[84] Although the conventional wisdom is that *S. typhi* is obtained from blood during the first week of illness more frequently than from the stool, whereas the reverse applies during the second and third weeks of the illness, the clinician should be reminded that the organism can be cultured from blood as late as the fifth week of the disease,[62] and the organism may be cultured from the stool throughout the disease. The organism is less frequently isolated from urine, but it is useful to determine whether a patient does excrete the organism in the urine because this could become a site for chronic carriage. Culture of bone marrow or skin snips taken from rose spots may yield the organism when it cannot be obtained from blood, stool or urine.[25] The organism can be cultured from the bone marrow in as many as 90% of patients even after antibiotics have already been given;[25] in one group of patients *S. typhi* was isolated from the blood in 40%, from the stool in 37% and from urine in 7%, but from rose spots in 63% of patients.[25] In a case of paratyphoid fever bone marrow culture yielded the organism even though antibiotics had been administered.[42] In general the administration to a patient with pyrexia of unknown origin of amoxycillin, ampicillin or co-trimoxazole inevitably hampers the diagnosis of typhoid fever.[8]

The liquid and solid media that are suitable for isolating *Salmonella typhi* and *S. paratyphi* are similar to those described in Chapter 3 for the diagnosis of salmonellosis. However strontium selenite broth is superior to selenite F broth for the isolation of *S. typhi* especially when relatively few typhoid bacilli are present in faeces, for example after antibiotic therapy or if stool specimens have been left for prolonged periods at room temperature;[13] and salmonella-shigella agar has been found to be superior to xylose lysine deoxycholate agar for the isolation of *S. typhi*. Modified bismuth sulphate agar is superior to deoxycholate agar for the growth of *Salmonella* sp., and is mandatory if the diagnosis of typhoid is very likely, or if a carrier is being investigated.[31]

In conclusion, although blood culture is most likely to yield the organism during the first week, or septicaemic phase of the illness, the clinician is advised to order blood, stool and urine cultures on one or more occasions to confirm or exclude the diagnosis.

Serological diagnosis

The Widal test has long been used as a serological aid in the diagnosis of typhoid fever. Two specimens of serum are required at an interval of 7–10 days and a four-fold rise in the titres of H (flagellar) or O (somatic) agglutinins indicates a strong likelihood of the disease. Previous TAB immunization may leave residual titres of H agglutinins, and a rise in O agglutinins may be more relevant in such patients. However even in immunized patients it is possible to get a rise only in H agglutinins and not in O agglutinins. The Widal test has the disadvantage that diagnosis is delayed until a second specimen is received. However, counter-immunoelectrophoresis (CIE) of a single specimen of serum to detect *S. typhi* O antigen can yield a positive result early in the disease; 96% of 52 sera from typhoid patients were positive with no false positives.[82] In another study in India, in 26 culturally proven patients with typhoid, CIE detected 25 out of 26 cases during the early stage — 24 positive for *S. typhi* antigen and one for antibody — and CIE was also found to be suitable for diagnosis in the chronic or late stages of typhoid fever.[30]

Salmonella typhi has also a Vi antigen, and antibodies to this antigen can be looked for in a patient's blood, but it has historically been used to diagnose a chronic carrier of *S. typhi*, as described below. *S. typhi* can be subdivided for useful epidemiological purposes by phage typing; there are 80 Vi phage types. To identify the source of an outbreak, Vi phage typing is required to establish identity of strain between source and patient.

The standard laboratory techniques of agglutinating isolates of Salmonella with O and H antisera are described in Chapter 3.

The Widal test can be performed on a single serum, particularly if CIE is not available; elevated titres of H and O agglutinins in unvaccinated subjects are strongly suggestive of *S. typhi* infection if the person comes from a non-endemic area or is a child less than 10 years old in an endemic area.[46]

COMPLICATIONS

Of all the complications of typhoid the two that are often an immediate threat to life are perforation and haemorrhage. They commonly occur during the third week of illness.

Perforation

In the pre-antibiotic days intestinal perforation commonly involving the distal ileum, was cited as a complication in approximately 1% of patients[80] but figures as high as 18% have been reported.[3] Chloramphenicol has had a major influence in achieving reduction in mortality from typhoid but regrettably did not reduce the incidence of perforation.[18] Perforation of a small bowel typhoid ulcer is regarded by Kuruvilla[43] as a surgical emergency. Any delay in diagnosis could well be responsible for higher mortality rates. Death rates following surgery have varied from 9.9% in South Korea[41] to 30% in Ghana[3] and 29% in South Africa.[2] The experience of Eggleston *et al.*,[18] working in the Punjab, and based on 78 cases, was that poor prognosis could be linked with the duration of illness, duration of perforation, shock, uraemia, encephalopathy and faecal peritonitis. The reported mortality rate from perforation was 32% in their series of 78 cases. They viewed surgery as the treatment of choice because in 96% of their cases they found either open perforation or gangrene.[18] Archampong[3] observed that the mortality rate rose 76% if operation was performed later than the fifth day after perforation. For the treatment of typhoid perforation when physical signs are localized and minimal and the general condition of the patient is good, intensive medical care is probably adequate.[43] For uncomplicated solitary perforation, simple closure surgically is adequate; with bleeding or multiple ulceration, resection is suggested.[43]

Haemorrhage

According to Nasrallah and Nassar[55] severe intestinal haemorrhage affects about 2% of patients. In most instances treatment should be conservative with the use of suitable antibiotics, blood transfusion and rest to the intestine. In cases where bleeding is persistent and very heavy and fails to respond to conservative measures, resection of the affected portion of intestine may need to be considered.[85]

TYPHOID HEPATITIS

Typhoid hepatitis is a term used by Ramchandran *et al.*,[63] from Sri Lanka, to describe hepatomegaly and jaundice occurring during the course of the disease. Hepatomegaly was detected in 27% of their patients but jaundice was observed in less than a third of those patients with hepatic enlargement. The incidence of hepatomegaly was slightly lower in cases of paratyphoid fever. SGPT levels were elevated in 35% of cases (*S. typhi* or *S. paratyphi*). In a large study of 360 cases of typhoid hepatic enlargement was reported in 25% of patients.[80]

DISSEMINATED INTRAVASCULAR COAGULATION

Disseminated intravascular coagulation (DIC) is a common occurrence in typhoid fever but is stated to be a subclinical event.[10]

HAEMOLYTIC-URAEMIC SYNDROME

Haemolytic-uraemic syndrome in typhoid fever was detected in 12.5% of 43 patients seen in Rhodesia.[4] In that area typhoid had to be considered as a precipitating cause of acute renal failure.

ACUTE HAEMOLYTIC ANAEMIA

Huckstep[37] maintains that mild haemolytic anaemia is not uncommon in very toxic patients. There have been occasional reports of more severe anaemia.[49]

MYOCARDITIS

Myocarditis is an uncommon complication of typhoid fever and was reported by Rowland[68] in nine out of 530 patients (1.2%).

MENINGITIS

Salmonella typhi meningitis is not common even in endemic areas. In Durban (South Africa) there were only seven cases in African children during the period 1964–76.[73]

ACUTE DISSEMINATED ENCEPHALOMYELITIS

This complication of typhoid fever has been documented by Ramchandran *et al.*[64] from Sri Lanka. The patient developed an encephalopathy with clinical features of brain stem involvement and died within 24 hours of the onset of neurological signs. Histology of brain disclosed lesions in midbrain and pons with the appearance of acute disseminated encephalomyelitis and demyelination of these areas.

OTHER COMPLICATIONS

These include dehydration, bedsores, typhoid abscesses, pneumonia, acute parotitis, osteomyelitis.[37]

UNCOMMON COMPLICATIONS

Myocarditis, meningitis, acute disseminated encephalomyelitis and granulomatous mastitis[11] and recurrent peritonitis[19] are included in this category.

TYPHOID CARRIERS

Carriers of *S. typhi* are either convalescent carriers who excrete the organism for a limited period of time after apparent clinical cure, or chronic carriers in whom persistent excretion of *S. typhi* in stool or urine can be detected a year after clinical illness. Chronic faecal carriers occur more commonly than do chronic urinary ones. The numbers of typhoid bacilli excreted in the stools of these cases may be inordinately large, each gram of faeces usually containing 10^6 or more viable organisms.[53]

Vi-ANTIBODY TESTS

Serological tests are used to screen people suspected of being chronic carriers of *Salmonella typhi*. The Vi-agglutination test has been used for many years and Bokkenheuser[6] has stated: 'The Vi test should not be used indiscriminately in screening populations for typhoid carriers, but may have limited usefulness in an attempt to trace suspected carriers in a closed group of individuals. A Vi reactor must be followed up by bacteriological investigation, but the chance of a reactor being a carrier is very small. The demonstration of a carrier among the reactors does not exclude the possibility of another carrier occurring among the non-reactors'.[6] Not more than 70% of chronic carriers of *S. typhi* have Vi agglutinating antibodies with titres in excess of 1:5.[7] 'False positive' reactions have been obtained from culture negative individuals.[14] The fluorescent Vi antibody test has been used to demonstrate significant serum antibody titres in 11 out of 12 typhoid carriers, with two out of 119 (1.7%) of culture-negative suspects also with significant antibody titres.[14] By counter-immunoelectrophoresis (CIE) and passive haemagglutination (HA) 13 out of 14 chronic typhoid carriers were detected, and solid phase radio-immunoassay studies showed that the antibodies were mainly of the IgG class.[89] Vi antibody was detected in 3% of 329 controls by HA but not by CIE. In 1030 hospitalized non-typhoid patients one chronic carrier was detected by CIE and one non-carrier gave a positive CIE test.[89] Successful treatment with amoxycillin in one carrier was followed after 6 months by a negative CIE result. A new haemagglutination assay for Vi antibodies, utilizing purified Vi antigen from *Citrobacter* to sensitize the red blood cells, is claimed to be as sensitive and specific as faecal culture in detecting symptom-free typhoid carriers.[59]

Gelatin capsule string test for detection of chronic faecal carriers

Because excretion of organisms in the faeces of chronic carriers is often inter-mittent, methods other than faecal culture have been devised to increase the chances of obtaining positive cultures. For many years culture of duodenal aspirates was used to increase diagnostic accuracy in patients suspected of being gallbladder carriers. More recently Gilman *et al.*[26] have suggested the use of a gelatin capsule containing a nylon string for collecting duodenal specimens in carriers of *S. typhi*. They found that duodenal contents obtained with either the string or duodenal tube were more often positive than were stool cultures. The string test has the additional advantage of avoiding the discomfort associated with passage of a duodenal tube.

Chronic urinary carriers

Farid *et al.*[22] refer to a high incidence of urinary salmonellae excreted in Egypt and state that this is related to the damaged urinary tract caused by *Schistosoma haematobium.* They studied 15 chronic urinary carriers, and ascertained that not only did the carriers excrete *S. typhi* or *S. paratyphi* A in the urine but periodically shed these organisms into the blood. All 15 patients had damaged urinary tracts due to schistosomal infection.

ANTIMICROBIAL THERAPY

For the treatment of the acute condition, a number of agents have been used — chloramphenicol, amoxycillin, cotrimoxazole and mecillinam. Microbiological procedures to determine the antibiotic sensitivities of the isolate of *S. typhi* from the patient are mandatory.

Chloramphenicol

In 1948, Woodward *et al.*[86] announced: 'A new antibiotic Chloromycetin has been clinically tested in the treatment of typhoid fever and has been found to exhibit significant chemotherapeutic effects . . .' There is little doubt that the introduction of this antibiotic in 1949 revolutionized the treatment of typhoid fever. Antibiotic treatment of typhoid fever cut the mortality rates from 12% to 4%.[87] It could not be expected that chloramphenicol would maintain an unblemished track record. It remained the linchpin of treatment for many years, but in 1973 widespread chloramphenicol resistance was reported in Mexico. There had been other isolated reports of chloramphenicol resistance.[9]

Chloramphenicol is given by mouth in a dose of 500 mg 6-hourly for 15 days. During the first few days a 4-hourly regimen is recommended until the temperature settles. However, Scragg *et al.*[75] maintained that a 21-day course of treatment was necessary in order to keep the relapse rate at a low level. Following a subsequent investigation, Scragg and Rubidge[74] stated: 'It is our impression, and that of others, that the response to chloramphenicol is not as satisfactory as formerly . . .' Hard on the heels of this statement came a report of an outbreak of typhoid fever due to a chloramphenicol-resistant strain of *S. typhi* in a village of Central Mexico during mid-1972.[27] With subsequent spread, over 10 000 substantiated cases of typhoid fever were documented in this part of Mexico[60] and almost all were chloramphenicol-resistant. Virtually all the organisms were resistant to sulphonamides, streptomycin and tetracycline and contained a self-transmissible plasmid. Resistance plasmids have been detected in many other enteric and non-enteric bacteria. Interestingly, the pendulum has now swung in the opposite direction with most *S. typhi* strains from Mexico being sensitive to chloramphenicol.[69]

Under certain circumstances, such as intestinal perforation, it may not be possible to give the antibiotic by the oral route and parenteral administration may be necessary. This gives rise to a paradoxical situation, inasmuch as blood chloramphenicol concentrations are significantly lower after this method of administration.[79] It was not surprising, therefore, that Snyder *et al.*[79] observed a shorter course of fever and a lower relapse rate in those taking oral chloramphenicol than in patients who had received the antibiotic by the parenteral route.

Transmissible drug resistance is 'plasmid-mediated'. It is often associated with the formation of a protein which may be in the nature of an inactivating enzyme.[54] In the case of chloramphenicol resistance, this is conferred by an acetylating enzyme known as chloramphenicol acetyltransferase.[76] Murray and Moellering,[54] in an extensive review of the literature on antibiotic resistance, assert that chloramphenicol acetyltransferase can be plasmid- or chromosomally-mediated but in some cases may be interlinked. In these cases, the gene for chloramphenicol can move from plasmid to chromosome and may indeed move back again by transposition or recombination.

RELAPSE

Relapse after treatment of typhoid will occur in a small percentage of patients, whether treatment has been given or not. Strangely, the percentage of patients relapsing after treatment with chloramphenicol is somewhat higher than in those who have received no treatment — approximately 20% in those given treatment as opposed to approximately 10% in the untreated group. As relapse may occur some weeks following apparently successful treatment, it is obviously advisable to review the progress of patients for several consecutive months.

Amoxycillin

Amoxycillin has gained wide acceptance as a suitable alternative to chloramphenicol in the treatment of typhoid fever. There is some evidence to suggest that this antibiotic could well prove the treatment of choice. Scragg[72] from Durban (South Africa), after carrying out a comparative trial in children, was able to show that amoxycillin gave better results than chloramphenicol. She referred to the fact that a satisfactory clinical response occurred within 5 days in 89% of patients taking the former antibiotic and 54% of those taking chloramphenicol — a difference regarded as highly significant. The adult dose of amoxycillin is 4 g daily (1 g 6-hourly) for 21 days. Alternatively the daily dosage can be worked out for both adults and children on the basis of 50–75 mg/kg. This regimen is given by Herzog[32] who advocated full doses, continuing for 2 days after defervescence and followed by half the dose for a minimum of another 10 days. This scheme for duration of treatment can be applied to other antibiotics in use against typhoid.

Parenteral amoxycillin has been used in the treatment of severely ill children. Thirty African children at King Edward VIII Hospital in Durban, and in whom the diagnosis of typhoid had been established by blood culture, were given sodium amoxycillin by intramuscular injection. The dose was 100 mg/kg in divided doses every 6 hours for the first 3 days followed by the same dose given by mouth for a further 18 days.[67] There were no relapses or carriers. There is now an intravenous preparation available and it can be anticipated that the intravenous route of administration will replace the more painful intramuscular one.

Amoxycillin has supplanted ampicillin. With the latter there is a longer period of fever and faecal excretion of *S. typhi* than with chloramphenicol.[79]

Cotrimoxazole

Cotrimoxazole is composed of trimethoprim and sulphamethoxazole; a standard tablet contains 80 mg of the former and 400 mg of the latter. The compound acts by sequential blockade of folic acid synthesis. The combination is alleged to make a bactericidal compound out of two individually bacteriostatic constituents. Its use is contra-indicated in patients with megaloblastic anaemia or megaloblastic marrow changes.[44] A trial in children with typhoid revealed that the response to cotrimoxazole was unsatisfactory with a bacteriological failure rate of 34%, and this bore no relationship to size of dose or duration of therapy.[74] The bacteriological failure rate with chloramphenicol was only 10%. However in Bombay, when cotrimoxazole was compared with chloramphenicol, response to treatment was good in both groups and there were no treatment failures.[39] Another trial in Chile showed that the majority of patients (79%) responded as well to cotrimoxazole as to chloramphenicol;[78] however, in the majority of patients who failed to respond after 11 days of treatment, neither drug levels nor *in vitro* sensitivities could account for the slowness of response. Treatment failure 'non-responsiveness' has also been reported from Sri Lanka in a little under 10% of cases treated with cotrimoxazole.[65] One of the advantages of cotrimoxazole is that it can be given intravenously.[28] The daily oral dosage is cited as 7–8 mg/kg for trimethoprim and 35–40 mg/kg for sulphamethoxazole.[32] The dose is continued at this level for 2 days after defervescence of fever and then half the dose is given for a further 10 days.

Trimethoprim

A preliminary trial in eight patients, seven with typhoid fever and one with *S. paratyphi* A has shown this substance to be well tolerated and effective when used on its own.[50]

Mecillinam

This antibiotic is derived from 6-aminopenicillanic acid (6-APA) which is the penicillin nucleus. It is not viewed as a true penicillin as it is an amidino-penicillinate as opposed to true penicillins which are acylaminopenicillinates.[45] Initial enthusiasm for this antibiotic in the treatment of typhoid fever has been shown to be unfounded; the drug is not an effective or consistent treatment for enteric fever.[51] Twelve patients with enteric fever were treated with mecillinam for 14 days; four continued to have fever and toxaemia for 7–9 days, and at that stage change of treatment to chloramphenicol proved beneficial.[51] Only 7 out of 12 patients were cured with mecillinam alone.

PIVMECILLINAM

This is the orally absorbed pivaloxymethylester of mecillinam. A study by Ball *et al.*[5] indicated that the clinical results of treatment were similar to those obtained with cotrimoxazole. Unlike the latter, relapses occurred with pivmecillinam while patients were still undergoing treatment. Furthermore the time taken to obtain negative stool specimens was stated to be a mean of 8.5 days longer with pivmecillinam than with cotrimoxazole. Uncomplicated recovery on primary therapy was stated to be 78% for the former and 72% for the latter.

TREATMENT OF CHRONIC ENTERIC CARRIERS

Any person who excretes *S. typhi* for 12 months or longer without clinical symptoms is regarded as a chronic enteric carrier. When ampicillin was used to treat typhoid carriers, the relapse was in the region of 40%.[40,77] With amoxycillin an overall cure rate of 73% was achieved in 15 chronic enteric carriers of *S. typhi*.[58] The dosage schedule was 2 g by mouth three times a day for 4 weeks. Cotrimoxazole can also be used in the treatment of chronic carriers. It is an accepted principle in the treatment of chronic typhoid carriers that the nidus of infection, which is usually the gallbladder, may require surgical removal before cure can be accomplished. Even then, the cure rate may only be 85%.[34]

PREVENTION OF TYPHOID

General measures suitable for all enteric illnesses are chlorinated water supplies and proper sewage disposal; and only foods that can be peeled, or are still hot, should be eaten by travellers in areas where hygienic standards are poor. Canned or bottled beverages are not always safe; the use of boiled water is recommended.[69] Specific measures may be employed, which include vaccination of travellers, which will decrease but not necessarily eliminate the risk of typhoid.[69] Rapid diagnosis and treatment of clinical cases and carriers limits the sources of infection. Carriers must be excluded from food handling, or working in schemes associated with water supplies. Phage types of all carriers should be known and recorded. Under epidemic circumstances, samples are taken from both piped water supply and sewerage, and phage typing is carried out on typhoid organisms isolated.

Typhoid vaccine

Immunization cannot replace the basic method of control. It will not guarantee freedom from an attack of typhoid fever. The latter may occur despite immunization if the inoculum is large.

Acetone-dried typhoid vaccine affords protection but needs to be given in two doses as one dose is less effective.[81] This vaccine is stated to give 70–85% protection for 3–4 years, which is a slightly higher protection rate than that given for example by heat-phenol inactivated vaccine.[83] A live oral vaccine (galactose epimerase-less) has been found to be safe and to give 87% protection in volunteers, but the results of an Egyptian field trial are still awaited.[83,88]

A full discussion of current and potential vaccines can be found in Chapter 12.

REFERENCES

1 Anderson K. E., Joseph S. W., Nasution R., Sunoto Butler T., van Peenen P. F. D., Irving G. S., Saroso J., Sulianti, Watten R. H. (1976) Febrile illnesses resulting in hospital admission: A bacteriological and serological study in Jakarta, Indonesia. *Am. J. Trop. Med. Hyg.* **25**, 116.

2 Angorn I. B., Pillay S. P., Hegarty M. and Baker L. W. (1975) Typhoid perforation of the ileum: A therapeutic dilemma. *South Afr. Med. J.* **49**, 781.

3 Archampong E. O. (1969) Operative treatment of typhoid perforation of the bowel. *Brit. Med. J.* **3**, 273.

4 Baker N. M., Mills A. E., Rachman I. and Thomas J. E. P. (1974) Haemolytic-uraemic syndrome in typhoid fever. *Brit. Med. J.* **2**, 84.

5 Ball A. P., Farrell I. D., Gillett A. P., Geddes A. M., Clarke P. D. and Ellis C. J. (1979) Enteric fever in Birmingham: Clinical features, laboratory investigation and comparison of treatment with pivmecillinam and co-trimoxazole. *J. Infect.* **1**, 353.

6 Bokkenheuser V. (1960) The interpretation of the Vi-tests. *South Afr. Med. J.* **34**, 601.

7 British Medical Journal (1978) Typhoid and its serology. *Br. Med. J.* **1**, 389.

8 British Medical Journal (1979) Typhoid fever. *Br. Med. J.* **1**, 213.

9 Butler T., Linh Nguyen Ngoc, Arnold K. and Pollak M. (1973) Chloramphenicol-resistant typhoid fever in Vietnam associated with R factor. *Lancet* **ii**, 983.

10 Butler T., Bell W. R., Levin J., Linh Nguyen Ngoc and Arnold K. (1978) Typhoid fever. Studies of blood coagulation, bacteremia and endotoxemia. *Arch. Int. Med.* **138**, 407.

11 Campbell F. C., Eriksson B. L. and Angorn I. B. (1980) Localised granulomatous mastitis — an unusual presentation of typhoid. A case report. *South Afr. Med. J.* **57**, 793.

12 Cassel R. and Koornhof H. J. (1977) Typhoid fever in Southern Africa. In: *Medicine in a Tropical Environment.* Proceedings of the International Symposium South Africa, 1976, published for the South African Medical Research Council by A.A. Balkema, Cape Town, Rotterdam.

13 Chau P. W. and Forrest C. R. (1972) Further study of strontium selenite and selenite F broths for the isolation of *Salmonella typhi. J. Clin. Path.* **25**, 966.

14 Chitkara Y. and Urquhart A. E. (1979) Fluorescent Vi antibody test in the screening of typhoid carriers. *Am. J. Clin. Path.* **71**, 87.

15　Cornes J. S. (1965) Number, size and distribution of Peyer's patches in the human small intestine. Part 1. The development of Peyer's patches. *Gut* **6**, 225.

16　Dukes C. and Bussey H. J. R. (1926) The number of lymphoid follicles of the large intestine. *J. Path. Bacteriol.* **29**, 111.

17　Edington G. M and Gilles H. M. (1976) *Pathology in the Tropics*, 2nd edn, Edward Arnold, London.

18　Eggleston F. C., Santoshi B. and Singh C. M. (1979) Typhoid perforation of the bowel. *Ann. Surgery* **190**, 31.

19　Eng R. H., Corrado M. L. and Cleri D. (1980) Recurrent *Salmonella typhi* peritonitis. *J. Am. Med. Assoc.* **243**, 363.

20　Epidemiological Comments. Department of Health, Pretoria. Republic of South Africa. December, 1979.

21　Evans N. (1979) Pathogenic mechanisms in bacterial diarrhoea. *Clin. Gastroenterol.* **8**, 599.

22　Farid Z., Bassily S., Kent D. C., Sanborn W. R., Hassan A., Abdel-Wahab M. F. and Lehman J. S. Jr (1970) Chronic urinary salmonella carriers with intermittent bacteraemia. *J. Trop. Med. Hyg.* **73**, 153.

23　Foote S. C. and Hook E. W. (1979) Salmonella species (including typhoid fever). In: *Principles and Practice of Infectious Diseases*, Eds Gerald L. Mandell, R. Gordon Douglas Jr and John E. Bennett, John Wiley and Sons, New York.

24　Geddes A. M. (1973) Enteric fever, salmonellosis and food poisoning. *Br. Med. J.* **1**, 98.

25　Gilman R. H., Terminel M., Levin M. M., Hernandez-Mendoza P. and Hornick R. B. (1975) Comparison of the relative efficacy of blood, urine, rectal swab, bone marrow and rose spot cultures for recovery of *Salmonella typhi* in typhoid fever. *Lancet* i, 1211.

26　Gilman R. H., Islam S., Rabbani H. and Ghosh H. (1979) Identification of gall bladder typhoid carriers by a string device. *Lancet* i, 795.

27　Gonzales-Cortes, Bessudo D., Sanchez-Leyva R., Fragoso R., Hinojosa M. and Becerril P. (1973) Waterborne transmission of chloramphenicol-resistant *Salmonella typhi* in Mexico. *Lancet* ii, 605.

28　Goodwin N. M. (1973) Intravenous Bactrim. *South Afr. Med. J.* **47**, 2159.

29　Gulati P. D., Saxena S. N., Gupta P. S. and Chuttani H. K. (1968) Changing pattern of typhoid fever. *Am. J. Med.* **45**, 544.

30　Gupta A. K. and Rao K. M. (1979) Simultaneous detection of *Salmonella typhi* anitgen and antibody in serum by counter-immunoelectrophoresis for an early and rapid diagnosis of typhoid fever. *J. Immunol. Methods* **30**, 349.

31　Harvey R. W. S. and Price T. H. (1979) Principles of Salmonella isolation. *J. Appl. Bacteriol.* **46**, 27.

32　Herzog C. (1980) New trends in the chemotherapy of typhoid fever. *Acta Tropica* **37**, 275.

33　Holmes M. B., Johnson D. L., Fiumara N. J. and McCormack W. M. (1980) Acquisition of typhoid fever from proficiency-testing specimens. *N. Eng. J. Med.* **303**, 519.

34　Hornick R. B., Greisman S. E., Woodward T. E., Du Pont H. L., Dawkins A. T. and Snyder M. J. (1970) Typhoid fever: Pathogenesis and immunological control (Parts I and II). *N. Eng. J. Med.* **283**, 686; **283**, 739.

35　Howard-Jones N. (1973) Gelsenkirchen typhoid epidemic of 1901, Robert Koch and the dead hand of Max von Pettenkofer. *Br. Med. J.* **1**, 103.

36　Huckstep R. L. (1962) Typhoid fever and other Salmonella infections. E. and S. Livingstone Ltd., Edinburgh.

37　Huckstep R. L. (1974) Typhoid fever and other Salmonella infections. In: *Medicine in the Tropics*, Ed. A. W. Woodruff, Churchill Livingstone, Edinburgh.

38　Jacobs M. R., Koornhof H. J., Crisp S. I., Palmhert H. L. and Fitzstephens A. (1978) Enteric fever caused by *Salmonella paratyphi* C in South and South West Africa. *South Afr. Med. J.* **54**, 434.

39　Kamat S. A. (1970) Evaluation of therapeutic efficacy of trimethoprim-sulfamethoxazole and chloramphenicol in enteric fever. *Br. Med. J.* **3**, 320.

40 Kaye D., Merselis J. G., Connolly C. S. and Hook E. W. (1967) Treatment of chronic enteric carriers of Salmonella typhosa. *Ann. N.Y. Acad. Sci.* **145**, 429.
41 Kim J. P., Oh S. K. and Jarrell F. (1975) Management of ileal perforation due to typhoid fever. *Ann. Surgery* **181**, 89.
42 Knowles G. K. and Murphy M. F. G. (1979) Paratyphoid A fever diagnosed from bone marrow culture after indiscriminate antibiotic treatment. *Br. Med. J.* **1**, 384.
43 Kuruvilla M. J. (1978) Role of resection in typhoid perforation. *Ann. Roy. Coll. Surgeons Eng.* **60**, 408.
44 Lancet (1973) Cotrimoxazole and blood. *Lancet* ii, 950.
45 Lancet (1976) Mecillinam. *Lancet* ii, 503.
46 Levine M. M., Grados O., Gilman R. H., Woodward W. E., Solis-Plaza R. and Waldman W. (1978) Diagnostic value of the Widal test in areas endemic for typhoid fever. *Am. J. Trop. Med. Hyg.* **27**, 795.
47 Liberman D. F. (1979) Occupational hazards. Illness in the microbiological laboratory. *Public Health Lab.* **37**, 118.
48 Morbidity and Mortality Weekly Report, 1980 Human *Salmonella* isolates — United States, 1978. **28**, 618.
49 McFadzyean A. J. S. and Choa G. H. (1953) Haemolytic anaemia in typhoid fever. A report of six cases, together with the effect of chloramphenicol and A.C.T.H. *Br. Med. J.* **2**, 360.
50 McKendrick M. W., Geddes A. M. and Farrell I. D. (1981) Trimethoprim in enteric fever. *Br. Med. J.* **282**, 364.
51 Mandal B. K., Ironside A. G. and Brennand J. (1979) Mecillinam in enteric fever. *Br. Med. J.* **1**, 586.
52 Meals R. A (1976) Paratyphoid fever: Report of 62 cases with several unusual findings and review of the literature. *Arch. Int. Med.* **136**, 1422.
53 Merselis J. G. Jr, Kay D., Connolly C. S. and Hook E. W. (1964) Quantitative bacteriology of the typhoid carrier state. *Am. J. Trop. Med. Hyg.* **13**, 425.
54 Murray B. E. and Moellering R. C. (1978) Patterns and mechanisms of antibiotic resistance. *Med. Clin. North Am.* **62**, 899.
55 Nasrallah S. M. and Nassar V. H. (1978) Enteric fever: A clinicopathologic study of 104 cases. *Am. J. Gastroenterol.* **69**, 63.
56 Neves J. and Martins N. R. da luz Lobo (1967) Long duration of septicaemic salmonellosis: 35 cases with 12 implicated species of salmonella. *Trans. R. Soc. Trop. Med. Hyg.* **61**, 541.
57 Neves J., Marinho R. P., Martins N. R. da luz Lobo, de Araujo P. K. and Lucciola J. (1969) Prolonged septicaemic salmonellosis: Treatment of intercurrent schistosomiasis with niridazole. *Trans. R. Soc Trop. Med. Hyg.* **63**, 79.
58 Nolan C. M. and White P. C. (1978) Treatment of typhoid carriers with amoxicillin. *J. Am. Med. Assoc.* **239**, 2352.
59 Nolan C. M., White P. C., Feeley J. C., Brown S. L., Hambie E. A. and Wong K. H. (1981) Vi serology in the detection of typhoid carriers. *Lancet* i, 583.
60 Olarte J. and Galindo E. (1972) *Salmonella typhi* resistant to chloramphenicol, ampicillin and other anti-microbial agents: strains isolated during an extensive typhoid fever epidemic in Mexico. *Antimicrob. Agents Chemother.* **4**, 597.
61 Onyemelukwe G. C., Mee J. Adesanya O. and Baksi A. (1979) Peripheral gangrene in *Salmonella paratyphi* septicaemia. *Trop. Geog. Med.* **31**, 297.
62 Popkiss M. E. E. (1980) Typhoid fever. A report on a point-source outbreak of 69 cases in Cape Town. *South Afr. Med. J.* **57**, 325.
63 Ramchandran S., Godfrey J. J. and Perera M. V. F. (1974) Typhoid hepatitis. *J. Am. Med. Assoc.* **230**, 236.
64 Ramchandran S., Wickremesinghe H. R. and Perera M. V. F. (1975) Acute disseminated encephalomyelitis in typhoid fever. *Br. Med. J.* **1**, 494.
65 Ramchandran S., Godfrey J. J. and Lionel N. D. W. (1978) A comparative trial of co-trimoxazole and chloramphenicol in typhoid and paratyphoid fever. *J. Trop. Med. Hyg.* **81**, 36.

66   Rice P. A., Baine W. B. and Gangarosa E. J. (1977) *Salmonella typhi* infections in the United States, 1967–72: Increasing importance of international travellers. *Am. J. Epidemiol.* **106**, 160.

67   Robinson O. P. W. and Scragg J. N. (1980) Parenteral amoxicillin therapy in typhoid fever. In: *Current Chemotherapy and Infectious Disease*, Volume 11. Proceedings of the 11th International Congress of Chemotherapy and the 19th Interscience Conference on Antimicrobial Agents and Chemotherapy, Boston. Massachusetts. 1–5 October, 1979, Eds John D. Nelson and Carlo Grassi, Am. Soc. Microbiol., Washington, DC.

68   Rowland H. A. K. (1961) The complications of typhoid fever. *J. Trop. Med. Hyg.* **64**, 143.

69   Ryder R. W. and Blake P. A (1979) Typhoid fever in the United States, 1975 and 1976. *J. Infect. Dis.* **139**, 124.

70   Sangster G. (1977) Diarrhoeal diseases. In: *A World Geography of Human Diseases*, Ed. G. Melvyn Howe, Academic Press, London.

71   Scottish Home and Health Department (1964) *The Aberdeen typhoid outbreak*, HMSO, Edinburgh.

72   Scragg J. N. (1976) Further experience with amoxycillin in typhoid fever in children. *Br. Med. J.* **2**, 1031.

73   Scragg J. N. and Appelbaum P. C. (1979) *Salmonella typhi* meningitis in children: report of 7 cases. *Trans. R. Soc. Trop. Med. Hyg.* **73**, 235.

74   Scragg N. J and Rubidge C. J. (1971) Trimethoprim and sulphamethoxazole in typhoid fever in children. *Br. Med. J.* **3**, 738.

75   Scragg J. N., Rubidge C. J. and Wallace H. L. (1969) Typhoid fever in African and Indian children in Durban. *Arch. Dis. Childh.* **44**, 18.

76   Shaw W. V. (1971) Comparative enzymology of chloramphenicol resistance. *Ann. N.Y. Acad. Sci.* **182**, 234.

77   Simon H. J. and Miller R. C. (1966) Ampicillin in the treatment of chronic typhoid carriers. *N. Eng. J. Med.* **274**, 807.

78   Snyder M. J., Perroni J., Gonzales O., Palomino C., Gonzalez C., Music S., Du Pont H. L., Hornick R. B. and Woodward T. E. (1973) Trimethoprim-sulfamethoxazole in the treatment of typhoid and paratyphoid fevers. *J. Infect. Dis.* **128** (Suppl); S734.

79   Snyder M. J., Perroni J., Gonzalez O., Woodward W. E., Palomino C., Gonzalez C., Music S. I., Du Pont H. L., Hornick R. B. and Woodward T. E. (1976) Comparative efficacy of chloramphenicol, ampicillin and cotrimoxazole in the treatment of typhoid fever. *Lancet* **ii**, 1155.

80   Stuart B. M. and Pullen R. L. (1946) Typhoid. Clinical analysis of three hundred and sixty cases. *Arch. Int. Med.* **78**, 629.

81   Tapa S. and Cvjetanovic B. (1975) Controlled field trial on the effectiveness of one and two doses of acetone-inactivated and dried typhoid vaccine. *Bull. WHO* **52**, 75.

82   Tsang R. S. and Chau P. Y. (1981) Serological diagnosis of typhoid fever by counterimmunoelectrophoresis. *Br. Med. J.* **282**, 1505.

83   WHO Memorandum (1979) Intestinal immunity and vaccine development. *Bull. WHO* **57**, 719.

84   Watson K. C. (1978) Laboratory and clinical investigation of recovery of *Salmonella typhi* from blood. *J. Clin. Microbiol.* **7**, 122.

85   Wong S. H. (1978) The emergency surgical management of massive and persistent intestinal haemorrhage due to typhoid fever: a report of 3 cases. *Br. J. Surgery* **65**, 74.

86   Woodward T. E., Smadel J. E., Ley H. L. Jnr, Green R. and Mankikar D. S. (1948) Preliminary report on the beneficial effect of chloromycetin in the treatment of typhoid fever. *Ann. Int. Med.* **29**, 131.

87   Woodward T. E. and Smadel J. E. (1964) Management of typhoid fever and its complications. *Ann. Int. Med.* **60**, 144.

88   Woodward W. E. (1980) Volunteer studies of typhoid fever and vaccines. *Trans. R. Soc. Trop. Med. Hyg.* **74**, 553.

89   Chau P. Y. and Tsang R. S. W. (1982) Vi serology in screening of typhoid carriers: improved specificity by detection of Vi anitbodies by counterimmunoelectrophoresis. *J. Hyg. (Camb.)* **89**, 261.

7 Gastroenteritis due to *Staphylococcus aureus, Clostridium perfringens* and *Bacillus cereus*

J. Schneider

Introduction   149
  The importance of an aetiological diagnosis   150
Staphylococcal gastroenteritis   150
  Epidemiology   150
  Pathogenesis   151
  Clinical features   151
  Laboratory diagnosis   151
  Prevention of staphylococcal gastroenteritis   152
Clostridial gastroenteritis   152
  Pathogenesis   153
  Clinical features   153
  Laboratory diagnosis   153
  Prevention of clostridial gastroenteritis   154
Bacillus cereus gastroenteritis   154
  Causative organism   154
  Epidemiology   154
  Pathogenesis   155
  Clinical features   155
  Laboratory diagnosis   155
  Control   156
References   156

INTRODUCTION

Gastroenteritis due to the bacteria considered in this chapter is commonly known as 'food poisoning'. Outbreaks of disease due to these organisms continue to occur in developed countries in spite of the fact that public health departments endeavour to disseminate and enforce safe methods of food preparation and storage. It is generally agreed that the official notifications of food poisoning outbreaks are a considerable underestimate of the actual incidence.[3,36] The common denominator linking these bacterial infections of the bowel is that their symptomatology depends upon the production of a toxin, and the infection is food-borne. Staphylococcal toxin and *Bacillus cereus* toxin are produced in the food, whereas the toxin of *Clostridium perfringens* is elaborated in the gut of the patient. The dominant initial symptom in staphylococcal food poisoning is vomiting. When *C. perfringens* is involved abdominal pain and diarrhoea are the major features. In the case of food poisoning due to *B. cereus* either vomiting or diarrhoea may predominate. Estimation of the incubation period is of considerable help when attempting to make a provisional aetiological diagnosis before results of laboratory tests become available. It can be assumed that most outbreaks of abdominal pain and gastroenteritis in which the median incubation period was less than 1 hour were of chemical aetiology. An outbreak in which the median incubation period was 1–7 hours was probably of staphylococcal aetiology, and one in which the median incubation period was 8–14 hours was probably caused by *C. perfringens*.[36]

The importance of an aetological diagnosis

The necessity for making a rapid and accurate diagnosis is underlined by the fact that this will enable measures to be taken to detect and protect contacts. Shigellosis and salmonellosis may pose a threat to infant or elderly contacts of a patient, whereas staphylococcal or *C. perfringens* food poisoning would not.[17] An accurate prediction of the subsequent course of the disease can often be given after specific diagnosis of the underlying cause has been made. The symptoms of staphylococcal and *C. perfringens* food poisoning would not be expected to last more than a day or two, whereas with shigella or salmonella infections symptoms could easily persist for a week or more.[17] Positive identification of the aetiological agent will help in tracing the source of infection. Any undue delay in submitting specimens will ruin the chances of identification. The rapid isolation of an offending organism, or toxin assay, allows one to institute appropriate specific or supportive treatment. The treatment of staphylococcal, *B. cereus* and *C. perfringens* infection is entirely supportive. The value of this type of treatment must not be underestimated. The occasional patient may become seriously ill.

STAPHYLOCOCCAL GASTROENTERITIS

Epidemiology

In most instances a protein-containing food appears to be the vehicle for *Staphylococcus aureus*, but dairy products are often implicated. In the USA in 1978 ham was the most common vehicle, being implicated in 28% of instances of staphylococcal food poisoning.[25] The important part played by food handlers in the spread of infection needs to be stressed. In an outbreak of staphylococcal food poisoning aboard a commercial aircraft ham was strongly incriminated as the vehicle of the outbreak, and the source appeared to have been a cook with staphylococcal lesions of his fingers. The attack rate was 86% for passengers who ate ham handled by the cook, and 0% for passengers who ate ham handled exclusively by another food preparer.[6] There are also dangers inherent in preparation of certain foods, such as salami meats. In the production of fermented sausage lightly-salted meat is intentionally temperature-controlled to allow lactobacilli to grow; these usually inhibit the growth of other organisms. However, if the procedure is not adequately monitored *S. aureus* may multiply on the surface of the sausage and produce enterotoxin. The curing period for sausages is usually 1–2 months, and during this time staphylococcal organisms tend to die, but the enterotoxin which causes human illness can remain.[24]

Pathogenesis

Five enterotoxins of *Staphylococcus aureus* have been recognized — A, B, C, D and E; they are all heat stable. Type B has a strong association with staphylococcal enterocolitis, but type A is the most frequently detected in food-borne illness.[7] The enterotoxins are heat stable and are produced by relatively few strains of *S. aureus*, often from phage group III.[25]

Clinical features

Certain features point to the possibility of food-borne disease being staphylococcal in origin. A mean incubation period varying between 2 and 7 hours and occurring in association with upper gastrointestinal symptoms is very likely to be staphylococcal food poisoning.[17] Vomiting is a prominent feature and may frequently be accompanied by diarrhoea. Fever occurs in a minority of instances.[9] There are, however, exceptions to every rule and an elevated temperature was recorded in almost 50% of the passengers who developed staphylococcal food poisoning during the course of a Japanese charter flight from Tokyo to Copenhagen;[5] 142 passengers had to be admitted to hospital. In a few patients blood was present in the stool. In this outbreak some of the complications that occasionally supervene were observed. One patient developed shock and anuria, and another manifested transient cerebral ischaemia with hemiparesis.[5] Both patients were discharged well, after 10 days in hospital.

In an outbreak of acute gastrointestinal disease due to *S. aureus* in Delaware (USA) 67 of 107 wedding guests became ill.[25] The incubation period ranged from 1.6–6.5 hours with a median period of 3.5 hours. Vomiting was the most frequent symptom in 85%, but diarrhoea occurred in 39%. Both nausea and abdominal cramps occurred more frequently than diarrhoea.[25] In another outbreak of staphylococcal food poisoning after a Thanksgiving dinner in Florida (USA) 54 of 350 students developed an illness marked by the acute onset of nausea and vomiting, followed by diarrhoea. Fever was not reported.[23]

Laboratory diagnosis

The incrimination of *Staphylococcus aureus* as the cause of an outbreak of gastroenteritis is not always easy, because this species may be regularly found on food and food handlers as a harmless commensal. The diagnosis is made on the basis of a large number of *S. aureus* in the suspected food, and if organisms can be isolated from the vomit or faeces they must be the same phage type as in the food, and should be found on the food handlers. In food a count of 10^5 *S. aureus*/g or greater is highly suggestive that this organism is aetiologically significant. However *S. aureus* can be destroyed by heat, while the enterotoxin is heat-stable, so that the offending phage type may not be isolated from the patients.

The demonstration of *S. aureus* in faeces does not necessarily mean that this organism is responsible for the food poisoning as it is a normal inhabitant of faeces in 25% of healthy individuals. However the detection of staphylococcal enterotoxin in the food would make the diagnosis highly likely. Direct or indirect methods to detect the enterotoxin are available. Enterotoxigenic staphylococci usually produce a thermostable deoxyribonuclease, and the estimation of this enzyme is an excellent screening test for the probable presence of staphylococcal enterotoxin. The test is rapid, reliable and a relatively simple screening method for enterotoxins in food including dairy products.[2] Direct detection of enterotoxin may be accomplished by the sophisticated techniques of immuno-diffusion and reverse passive haemagglutination with specific antitoxin.

To isolate *S. aureus* from foodstuffs the medium of Baird-Parker may be used; this contains potassium tellurite to inhibit Gram-negative bacteria, and it also contains egg yolk which makes the medium opaque. *S. aureus* and some strains of *S. saprophyticus* produce clear zones by lipolysis or proteolysis of the egg yolk lipoproteins.

Prevention of staphylococcal gastroenteritis

There are two main principles. Food handlers must be free of any source of infection, especially infected lesions on the fingers; such lesions constitute a common source of staphylococcal contamination. Secondly, the role of temperature is critical, and overgrowth of organisms can be prevented by storage at a low temperature.[6] The hazard of incapacitating illness amongst the cockpit crew of an aeroplane is obvious.[6] Individual members of the crew should eat meals prepared by different members of the cabin staff.

CLOSTRIDIAL GASTROENTERITIS

Since the authoritative report by Hobbs *et al.*[15] in 1953 gastroenteritis due to *Clostridium perfringens* has been diagnosed with ever-increasing frequency. There have been alarming reports of food poisoning due to *C. perfringens* in hospitals.[18] From 1973–77 *C. perfringens* predominated (62%) in 50 outbreaks of acute food poisoning in Scottish hospitals.[28] In England and Wales from 1973–75, out of 202 outbreaks of food poisoning and salmonella infections in hospital, 22% were due to *C. perfringens*.[18] Meat dishes, especially minced meat cooked in institutions, usually are the vehicles for the organism. The meat is contaminated by spores from the faeces of animals at the time of slaughter, or from human faeces. The dish may be cooked on one day and reheated the next day, with inadequate cooling overnight.[28]

Necrotizing enterocolitis, which may be due to *C. perfringens* is discussed in Chapter 1.

Pathogenesis

Clostridium perfringens produce an alpha enterotoxin which has been characterized as a heat-labile protein with a molecular weight in the region of 36 000 daltons.[14,30] This enterotoxin is produced by type A2; type A strains produce alpha toxin only. Isolates of *C. perfringens* that produce such an alpha toxin are usually non-haemolytic on horse blood agar, and have spores that are markedly heat resistant.[15] However food poisoning can also be produced by the A1 strain which has relatively heat-sensitive spores.[31] *C. perfringens* enterotoxin has been shown to stimulate adenylate cyclase activity.[8] The enterotoxin can cause accumulation of fluid and electrolytes in the ligated ileal loop;[20] the enterotoxin acts by producing membrane damage to the microvillus brush borders of individual cells as well as by affecting the basic function of macromolecular synthesis.[21] There is also a beta toxin which has been shown to produce haemorrhagic necrotizing enteritis;[19,27] it has a molecular weight of about 48 000 daltons.[19] The organism producing this toxin is known as *Clostridium perfringens* type C, it forms not only beta toxin but alpha toxin as well. A close relationship has been shown between spore formation and enterotoxin production.[4]

Clinical features

Colicky abdominal pain, often in the upper abdomen, and diarrhoea are the cardinal symptoms of *C. perfringens* infection. The incubation period varies between 8 and 24 hours. It is uncommon for symptoms to persist for longer than 1 day. Constitutional symptoms are not usual.

Laboratory diagnosis

Standard laboratory methods to detect *C. perfringens* include culture of food and faeces on medium containing lecithin; the lecithinase of *C. perfringens* produces a large zone around the colony, and this lecithinase action can be inhibited by specific antitoxin. Serotyping of organisms isolated from faeces of patients and from infected food is required. The same serotype should be isolated from the affected patients and from food. If a group of people have not suffered clinical symptoms, then the serotype should not be obtained from their stools.[17] Although *C. perfringens* are part of the normal bowel flora, they are usually present in a count not in excess of 10^5 organisms/gram of faeces. In a patient with food poisoning due to *C. perfringens* the organism may be obtained in faeces in a count as high as 10^9 organisms/gram.[10]

Enterotoxin can be demonstrated in the stools of patients using a reverse passive haemagglutination test. This is very sensitive and capable of detecting 1 ng/ml.[11] A second technique is counterimmunoelectrophoresis which can detect 0.2 ng enterotoxin/ml.[26] Enterotoxin production can be enhanced in some strains by subjecting the strains to heat treatment before incubation in a sporulation medium.[35]

Prevention of clostridial gastroenteritis

Basic principles for the prevention of food poisoning were enunciated by Hobbs and Gilbert.[16] Raw and cooked food should be handled in separate areas to prevent cross-contamination. Secondly, all food which has not been consumed should be quickly cooled and refrigerated, because some spores may not have been killed by cooking or processing. Ideally food should not be prepared for many hours before being served.[37] If meat is to be reheated a minimum internal temperature of 74° C must be achieved. Food which is to be served hot should be kept at temperatures above 60° C. The practice of allowing hot food to cool down slowly in room temperature before being put in a refrigerator is condemned. Immediate refrigeration is necessary after cooking.[37] To prevent human spores of *C. perfringens* contaminating a meat dish scrupulous attention to handwashing after defaecation is required by food handlers.

A report from the Australian Department of Health has indicated how the microbiological examination of food can aid preventive measures.[1] In 1979 the New Zealand Department of Health detected *C. perfringens* the toxin of which was lethal to mice, in shipments from Hong Kong of imported fish, canned, dried, and salted in oil.[1] Many of these stocks were 3 years old.

BACILLUS CEREUS GASTROENTERITIS

Causative organism

In recent years *Bacillus cereus* has assumed increasing importance as a cause of food poisoning. The organism is an aerobic motile Gram-positive rod with the ability to form spores. Not only can it cause diarrhoea but it can also cause infective endocarditis and osteomyelitis. The organism may be found in the faeces of healthy adults; it was found in 14% of 711 adults in England.[12]

Epidemiology

Food poisoning due to *Bacillus cereus* became common after the increase in the number of Chinese restaurants in western countries. In such establishments large quantities of rice are cooked the previous evening and stored at room temperature overnight. The spores of *B. cereus* are blown in dust and easily contaminate rice, and the warm temperature overnight allows the spores to germinate and multiply. During 1971–74, in Britain, more than 30 separate incidents of food poisoning linked with cooked rice were reported.[13] The number of *B. cereus* organisms necessary to produce food poisoning is usually greater than 10^5 organisms/gram. In addition to rice other foods such as meats, vegetables, poultry and sauces have been found to be contaminated with *B. cereus*.[22]

Pathogenesis

B. cereus produces at least two enterotoxins one of which is heat stable and produces vomiting;[32] the other is heat-labile and is responsible for diarrhoeal symptoms.[34] The heat-labile toxin probably acts like cholera-enterotoxin in that it stimulates adenylate cyclase and formation of cyclic AMP in intestinal epithelial cells.[29,33] The heat-stable toxin causes accumulation of fluid in rabbit ileal loops.[29] In some instances of gastroenteritis due to this organism one or other of these toxins may predominate or both may be present. Therefore if the toxin responsible for vomiting predominates, the gastroenteritis may mimic staphylococcal food poisoning, but if the diarrhoea-enterotoxin predominates the disease may appear similar to gastroenteritis due to *C. perfringens*.

Clinical features

The two clinical syndromes that were discerned by Turnbull[33] can be understood in terms of which enterotoxin predominates. One syndrome is characterized by nausea and vomiting which occurs 1–5 hours after eating contaminated material.[32] Only 33% of patients may have diarrhoea, and the duration of the illness is only 8–10 hours. The other syndrome, associated with abdominal pain and diarrhoea develops 8–16 hours after ingestion of contaminated food. Vomiting occurs in only 23% of patients and the duration of illness is up to 36 hours. Ten outbreaks involving 133 people were reported in the USA during the years 1966–75.[32] Again two syndromes were detected, one in which diarrhoea was the most important symptom and the other in which vomiting was the cardinal feature.[32]

Laboratory diagnosis

For the isolation of *B. cereus* in foodstuffs a medium is used that contains polymyxin B to inhibit the growth of Gram-negative bacteria; it also contains egg yolk to provide lecithin, and it contains phenol red. *Bacillus cereus* produces a lecithinase; its pink colonies are surrounded by a zone of opacity. Biochemical tests are used to identify *B. cereus* which produces acid in arabinose, xylose and mannitol. To incriminate *B. cereus* in food over 10^5 organisms/gram of food should be obtained. Serotyping is not commonly available.

Control

In food shops or restaurants that sell large amounts of cooked rice the incidence of *B. cereus* food poisoning can be cut drastically by the simple expedient of keeping all cooked rice in the refrigerator. Other practical suggestions have been made,[13] rice should be boiled in smaller amounts on several occasions during the day so that storage time before frying can be reduced. After boiling, rice should be kept hot with a temperature in excess of 63° C or, alternatively, should be cooled rapidly and placed in a refrigerator within 2 hours of cooling. Neither boiled nor fried rice should be kept at temperatures between 15 and 50° C.

REFERENCES

1 Australia Communicable Diseases Intelligence (1979) Contaminated imported canned dried fish in oil. Bulletin Number 79/20 (12 October 1979).
2 Batish V. K., Ghodekar D. R. and Ranganathan B. (1978) The thermostable deoxyribonuclease (DNase) test as a rapid screening method for the detection of staphylococcal enterotoxin in milk and milk products. *Microbiol. Immunol.* **22**, 437.
3 Bostock A. D. (1979) Food Hygiene. *J. R. Soc. Med.* **72**, 481.
4 Duncan C. L., Strong D. H. and Sebald M. (1972) Sporulation and enterotoxin production by mutants of *Clostridium perfringens. J. Bacteriol.* **110**, 378.
5 Effersøe P. and Kjerulf K. (1975) Clinical aspects of outbreaks of staphylococcal food poisoning during air travel. *Lancet* **ii**, 599.
6 Eisenberg M. S., Gaarslev K., Brown W., Horwitz M. and Hill D. (1975) Staphylococcal food poisoning aboard a commercial aircraft. *Lancet* **ii**, 595.
7 Evans N. (1979) Pathogenic mechanisms in bacterial diarrhoea. *Clin. Gastroenterol.* **8**, 599.
8 Evans D. J., Chen L. C., Curlin G. R. and Evans D. G. (1972) Stimulation of adenyl cyclase by *Escherichia coli* enterotoxin. *Nature New Biology* **236**, 137.
9 Feig M. (1950) Staphylococcal food poisoning. A report of two related outbreaks and a discussion of the data presented. *Am. J. Public Health* **40**, 279.
10 Fraser A. G. and Collee J. G. (1979) Food poisoning caused by *Clostridium perfringens* (*C. welchii*) type A. *Papua New Guinea Med. J.* **22**, 87.
11 Genigeorgis C., Sakaguchi G. and Riemann H. (1973) Assay methods for *Clostridium perfringens* type A enterotoxin *Appl. Microbiol.* **26**, 111.
12 Ghosh A. C. (1978) Prevalence of *Bacillus cereus* in the faeces of healthy adults. *J. Hyg. (Camb.)* **80**, 233.
13 Gilbert R. J., Stringer M. F. and Peace T. C. (1974) The survival and growth of *Bacillus cereus* in boiled and fried rice in relation to outbreaks of food poisoning. *J. Hyg. (Camb.)* **73**, 433.
14 Hauschild A. H. W., Hilsheimer R. and Martin W. G. (1973) Improved purification of *Clostridium perfringens* type A enterotoxin. *Can. J. Microbiol.* **19**, 1379.
15 Hobbs B. C., Smith M. E., Oakley C. L., Warrack G. H. and Cruickshank J. C. (1953) *Clostridium welchii* food poisoning. *J. Hyg. (Camb.)* **51**, 75.

16   Hobbs B. C. and Gilbert R. J. (1978) *Food Poisoning and Food Hygiene*, Edward Arnold, London.

17   Horwitz M. A. (1977) Specific diagnosis of foodborne disease. *Gastroenterology* **73**, 375.

18   Lancet (1980) Food poisoning in hospitals. *Lancet* **i**, 576.

19   Lawrence G., Watt S. and Basten A. (1979) Purification and some effects of *Clostridium welchii* type C beta toxin. *Papua New Guinea Med. J.* **22**, 79.

20   McDonel J. L. and Duncan C. L. (1977) Regional localisation of aetiology of *Clostridium perfringens* type A enterotoxin in the rabbit ileum, jejunum and duodenum. *J. Infect. Dis.* **136**, 661.

21   McDonel J. R. (1979) The molecular mode of action of *Clostridium perfringens* enterotoxin. *Am. J. Clin. Nutr.* **32**, 210.

22   Melling J., Capel B. J., Turnbull P. C. B. and Gilbert R. J. (1976) Identification of a novel enterotoxigenic activity association with *Bacillus cereus. J. Clin. Pathol.* **29**, 938.

23   Morbidity and Mortality Weekly Report, Center for Disease Control (1979) Staphylococcal food poisoning — Florida. *M.M.W.R.* **28**, 153.

24   Morbidity and Mortality Weekly Report, Center for Disease Control (1979) Staphylococcal food poisoning associated with Genoa and hard salami, United States. *M.M.W.R.* **28**, 179.

25   Morbidity and Mortality Weekly Report, Center for Disease Control (1979) Staphylococcal food poisoning — Delaware. *M.M.W.R.* **28**, 445.

26   Naik H. S. and Duncan C. L. (1977) Rapid detection and quantitation of *Clostridium perfringens* enterotoxin by counterimmunoelectrophoresis. *Appl. Environ. Microbiol.* **34**, 125.

27   Sakurai J. and Duncan C. L. (1978) Some properties of Beta-toxin produced by *Clostridium perfringens* type C. *Infect. Immun.* **21**, 678.

28   Sharp J. C. M., Collier P. W. and Gilbert R. J. (1979) Food poisoning in hospitals in Scotland. *J. Hyg. (Camb.)* **83**, 231.

29   Spira W. M. and Goepfert J. M. (1972) An enterotoxic factor produced by *Bacillus cereus* and assayed in the ligated loop of rabbits. Abstracts of the Annual Meeting of the American Society of Microbiology, Washington DC, (1972), American Soc. of Microbiology, p. 23.

30   Stark R. L. and Duncan C. L. (1972) Purification and biochemical properties of *Clostridium perfringens* Type A enterotoxin. *Infect. Immun.* **6**, 662.

31   Sutton R. G. A. and Hobbs B. C. (1969) Food poisoning caused by heat-sensitive *Clostridium welchii*. A report of five recent outbreaks. *J. Hyg. (Camb.)* **66**, 135.

32   Terranova W. and Blake P. A. (1978) *Bacillus cereus* food poisoning. *N. Eng. J. Med.* **298**, 143.

33   Turnbull P. C. B. (1976) Studies on the production of enterotoxins by *Bacillus cereus. J. Clin. Pathol.* **29**, 941.

34   Turnbull P. C. B, Kramer J. M., Jorgensen K., Gilbert R. J. and Melling J. (1979) Properties and production characteristics of vomiting, diarrhoeal and necrotizing toxins of *Bacillus cereus. Am. J. Clin. Nutr.* **32**, 219.

35   Uemura T. (1978) Incidence of enterotoxigenic *Clostridium perfringens* in healthy humans in relation to the enhancement of enterotoxin production by heat treatment. *J. Appl. Bacteriol.* **44**, 411.

36   WHO Weekly Epidemiological Record No. 23 — 6 June 1980, p. 173. Confirmed foodborne disease outbreaks and cases by etiology, United States of America, 1977.

37   Zottola E. A. (1979) Contemporary nutrition. Foodborne disease. *N.Y. State J. Med.* **79**, 146.

8 The virology of acute infectious diarrhoea

T. H. Flewett

Introduction   159
   Clinical features   160
   Pathogenesis   160
   Effect of virus dose   161
   Recovery   165
Detection of viruses in diarrhoea   165
   The Norwalk agent   166
Rotaviruses   166
   Epidemiology   168
   Transmission   168
   Immunity and prevention   169
Adenoviruses   170
Coronaviruses   172
Astroviruses   172
Caliciviruses   173
Parvoviruses   174
Appendix   174
   Methods for detecting viruses in faeces by direct electron microscopy   174
   Immunoelectron microscopy   175
   Isolation in tissue culture   177
   Tissue culture methods   178
   Serological reactions of rotaviruses   179
   Titration of antibodies by immunofluorescence   179
   Detection of rotavirus in faeces by the ELISA test   180
   Serotypes   182
   Typing of rotaviruses by electrophoresis of genome segments 182
References   183

INTRODUCTION

The most important single cause of acute infectious diarrhoea of young children is infection by rotaviruses. Adenoviruses — at least in the UK — are the next most important viral pathogens. Other viruses — coronaviruses, astroviruses and undifferentiated small round viruses — are less important. Episodes of 'winter vomiting disease' in older children appear mainly to be caused by the 'Norwalk' group of viruses and caliciviruses. This chapter describes the clinical features, and virology of this group of infections, and the technical procedures for their investigation.

Clinical features

After an incubation period of 2–4 days early symptoms in children are vomiting — occasionally projectile, more usually simple regurgitation. Some children vomit only on the first day, others continue to vomit throughout the illness. Diarrhoea begins with semi-formed stools on the first day, and is usually at its most profuse 2–4 days after onset; without treatment, in those who recover, it usually clears up after 7–9 days. A wide variation in severity may be found, from subclinical, through to mild and unimportant (probably the commonest form) to severe dehydration in young children requiring urgent parenteral rehydration in hospital, or even to death. Pharyngitis has been associated with rotavirus diarrhoea; respiratory tract inflammation and otitis media are frequent complications in young children, probably because of vomit irritating the pharynx and travelling up the nose and into the Eustachian tube.[17] These are often the first symptoms in rotavirus infection, much more so than in diarrhoea of bacterial cause. Fever is variable, usually insignificant or absent in mild cases; but severely ill children and adults may have fever of 38–39° C, or up to 40° C if dehydration is severe. Stopping milk and giving an appropriate oral rehydration saline-glucose mixture by mouth causes rapid improvement and the patient's illness and virus excretion usually both cease completely in 5–8 days. Intravenous therapy is rarely necessary for children treated in good time. These remarks apply not only to rotavirus infections, but, as far as is known, to the acute gastroenteritis associated with other viruses. Certainly subclinical infections have been described for rotaviruses, caliciviruses, astroviruses and coronaviruses (q.v.); in the case of caliciviruses and astroviruses it may be that symptomatic infections are in the minority. Pharyngitis was a prominent symptom in one outbreak of coronavirus-associated vomiting and diarrhoea in apprentices.[2]

Pathogenesis

Infection is by the *oral* route; there is no evidence for any other. All the viruses known to cause acute gastroenteritis in man and animals are resistant to low pH; e.g. pH 4 for 1 hour does not cause more than a moderate loss of titre. Although resistance to acid is not essential for an enteropathic agent (*Vibrio cholerae* is acid sensitive) acid resistance must be advantageous to any virus which has to pass through the stomach on its way to its target organ.

The target organ for the diarrhoea viruses is the epithelium lining the small bowel, on the sides and tips of the villi, but not the epithelium in the crypts of Lieberkuhn. This target epithelium is constantly renewed; new cells are generated by mitoses in the crypts, and are pushed towards the lumen, moving up the sides of the villi towards the tip and differentiating to acquire a brush border, and finally being shed into the lumen when they reach the tip of their villus. Probably not many viruses have the capacity for easy multiplication in high titre in these cells, but for those which have — the rotaviruses, some adenoviruses, coronaviruses, astroviruses, caliciviruses, some parvoviruses and undifferentiated small round viruses — the enormous convoluted epithelial surface of the small bowel enables these viruses to reproduce in enormous numbers. Particle counts up to 10^{11}/g of faeces are not unusual for rotaviruses and adenoviruses, and we have seen parvovirus-like particles, associated with adenoviruses, at 10^{13}/g of faeces.[7] This is fortunate for virologists, because most of these viruses have a characteristic morphology and diagnosis can easily be made by direct electron microscopy of faecal extracts (see Appendix p.174).

Effect of virus dose

This cannot ethically be investigated in children; but in gnotobiotic calves given high doses of rotavirus, symptoms begin as early as 18 hours after infection. The incubation period for rotavirus and calicivirus infections in children is 1–4 days, usually about 48 hours.[9] For adenovirus diarrhoea it is 8–10 days.[22] The infectivity/virus particle ratio is not known for animals or man (except possibly the mouse); but piglet faeces had a lethal infectivity titre of 10^7 infective doses/g of faeces in experimental piglets.[30] Some human faeces probably have similar infective titres.

Infection by most of these viruses is completely confined to the small bowel; but coronavirus infection in experimentally infected piglets gives rise to scattered lesions in the colon and lung also. The site of multiplication of human coronavirus-like particles is not known.

An early consequence of many virus infections is a change in plasma membrane permeability of infected cells. This probably explains the occurrence of diarrhoea in experimental animals less than 24 hours postinfection when damage to the brush-border epithelium disturbs the mechanism of electrolyte transport between the cells and the lumen. Experiments by Hamilton and his colleagues in Toronto on experimentally infected piglets revealed that the normal Na^+ ion transport across the membrane from the lumen to the extracellular fluid was diminished.[5] Furthermore, while in the normal animal this flux was increased by the presence of glucose, in the infected animal glucose had much less effect. And because in the infected bowel lactose is not being split by lactase, less glucose is available in any case.

The physiological consequences of infection and destruction of the brush-bordered epithelial layer of the small bowel are related to its functions. The brush-border itself is the site of production and activity of lactase and other disaccharidases. Disaccharides are not absorbed through the bowel wall into the bloodstream; they must first be broken down to monosaccharides. An early consequence, therefore, of infection by rotaviruses, coronaviruses and the 'Norwalk agent' and some adenoviruses, is reduction of lactase activity. This is an important mechanism of pathogenesis. Human milk contains 71 g/l of lactose. This concentration of lactose alone is almost isotonic. If not dissociated, the lactose remains in the lumen and so this osmotic effect is added to the osmotic effect of the other constituents of the chyme, and tends to prevent absorption of water from the small bowel. Even cow's milk contains about 56 g/l lactose; but

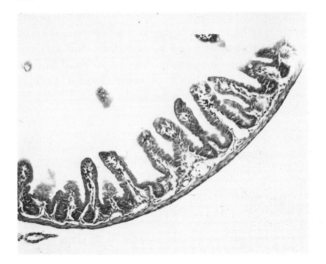

Fig. 8.1 Normal small intestinal villi. The epithelial surface is smooth and bears a brush-border (H and E)

before being given by bottle to infants it is usually 'humanized' by having extra sucrose or lactose added to it, so that the same osmotic effect still occurs. Thus, the volume of the contents of the small bowel is larger than in health. But the effect is compounded in the large bowel. The colon contains a rich flora of lactose-fermenting bacteria, which can rapidly split one molecule of lactose into up to six molecules of short-chain acids, thus increasing the osmolarity of the large bowel contents by up to 1000 mosmols, quite enough to cause water to drain from the body into the large bowel instead of flowing the other way, as it does from the healthy colon. The effect is comparable to that of a dose of Epsom salts.[7]

When the cells are damaged or killed an inflammatory response usually takes place. Biopsy studies in children and a rotavirus-infected man, and autopsies of experimentally infected rotavirus infected piglets and calves at various stages have shown that the brush-bordered epithelium is stripped off, and the villi become oedematous, shortened, and infiltrated with inflammatory cells (Figs 8.1 and 8.2). On the remaining infected epithelial cells the microvilli of the brush-border are shortened, distorted or absent (Figs 8.3 and 8.4). The cells contain vacuoles in which can be seen large numbers of virus particles. In calves with coronavirus infection cell damage in the colon may not be obvious, although many cells are infected (Fig. 8.5).

Increased volume within the lumen increases peristalsis; the more rapidly the contents move, the less time there is for the disaccharidases in the surviving cells to split the lactose or sucrose and also the less time for fluid resorption; so the less fluid is absorbed from the small bowel, the more lactose is left to be broken down in the large bowel, and so the faster dehydration sets in — a splendid example of a positive feedback system or 'vicious cycle'.

A simple and effective treatment is to discontinue milk supply and give by mouth about one-third normal saline, bicarbonate-buffered with a little added potassium, and containing a little glucose.[26] In children and young animals alike,

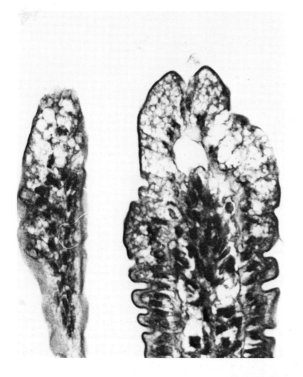

Fig. 8.2 Infection with rotaviruses. The villus is shortened, oedematous and infiltrated with inflammatory cells. The epithelium is in parts vacuolated and necrotic, in places missing (H and E)

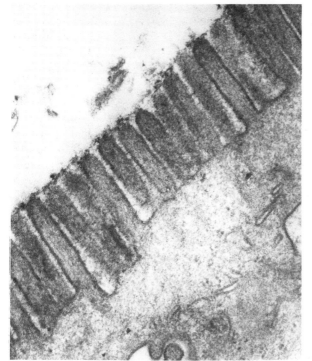

Fig. 8.3 Normal brush-border. Electron micrograph of thin section

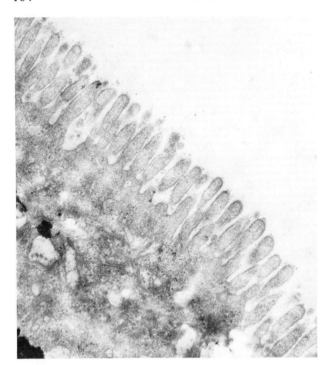

Fig. 8.4 Experimentally infected brush-bordered epithelium. The cytoplasm is vacuolated; the vacuoles contain rotavirus particles. The microvilli of the brush-border are stunted and disrupted

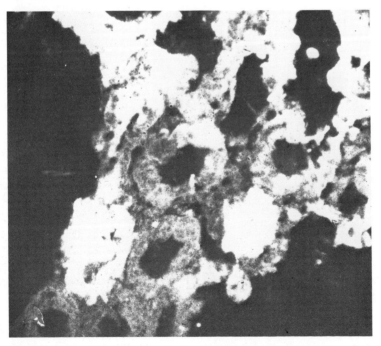

Fig. 8.5 Coronavirus infection of colon epithelium; a natural infection of a calf; infected cells are shown by immunofluorescence

this is usually enough to break the vicious cycle, rehydrating almost immediately and often saving life. Various saline mixtures have been proposed. The World Health Organization has designed a simple mixture suitable for both adults and children. This contains: NaCl 3.5 g/l, KCl 1.5 g/l, NaHCO$_3$ 2.5 g/l, Glucose 20.0 g/l (see also p.202).

RECOVERY

Viral diarrhoea in untreated patients can be fatal; but usually the loss of ileal epithelium is not fatal; new uninfected cells grow up from the crypts of Lieberkuhn, and within 8 days or so normal function returns, and diarrhoea and virus excretion cease.[3,7,25] Why are these new cells not infected? Antibody (mostly IgM at first) can be detected in patients' sera as soon as 3 days after the onset of symptoms, and IgA is at the same time being produced locally in the small bowel. Interferon also is probably being produced; experimental evidence of this would be difficult to obtain, at least in children. Nothing is known of the effects of interferon in diarrhoea; the calf rotavirus is said to be not very sensitive.

Sometimes recovery is slow and incomplete. A very small proportion of children continue to have diarrhoea and to excrete virus for 3 or 4 weeks. Presumably, in these patients, cell regeneration is retarded, or the local antibody response fails. Lactose intolerance may persist for months. Very occasionally a child may require intravenous feeding for months, but such cases are perhaps more often seen in outbreaks of diarrhoea associated with enteropathic *E. coli* infection. These organisms and rotaviruses sometimes occur together. Perhaps they exert a synergistic effect; but so far experimental evidence for this is lacking.

DETECTION OF VIRUSES IN DIARRHOEA

Enteropathic or enterotoxic strains of *E. coli* could be isolated only in a proportion of cases and outbreaks of acute gastroenteritis in children, though they have been much more frequently implicated in traveller's diarrhoea of adults. It seemed likely that viruses might be important, and for many years workers had endeavoured to isolate viruses by inoculation of animals with bacterium-free filtrates of faeces from human cases. These attempts mostly failed. Although Light and Hodes[18] reported successful infection of calves, others, with one exception, were not able to confirm their results; from recent examination of their stored material and recent similar experiments it now seems that they did succeed, although even now their results cannot always be reproduced. Gerald Woode and I failed in 1974 to infect English gnotobiotic calves with an English rotavirus. Perhaps it was the wrong serotype.

From 1945 onwards various workers succeeded in transmitting acute gastro-enteritis to human volunteers by feeding them with filtrates of patients' faeces. In this way the 'Norwalk agent' was isolated.

The 'Norwalk agent'

Filtrates of patients' faeces from an outbreak of epidemic 'winter vomiting disease' — acute gastroenteritis with vomiting and diarrhoea affecting schools in winter-time — were fed to adult volunteers. After an incubation period of 2–3 days volunteers developed symptoms of vomiting and/or diarrhoea lasting usually only 2–3 days. In their faeces could be found particles about 28 nm in diameter, density 1.4 g/ml; these could be agglutinated by volunteers' convalescent sera, although antibodies were detected also in prechallenge sera suggesting that most volunteers had had previous experience of such infections.[14] Further work has shown that there are at least three serotypes of this virus. Intestinal biopsies were taken from the volunteers; damage to the brush-bordered epithelium, and shortening and oedema of the villi was found. A transient deficiency in lactose absorption occurred at the time of symptoms (see also under 'pathogenesis').

All attempts to transmit 'Norwalk agent' to experimental animals or to tissue cultures have so far failed. Its taxonomic position among the viruses has not been established at the time of writing, but it is probably a calicivirus (see also under 'caliciviruses').

Outbreaks of 'winter vomiting disease' attributable to the Norwalk agent have occurred in many parts of the world;[12] in a large epidemic in Australia these viruses were transmitted by way of infected oysters. In an underdeveloped country (Bangladesh) infection as determined by seroconversion in the first months of life was common, but did not appear to be associated with much illness.

ROTAVIRUSES

Electron microscopy of faeces in recent years has revealed several different kinds of virus which may cause gastroenteritis of children. The most important of these are the rotaviruses, so called because they resemble, in negatively stained preparations, little wheels with a wide hub, short spokes, and a clearly defined circular rim, about 65 nm in diameter (Fig. 8.6). They were found independently in 1973 by workers in Birmingham, Melbourne and Toronto; the Melbourne workers found them first in ultrathin sections of biopsies of duodenal mucosa from young children.[11]

STRUCTURE

The virus particles consist of a core, diameter 38 nm, containing 11 segments of double-stranded nucleic acid, of molecular weights ranging from 24 000 to 2.2×10^6. This core is surrounded by a double-layered capsid; the inner layer is composed of short cylindrical hollow capsomeres disposed radially; the outer capsid layer is superimposed upon these at right-angles, like T-pieces upon up-

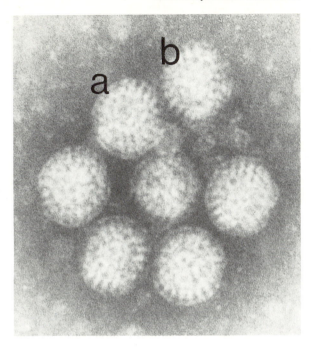

Fig. 8.6 Rotaviruses. These are found both with (a) and without (b) the outer capsid layer which gives the appearance of a smooth rim. Negatively stained with phosphotungstate (x 252 000)

rights, giving in negatively stained preparations a smooth, clearly defined outer layer or rim (Fig. 8.7). The inner layer of capsomeres is so disposed as to give, when seen end-on, an appearance of six-sided or sometimes five-sided rings about 10 nm in diameter. These, in any preparation, are visible on some particles and not on others. It all depends on how the particle happens to be lying; if a ring on the upper surface is situated directly above a ring on the lower surface it is clearly delineated, because in negatively stained preparations the image of the one side of a virion is usually superimposed on the image of the other side. This ring pattern can be revealed on any virion by tilting the preparation in a goniometer stage up to 3°. On further tilting it disappears and other ring patterns appear.

The outer capsid layer is absent from many of the virus particles seen in most extracts of faeces; the particles then are about 55 nm in diameter and have a spiky irregular outline.

These two kinds of particle can be separated in caesium chloride gradients. The complete particles have a density of 1.36 g/ml, the incomplete a density of 1.38 g/ml. Only the complete particles are infectious, at least for tissue cultures. This may not, however, apply to all rotaviruses; 'complete' mouse rotavirus particles are very hard to find in many highly mouse-infectious preparations.

The methods for detecting rotaviruses in faeces by direct electron microscopy, by immunoelectron microscopy, by the ELISA test and by isolation in tissue culture, are delineated and discussed in the appendix to this chapter. The appendix also contains a discussion of rotavirus antibodies and their detection, and the typing of rotaviruses by ELISA serotyping and by electrophoresis of genome segments.

Epidemiology

Rotavirus infections are usually prevalent in the winter months, at least in temperate countries. This has been found both north and south of the equator, in North America, Europe and Japan. In most tropical countries the relative importance of rotavirus as a cause of diarrhoea is unknown; much epidemiological research remains to be done. Rotaviruses have been recovered from faeces of children in Bangladesh and Lucknow; in Vellore (South India), Professor Mathan (personal communication) has found them prevalent in August and September; they were found in most children with diarrhoea throughout the year in a parallel study in Calicut, on the west coast of India at the same latitude as Vellore, but having a very different climate. Diarrhoea other than that attributable to recognized bacterial pathogens, kills more than 1 million infants a year in India alone; an annual toll of 600 000 has been estimated for Indonesia; probably at least 5 million deaths worldwide.

Transmission

When a stable virus is excreted in enormous numbers, ample opportunity exists for passive transfer from faeces to patient on a nurse's or a parent's hands, or to food via untreated sewage. In addition, evidence is accumulating that adults may acquire subclinical infection and excrete the virus in their faeces. A parent — or a

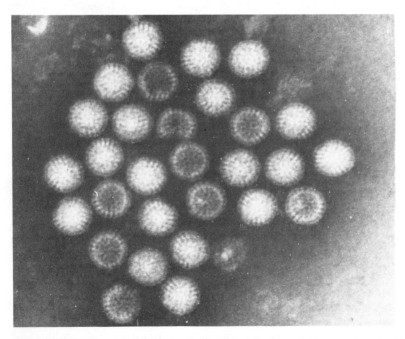

Fig. 8.7   Rotaviruses agglutinated with antibody in convalescent serum. Negatively stained with phosphotungstate (x 185 000)

nurse — may easily contaminate a hand, fail to remove virus by a perfunctory wash (or no wash at all) and contaminate food or one of the many articles which an inquisitive infant may put into its mouth.

Ward infections by rotaviruses causing diarrhoea have been described by several authors. Rotaviruses are known to retain their infectivity in liquid faeces at room temperature for months. They are excreted in faeces in such great numbers that even with a high standard of nursing care, infection must easily be transmitted mechanically. Few studies have been done on the effect of disinfectants, but antiseptics containing free chlorine, (e.g. 'Chloros'), are believed to be rapidly effective; formaldehyde and glutaraldehyde are effective, but act more slowly. Phenolic disinfectants may not be effective. It could be that animals might be a source of infection. In many parts of the world people live in close contact with their farm animals, the young of which enter freely into houses, are not house-trained, and could be a source of infection for a crawling infant. Human rotaviruses can infect pigs and calves: the experiment to see whether pig or calf rotavirus may infect children has not yet been made.

Immunity and prevention

Almost everyone has antibodies to rotaviruses by the age of 7. Second attacks are known, and infections of adults, usually infected by contact with children, are now known. Immunity to such infections classically is believed to depend upon IgA antibodies produced in the gut wall. Piglets experimentally infected with transmissible gastroenteritis (TGE) are not protected by circulating antibody of maternal origin, but are protected by antibodies in milk. Although a piglet may have high levels of circulating IgG, if prevented from suckling for only 24 hours it becomes fully susceptible to TGE although completely protected while suckling.

Human infants, however, certainly can get rotavirus infection, even though breast-fed. Subclinical infections in nurseries in maternity hospitals have been described. Can it be that human maternal antibody transmitted across the placenta protects? If so, the immunological mechanisms must be different in man. A parenteral killed vaccine might then protect. If, however, these were just examples of infection by strains of low virulence, the theory that bloodstream antibody is protective loses its force. If so, a vaccine given parenterally probably would not protect. This point needs to be settled.

As there is little cross-reaction by neutralization tests between rotaviruses of different species, one would have to use a human strain of virus to make a human vaccine. To confer immunity by feeding, it would have to be a live attenuated vaccine.

The problem, for long insoluble, of persuading the human rotavirus to multiply in tissue culture has now been solved. The most commonly occurring serotype has been adapted to grow in tissue culture by first being taken through 11 serial passages in gnotobiotic piglets. After this, it was found that with the aid of trypsin in the culture medium, it would multiply serially in tissue cultures of

African green monkey kidney cells and also that it could form plaques, which was a great help in infectivity assays.[31]

Serotype 2 of the human rotavirus posed a much more difficult problem because it hardly multiplies at all in the intestinal tract of gnotobiotic piglets. However, the bovine rotavirus was adapted to tissue culture many years ago and temperature sensitive mutants were made from this. By doubly infecting cells with the temperature-sensitive mutant of the bovine virus and with serotype 2, human rotavirus recombinants were obtained that would grow at the nonpermissive temperature and could be serially propagated. Some of these had the capacity of the bovine virus to grow serially in tissue culture and had the immunogenic property of the human virus eliciting, when injected into animals, neutralizing antibodies specific for the human strain.[13] Thus a technique has become available for preparing rotaviruses from any species which will grow in tissue culture, having the desired immunogenic capacity. The question still remains to be solved — will such tissue culture-adapted strains be nonpathogenic in babies and young children and if so, will they confer protection? As there is no suitable experimental animal model — virulent human rotaviruses have little or no virulence for baby pigs for example — the experiment will have to be tried in humans. First experiments should be with susceptible adults, those having no neutralizing antibodies for the strain concerned. After this, experiments could be done with teenagers and then younger children until the virus can be tried in babies.[15] If the virus appears to be avirulent in all these age groups, then field trials may eventually become possible. Will such a virus confer effective immunity? Nobody knows. A live attenuated culture-adapted calf rotavirus has been on sale for some time and opinions about its efficacy are, to put it politely, controversial.

But perhaps an inactivated, parenterally-given vaccine would work after all. Contrary to everyone's expectation, the introduction of the killed Salk polio vaccine was followed by the almost complete disappearance of wild strains. It might be the same with rotaviruses.

The other well established method of controlling enteric infection is by applying the principles of good hygiene. But the prospects here do not look good. Virus particles are excreted in enormous numbers; they are very stable, retaining infectivity in faeces almost indefinitely at room temperature. If washing and disinfection reduce infectivity of the environment by 100 000-fold — a very meritorious performance seldom achieved in practice — there may still be considerable infectivity left, as faeces are infective at a dilution of 1 in 10^7. Hygienic measures have not eliminated Sonne dysentery from infant nurseries and schools, and probably have as little effect on the diarrhoea viruses. Control of the virus diarrhoea is not going to be easy.

ADENOVIRUSES

These can frequently be isolated from faeces when respiratory infections due to these viruses are prevalent, and very frequently from faeces of very young children. In about half of these samples of faeces, scanty adenoviruses can be found by direct electron microscopy. But in certain cases of acute diarrhoea and vomiting, mainly in young children, but also in adults, enormous numbers of adenoviruses can be found in the faeces by electron microscopy; the numbers are such that often one does not have to search for them, many particles being found in every field (Fig. 8.8). The incubation period is 8–10 days, much longer than for rotavirus infections,[22] (Boxall, personal communication). The cases were first observed in an outbreak in a long-stay children's ward in Shropshire, but similar cases have been found in Africa, Asia, North America and elsewhere. Usually it has not been possible to isolate the viruses in tissue culture; although human fibroblasts can sometimes be infected by the original inoculum, subcultures are not possible. It seems to be the case with these, as with other diarrhoea viruses, that viruses capable of infecting the small bowel are not readily isolated in mono-layer tissue cultures. Some strains have, however, been isolated in Chang cells.[16] Some isolations have been made in ordinary tissue cultures, but usually these have been of types 1 or 2, viruses which are commonly present in the faeces of young children; the virus isolated may not have been the virus which was causing the diarrhoea.

Whitelaw, Davies and Perry[28] described a case of fatal adenovirus enteritis in which large numbers of adenoviruses were found in nuclei of the small intestinal epithelium. Dr Homola, of Melbourne, told me of another fatal human case there. In that case too, adenovirus particles were observed in thin sections of infected brush-border epithelium in the small bowel; numerous nuclei contained inclusion bodies consisting of crystalline aggregates of virus particles.

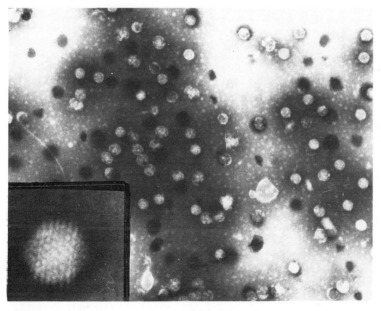

Fig. 8.8 Adenoviruses in faeces in great numbers. Inset — a single adenovirus. Phospho-tungstate (x 270 000)

CORONAVIRUSES

Coronaviruses (Fig. 8.9) have long been known to cause transmissible gastroenteritis of piglets (TGE), a disease with a mortality sometimes reaching 100%. More recently coronavirus enteritis of calves has been described.[20] The incubation period is from 18 to 96 hours, depending on dose. Young pigs suffer severe vomiting and watery diarrhoea. Coronaviruses in human cases of acute gastroenteritis were first described in India and Bristol in 1975.[2,19] There was an explosive outbreak of acute diarrhoea and vomiting, sometimes accompanied by fever and pharyngitis, among apprentices in an aircraft factory. Other outbreaks in closed communities such as nurses' homes have since been reported. The incubation period is not known. Virus particles are sometimes very numerous in the faeces (Fig. 8.9) and have been isolated in organ cultures of human embryo small bowel, from which they have been adapted to subculture in human embryo kidney monolayers.

Coronaviruses have also been found in great numbers in faeces of healthy persons — children and adults, but not in infants — in villagers around Vellore in South India,[19] and more recently in nomads in the Sahara (Puel, personal communication). They were not prevalent among town dwellers. They were not apparently usually associated with disease.

ASTROVIRUSES

This name was given by Dr Madeley of Glasgow to small viruses, about 28 nm in diameter, occurring in great numbers in faeces of young children with acute

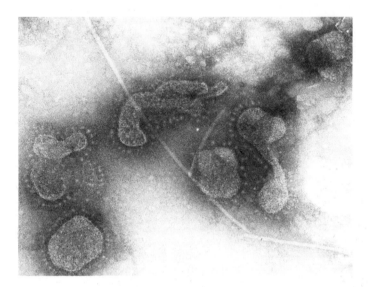

Fig. 8.9 Coronaviruses in faeces. The virus body is pleomorphic and is surrounded by a 'corona' of short stalks bearing clubbed ends. Ammonium molybdate (x 95 200)

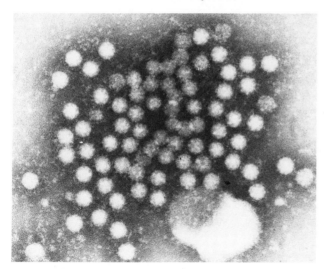

Fig. 8.10 Astroviruses in faeces. A five or six-pointed star pattern can be seen on some particles (x 108 000)

gastroenteritis, because of a radiating starry pattern often seen upon their surface (Fig. 8.10). These viruses can thus be distinguished from the ordinary entero-viruses which are about the same size but which do not show this appearance. Although these particles have indeed been found associated with several outbreaks of diarrhoea and vomiting and could be agglutinated by convalescent sera, they have also been found in faeces of normal children. They are most commonly found in neonates, but may even infect adults. These viruses have not yet been established as pathogens with certainty, though the available evidence suggests that they sometimes cause disease. Astroviruses have also been found in lambs and turkeys, where they cause some disease, and in calves, where they do not seem to be important pathogens.

CALICIVIRUSES

These, until recently, were known only as pathogens in kittens, where they cause enteric and respiratory tract infections; in pigs, where they cause a disease resembling foot-and-mouth disease; and in sea-lions and seals, where they cause a vesicular eruption on the flippers and sometimes abortion. Characteristic in their morphology (Fig. 8.11) these viruses have recently been detected in faeces both from patients with gastroenteritis and from healthy children. Caliciviruses can be very difficult to recognize in negatively stained preparations of faeces, and are sometimes even more difficult to recognize after segregation in a caesium chloride density gradient. They are most easily recognized if some are penetrated by the negative stain; the ring of projecting capsomeres (about 10 usually show) gives them away.[4] The human caliciviruses have not yet been isolated in tissue culture. The 'Norwalk agent', transmitted to human volunteers in 1972, is probably a calicivirus. At least five different human serotypes exist (Cubitt, personal communication).

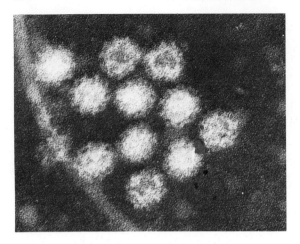

Fig. 8.11 Caliciviruses. These are often difficult to recognize. The ring of points around particles by the negative stain is an aid to identification. Phosphotungstate (x 298 800)

PARVOVIRUSES

In a very small proportion of cases of gastroenteritis very large numbers of small isometric particles (up to 10^{13}/g of faeces) are found (Fig. 8.12). These particles are about 22 nm in diameter, density 1.4 g/ml, and hexagonal in outline. Thus they are morphologically identical to the known parvoviruses. Such particles can often be found in small numbers in faeces of normal children, but not in great numbers. In faeces from patients containing these particles in great numbers adenoviruses are usually also present, and so it has been suggested that the small ones are probably adeno-associated viruses; but this has not so far been formally confirmed, nor even that these small particles are pathogens. Parvoviruses do cause a severe diarrhoea in cats and dogs, but are not usually associated with adenoviruses.

APPENDIX

Methods for detecting viruses in faeces by direct electron microscopy

It was for long supposed that faeces would be too dirty to allow detection of viruses by direct electron microscopy, but this is not so. Viruses can be separated fairly simply from most of the other components of faeces. A suspension of about 1 part faeces in 4 of water or saline is centrifuged to deposit the bacteria and to bring to the surface the unsplit fat which is often found in diarrhoeic faeces of young children. 7000 rev/min for 15 minutes in an angle rotor suffices (3000 rev/min for 20 minutes is usually enough, but does not provide as 'clean' a preparation). After centrifugation of the resultant supernatant at 50 000 rev/min for 1 hour, the pellet containing the viruses is resuspended in a few drops of distilled water. A few seconds' exposure to vibration in an ultrasonic cleaning bath helps to resuspend small viruses. A drop of the liquid containing the

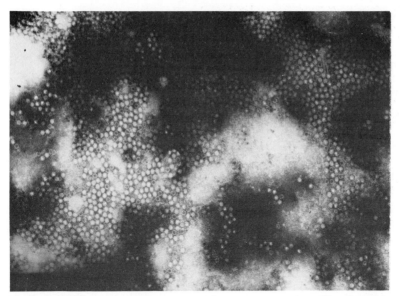

Fig. 8.12   Parvoviruses. These are present in enormous numbers. They have a hexagonal outline. Phosphotungstate (x 168 000)

resuspended viruses is allowed almost to dry on an electron microscope grid bearing a formvar membrane reinforced with carbon. Whilst still visibly just wet, the grid is rinsed thrice in distilled water, excess water being removed with filter paper between each rinse. It is then negatively stained with 2% potassium phosphotungstate, removing the excess after a few seconds, and allowed to dry. Other negative stains, e.g. ammonium molybdate, sodium tungstate, can also be used; uranium formate shows up coronavirus surface projections particularly well.

This procedure concentrates the virus in the faeces about 20-fold. To have one virus particle per grid square, assuming none is lost in the washing, 10^6/ml must be present in the virus suspension. Sometimes virus particles are very much more abundant than that, so that a very rapid diagnosis may be achieved without centrifugation, simply by putting a drop of 20% suspension of faeces on to a grid, allowing most of the liquid to evaporate, and washing and staining as above. The whole procedure takes only about 10 minutes. It may allow some virus clumps, otherwise deposited in the first centrifugation, to be detected. Most cases of rotavirus infection may be diagnosed in this way, though concentration in the ultracentrifuge is required for some specimens.

PRECAUTION

Rotaviruses, and probably other viruses, can also cause acute diarrhoea in adults. Samples of faeces may contain any kind of pathogen; and negative staining does not kill either viruses or bacteria. It is, therefore, essential to make sure that accidental laboratory infections do not take place; prepare grids in an inoculation cabinet; sterilize forceps after use, and keep their points sheathed. Grids should be sterilized by exposure on both sides to a tested source of ultraviolet light before taking them to the microscope. Dirty forceps can transfer virus from one grid to another and so cause false positive results.

Immunoelectron microscopy

This technique has been used to demonstrate that there are different antibodies for the internal and external capsid layers. Antibodies can be detected in serum by this method as early as 3 days after the onset of symptoms; early sera agglutinate particles into clumps (Fig. 8.12). Antibodies, found in sera taken a few weeks later, invest virus particles heavily, covering them with a 'fuzz' of globulin molecules. A convalescent serum from any species contains antibodies which react with the inner capsid layer of rotaviruses from its own or any other species but contains antibodies which will react with the outer capsid layer of viruses from its own species, but not necessarily of viruses from other species. Thus, human antibodies react with the inner and outer capsid layers of both human and calf rotavirus, whereas calf sera react with the inner but not with the outer capsid layer of the human rotavirus. Viruses with the outer layer complete are referred to as 'smooth' or 'S' forms; those which have lost their outer capsid are known as 'rough' or 'R' forms.[8,29] A 'one-way' cross-reaction, similar to that found between the human and calf antisera and their respective viruses, has also been found between reoviruses by immunoelectron microscopy. So it may be that reactions of this kind are a general feature of doubly capsidated viruses. However, a 'new' pig rotavirus has recently been isolated in America which has no serological cross-section with other rotaviruses.[24] Perhaps similar 'human' rotaviruses may exist. Faeces contain many bacteria; bacteria have their own viruses, and these are frequently encountered. Some are recognizable as such by their tails. But others are small and round and morphologically indistinguishable from viruses of mammalian cells. Small viruses can be identified if they are aggregated with a specific antiserum. This method has been applied particularly to detection of hepatitis A and B particles, but is applicable to other viruses also.

METHOD

To 1–4 ml of virus suspension is added 0.1–0.4 ml of antiserum; high titre antisera need to be diluted to give the best results; each antiserum must be tested against a known positive preparation to determine its best working dilution. The mixture is left for 1–2 hours, or overnight at 4° C, then made up to 5 ml with saline, and centrifuged at 18 000 rev/min. The tube is inverted to drain, and the deposit resuspended in about 0.25 ml distilled water and prepared for electron microscopy as described above. But for the method really to be of value a *specific* antiserum is required. These are best prepared by inoculation of a susceptible gnotobiotic animal with the organism under investigation, choosing a species of animal in which antibodies are not transmitted through the placenta to the fetus.

Another method of immunoelectron microscopy is to attach antibodies to an electron microscope grid and to float this upon liquid containing viruses in suspension. The antibody will specifically attract viruses and these will stick to the grid. Nicolaieff *et al.*[21] claim that this method greatly increases the sensitivity of electron microscopy as a technique for detecting viruses in suspension. The method was first developed for detecting plant viruses, but has subsequently been adapted for detecting rotaviruses in faeces. It is claimed to be a much more sensitive technique for detecting viruses than direct electron microscopy on material concentrated by differential ultracentrifugation.

METHOD

Electron microscope (EM) grids coated with formvar carbon are floated on 50 µl drops of protein A solution (20 µg/ml) for 4 minutes; then placed on drops of 0.1M sodium phosphate buffer, pH 7.0, and floated for 10 minutes on 50 µl drops of rabbit anti-rota serum diluted 1/500. Grids are then rinsed in phosphate buffer and left overnight on drops of centrifuged (5000 revs) 25% stool extract in distilled water mixed with an equal volume of 0.2M phosphate buffer. After rinsing three times and staining for 2 minutes in 1% uranyl acetate in 45% ethanol for 2 minutes, or in phosphotungstate, they can be examined in the electron microscope.

Isolation in tissue culture

Although many different viruses have been isolated by conventional tissue culture methods from patients with gastroenteritis none of these has been found specifically associated with the disease. The viruses described above recently discovered as causes or suspected causes of acute gastroenteritis have all hitherto proved either very difficult or impossible to isolate in conventional monolayer tissue cultures of human or other mammalian cells.

However, the rotavirus of calves discovered by Professor Mebus in Nebraska in 1969 was found to infect monolayer cultures of calf kidney cells. Infection could be detected after 48 hour incubation of cultures grown on coverslips by reacting them with a serum from a convalescent gnotobiotic calf, using an immunofluorescent reaction to detect infected cells. Usually serial subculture in monolayer tissue culture has failed, but numerous strains have been adapted to continuous subculture. The addition of 5 µ/ml of crystalline trypsin to the culture medium makes isolation easier and increases the virus yield from adapted strains. Rotaviruses from several species can be isolated in primary or secondary monolayer tissue cultures of monkey, calf, or human embryo kidney. Some infected cells can usually be found on the first or even second subculture but no virus growth usually appears in subsequent subcultures. Wyatt and his colleagues in Bethesda have succeeded in making up to 14 subcultures of the human virus in human embryo kidney, and Murphy in Australia has achieved up to six, but these results have not been reproducible. Banatvala showed that the infectivity of human virus for monolayer tissue cultures could be greatly increased by centrifuging the virus together with the cell cultures. Workers in my own laboratory have found that this method can be applied to rotaviruses from several species and that it can be used both for diagnostic isolation and also for titrating neutralizing antibodies in sera. LLC MK2 cells, a line of subtetraploid cells derived from rhesus monkey kidney epithelium, have been found to be the most susceptible for most of the rotaviruses, including those of man, horse, calf, pig, sheep, mouse and rabbit.[1]

Tissue culture methods

METHOD (a)

Monolayer LLC MK2 cells are grown upon circular coverslips 12 mm in diameter; a medium consisting of Eagle's minimal essential medium (MEM) with the addition of 10% fetal calf serum has been found satisfactory. The coverslips are placed on the flat bottom of screw-capped tubes. To 1 ml of maintenance medium (Eagle's MEM + 2% fetal calf serum is added 0.1 ml of suspension of faeces previously clarified by centrifugation at 3000 rev/min for 30 min. The tubes are centrifuged for 75 minutes at a speed to give 2100 g and incubated for 20–24 hours. The coverslips are removed, rinsed in saline, fixed in acetone, reacted with a serum containing rotavirus antibodies, washed again and 'stained' with a fluorescein-labelled antiglobulin serum.

METHOD (b)

This method is especially convenient for the examination of large numbers of specimens and for performing replicate titrations of virus or antibody.

Confluent monolayer cultures of LLC MK2 cells are established in 'microtitre' plastic plates with flat-bottomed wells. 50 000 cells/well are inoculated; they form a monolayer in 24 hours. An atmosphere containing 5% CO_2 is required. 0.5 ml of maintenance medium and 0.1 ml inoculum are added to each well. The wells are sealed with Sellotape and the plates centrifuged in swing-out holders at a speed to give 1200 g for 75 minutes. The plates are incubated for 20–24 hours at 37° C; then, after rinsing in phosphate buffered saline, pH 7.2, the cells are fixed for 1–2 min with methanol previously chilled to $-4°$ C (acetone dissolves the plastic of the plates), and infected cells are then 'stained' by the indirect immuno-fluorescence method as above. Infected cells can be observed by examining the inverted plates through a microscope fitted with a vertical illuminator designed for blue light fluorescence. A 50 or 200 watt mercury vapour lamp gives the best results, but a 100 watt quartz-iodine lamp can be used with the appropriate interference filters. Provided care is taken when pipetting inocula, cross-infection from one well to another does not readily occur and the method is much less laborious than using the corresponding number of tubes and coverslips. As a means of detecting human rotaviruses in faeces it is comparable in sensitivity with electron microscopy, and for detecting some animal rotaviruses it is probably even more sensitive.

So far, the method has been used for detecting rotaviruses only; it may well be useful for detecting other viruses also, provided that antisera to them are available.

Serological reactions of rotaviruses

Antibodies to rotaviruses can be detected by using a complement fixation test, by immunofluorescence, by neutralization, or by immunoelectron microscopy. Enzyme-linked immunosorbent assay (ELISA), radioimmunoassay (RIA), immune adherence methods and immunoelectroosmophoresis have also been used.

Complement fixing antibodies can be prepared firstly by concentrating virus from patients' stools. A stool, rich in virus particles by electron microscopy, is used. A 20% saline suspension is centrifuged to remove bacteria and an equal volume of Arcton 113 (ICI Ltd.) or Arklone (ICI Ltd.) is added. The mixture is shaken thoroughly for 1 hour. The aqueous phase may be used as the antigen without further treatment if the titre is adequate; or it may be concentrated by centrifuging the virus particles and protein at 50 000 rev/min for 1 hour and resuspending the deposit in veronal buffered saline (VBS) to one-fifth the original volume. Secondly, an excellent antigen may be made from the intestinal tracts removed from mouselings that have been inoculated 4 days previously by mouth with mouse (EDIM) rotavirus. Infected small and large bowels are removed, pooled, homogenized in four times their volume of VBS and treated with Arcton or Arklone, as above. Antigens prepared from human faeces are sometimes anticomplementary; this effect however can often be removed by adding heated guinea pig serum. Complement fixing antigen may also be prepared by propagating tissue culture-adapted calf rotavirus in calf-kidney tissue cultures — and concentrating the virus yield by ultracentrifugation.

IgM and complement fixing antibodies in rotavirus infection appear within 5–10 days of the onset of symptoms and thereafter diminish comparatively rapidly. These antibodies usually are not present in sera from children more than a few years old, unlike antibodies detectable by immunofluorescence or virus neutralization.

Titration of antibodies by immunofluorescence

This is most conveniently done using the tissue culture-adapted calf rotavirus, but can be done using rotavirus present in the faeces of an animal of any species to infect tissue culture cells; primary or secondary cultures of calf kidney, monkey kidney or human embryo kidney may be used; or LLC MK2 cells can be used. Rotaviruses will often infect cells after conventional inoculation of the tissue culture, but a much higher proportion of cells can be infected by the centrifugation technique described under 'tissue culture methods'. Cultures are then incubated for 24 hours after inoculation with virus from faeces, or for up to 5 days after inoculation with the adapted calf virus.

Fixation and 'staining' are performed as described under 'tissue culture methods'.

Rotavirus antibodies in an animal of one species react equally with cells infected with a rotavirus from the same or any other species, but not with the 'new' pig rotavirus mentioned above. Therefore, immunofluorescence can be used to detect rotavirus antibodies in any animal, whether a virus is known in that species or not. All one needs is a fluorescein-conjugated serum specific for the globulin of the species in question. Thus, rotavirus antibodies were found in rabbits before the rabbit rotavirus was found in rabbit faeces. The method has been used to determine the prevalence of antibodies in different age-groups of the population.[6]

NEUTRALIZING ANTIBODIES

These can be titrated using tissue cultures grown in flat-bottomed wells of microtitre plates. A suspension of virus is diluted to give 100–200 infective foci per well. Volumes of this dilution are mixed with equal volumes of serial dilutions of the serum to be tested and these mixtures are inoculated into tissue cultures in the wells in the microtitre plates. The dilutions of serum giving 50% reduction in the number of fluorescent foci is taken as the end-point. Controls in this, as in other methods, are essential.

This method has been used to compare rotaviruses from different species. Although cross-reactions occur, the titres of convalescent sera against the homologous virus are 16–32–fold higher than against rotaviruses from other species. It may thus be possible to identify the species of origin of a rotavirus provided that one has a set of convalescent or hyperimmune sera raised against rotaviruses from different species. Table 8.1 illustrates homotypic and heterotypic reactions.[29] Neutralizing antibody titres rise more slowly than antibodies detected by immunofluorescence or immune electron microscopy, although the titres eventually reached are similar.

Detection of rotavirus in faeces by the ELISA test

Electron microscopy is the only technique so far available which can detect all the known diarrhoea viruses. If, as with the rotaviruses, an antigen can be defined, then an antigen-antibody reaction can be used to detect virus in faeces. Complement fixation, immunoelectrophoresis or immune adherence can be

Table 8.1 Neutralization titres given by convalescent sera from children and young animals with rotaviruses from different species. The homologous neutralization titre is always 16-fold or more higher than neutralization titres against viruses from other species

Serum		Rotavirus Human	Calf	Piglet	Foal	Lamb	Mouse	Rabbit
Human	A	80	< 10	20	NT	NT	40	NT
	E	160	< 10	20	10	10	40	NT
	F	320	20	20	10	< 10	NT	10
Calf	D	10	160	10	10	< 10	20	10
	C	80	1280	160	80	80	160	80
Piglet	A	10	10	160	< 10	< 10	40	10
	B	10	10	320	< 10	20	40	10
Foal	B	10	10	10	80	10	40	20
Lamb	A	< 10	< 10	< 10	< 10	320	40	< 10
Mouse	C	< 10	< 10	< 10	< 10	10	160	NT
	D	< 10	< 10	< 10	< 10	20	160	NT
Rabbit*	A	< 20	< 20	< 20	< 20	< 20	< 20	320

The numbers represent the reciprocal of the serum dilution giving a 50% reduction in the number of fluorescent foci. * The lowest dilution of this serum tested was 1/20. NT not tested against that particular antigen.

used; but most useful is the ELISA test reaction. If the faecal antigen is applied directly to the 'solid phase' of a microtitre plate, a strong, unacceptable nonspecific reaction often occurs; hence it is necessary first to coat the microtitre plate with a 'capture' antibody; a suspension of faeces diluted about 1:40 is then added. Higher concentrations often give a prozone effect and the reaction is then less sensitive. Rotavirus antigen then adheres to the 'capture' antibody. It is detected by adding a 'detecting' antibody which has to be raised in a different species from that supplying the 'capture' antibody. If antigen is captured then the 'detecting' antibody adheres. This reaction in turn is signalled by adding an enzyme-labelled antiglobulin which, with its substrate, yields a visible colour. One disadvantage of this method lies in the presence of rheumatoid factor-like substances in some faeces. These combine nonspecifically both with the 'capture' antibody and with the enzyme-labelled antiglobulin conjugate, thus causing false positive reactions. Another disadvantage is that sera from two different species are required and each must have complete antibody coverage for every serotype of rotavirus which might have to be detected. This is made easier if EDTA is included in the diluent for the faeces; Ca^{++} ions are required to attach the outer capsid layer on to rotaviruses, and if these are chelated the outer layer becomes detached revealing the group-specific inner capsid proteins.

Rheumatoid factor can be removed by treating the faeces with N-acetyl cysteine.[32] However, if the 'detecting' antibody can be labelled directly with enzyme, antibody from the same species can also be used as 'capturing' antibody, and the nonspecific effect of rheumatoid factor-like substances in faeces is greatly reduced. Two commercially available diagnostic kits employ enzyme-labelled detecting antibody in this way. A truly group-specific monoclonal antibody reacting with all rotavirus serotypes would be ideal as a diagnostic tool.

Establishment of serotypes is of value firstly as an epidemiological tool, enabling one to trace the source and development of epidemics; electropherotyping of rotaviruses is also useful for this (see below). Secondly serotyping could indicate the extent to which immunity to one strain of virus is likely to confer immunity to others.

Serotypes

If rotaviruses are centrifuged to equilibrium in a caesium chloride gradient, three layers are formed; the first, at a density of about 1.3 g/ml, is virus protein, mostly empty capsids. The second, density 1.36 g/ml, is composed of complete virus particles, possessing inner and outer capsid layers; only this layer contains infectious virions. A third layer, density 1.38 g/ml, contains infectious virions which have lost their outer capsid layer; these are not infectious. If the infectious layer is injected, mixed with an adjuvant, into animals (which must be previously free of any rotavirus antibody), type-specific antibodies are made. This reaction with viruses in faeces can be demonstrated by the ELISA, complement fixation or neutralization tests. The last is tedious and requires infectious viruses in the faeces; we prefer the ELISA method. At least three, probably four, and possibly five serotypes exist.[10,27]

Typing of rotaviruses by electrophoresis of genome segments

The rotavirus RNA genome is contained within the virion as 11 separate segments. These can quite easily be extracted from faeces and separated by electrophoresis in polyacrylamide gels.[23] The details of the method are as follows:

Faeces containing rotaviruses are suspended in a sodium chloride-tris-EDTA buffer and centrifuged to remove bacteria and other debris. Sodium dodecyl sulphate (10%) is added to a final concentration of 1%; the mixture is incubated at 37° C for 30 min. RNA is extracted by adding an equal volume of water-saturated redistilled phenol; and then precipitated with ethanol; after centrifuging, the deposit is dissolved in 100 μl of 'sample' buffer and electrophoresed in polyacrylamide gel. 'Sample' buffer contains: glycerol 40%; 2-mercaptoethanol 0.5%; sodium dodecyl sulphate 0.3%; TRIS-HCl 0.5-M; bromophenol blue 0.002%. The gel is stained with ethidium bromide. The bands are then visible when the gel is illuminated with ultraviolet light, and can be photographed using very fast film. Major differences between strains are obvious upon inspection of photographs (Fig. 8.13a, b) but to establish minor differences it is necessary to mix RNA extracts from two different samples of faeces and electrophorese the mixture. RNA bands of different molecular weight of the two viruses appear in different places, but bands of identical molecular weight are superimposed (Fig.

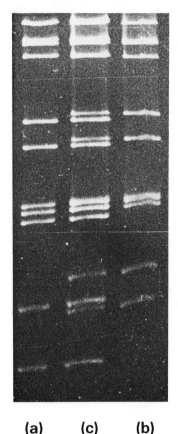

(a)   (c)   (b)

Fig. 8.13 (a) and (b) are electrophoretype patterns of rotavirus RNA genomic segments from subgroups 2 and 1 respectively. (c) is a 'co-run' of a mixture of both. Segments of identical molecular weight run together to the same position, but those which are different can easily be seen because they appear separately

8.13c). This method is an extremely accurate tool for detecting minor differences between strains, and has shown that human rotaviruses occur in two main subgroups, a common 'long' form (Fig. 8.13a) and a less common 'short' form (Fig. 8.13b). Subgroup 1 is a 'short' form and subgroup 2 is a 'long' form.

REFERENCES

1   Bryden A. S., Davies H., Thouless M. E. and Flewett T. H. (1977) Diagnosis of rotavirus by cell culture. *J. Med. Microbiol.* **10**, 121.
2   Caul E., Paver W. K. and Clarke S. K. R. (1975) Coronavirus particles in faeces from patients with gastroenteritis. *Lancet* **i**, 1192.
3   Coelho K. I. R., Bryden A. S., Hall Cheryl and Flewett T. H (1981) Pathology of rotavirus infection in suckling mice: A study by conventional histology; immunofluorescence, ultrathin sections, and scanning electron microscopy. *Ultrastruct. Pathol.* **2**, 59.
4   Cubitt W. D., McSwiggan D. A. and Moore W. (1979) Winter vomiting disease caused by caliciviruses. *J. Clin. Pathol.* **32**, 786.
5   Davidson G. P., Dall D. G., Petric M., Butler D. G and Hamilton J. R. (1977) Human rotavirus enteritis induced in conventional piglets. *J. Clin. Invest.* **60**, 1402.

6   Elias M. M (1977) Distribution and titres of rotavirus antibodies in different age groups. *J. Hyg.* **79**, 373.

7   Flewett T. H (1977) Acute non-bacterial infectious gastroenteritis, An essay in comparative virology. In: *Recent Advances in Clinical Virology 1*, Ed. Waterson A. P., Churchill-Livingstone, Edinburgh.

8   Flewett T. H., Bryden A. S., Davies H., Woode G. N., Bridger J. C. and Derrick J. M. (1974) Relation between viruses from acute gastroenteritis of children and newborn calves. *Lancet* **ii**, 61.

9   Flewett T. H., Bryden A. S., Davies H. A. and Morris C. A. (1975) Epidemic viral enteritis in a long-stay children's ward. *Lancet* **i**, 4

10   Flewett T. H., Thouless M. E., Pilford J. N., Bryden A. S. and Candeias J. A. N. (1978) More serotypes of human rotavirus. *Lancet* **ii**, 632.

11   Flewett T. H. and Woode G. N. (1978) The rotaviruses. Brief Review. *Arch. Virol.* **57**, 1.

12   Greenberg H. B., Wyatt R. G., Kalica A. R., Yolken R. H., Black R., Kapikian A. Z. and Chanock R. M. (1980) New insights in viral gastroenteritis. In: *Perspectives in Virology*, M. Pollard (ed.), vol. 11, Raven Press, New York.

13   Greenberg H. B., Kalica A. R., Wyatt R. G., Jones R. W., Kapikian A. Z. and Chanock R. M. (1981) Rescue of uncultivable human rotavirus by gene reassortment during mixed infection with ts mutants of a cultivable bovine rotavirus. *Proc. Natl Acad. Sci. USA* **78**, 420.

14   Kapikian A. Z., Wyatt R. G., Dolin R., Thornhill T. W., Kalica A. R. and Chanock R. M. (1972) Visualization by immune electron microscopy of a 27-nm particle associated with acute infectious nonbacterial gastroenteritis. *J. Virol.* **10**, 1075.

15   Kapikian A. Z., Wyatt R. G., Greenberg H. B., Kalica A. R., Kim Hyun Wha, Brandt Carl D., Rodriguez W. J., Parrott R. H and Chanock R. M. (1980) Approaches to immunization of infants and young children against gasteroenteritis due to rotaviruses. *Rev. Infect. Dis.* **2**, 459.

16   Kidd A. and Madeley C. R. (1981) *In vitro* growth of some fastidious adenoviruses from stool specimens. *J. Clin. Path.* **34**, 213–16.

17   Lewis H. M., Parry J. V., Davies H. A., Parry R. P., Mott A., Dourmashkin R. R., Sanderson P. J., Tyrrell D. A. J. and Valman H. B. (1979) A year's experience of the rotavirus syndrome and its association with respiratory illness. *Arch. Dis. Child.* **54**, 339.

18   Light J. S. and Hodes H. L. (1949) Isolation from cases of infantile diarrhoea of a filterable agent causing diarrhoea in calves. *J. Exp. Med.* **90**, 113.

19   Mathan M., Mathan V. I., Swaminathan S. P., Yesudoss S. and Baker S. J. (1975) Pleomorphic virus-like particles in human faeces. *Lancet* **i**, 1068.

20   Mebus C. A., Stair E. L., Rhodes M. B. and Twiehaus M. J. (1973) Pathology of neonatal calf diarrhoea induced by a corona-like agent. *Vet. Pathol.* **10**, 45.

21   Nicolaieff A., Obert G. and van Regenmortal M. H. (1980) Detection of rotavirus by serological trapping on antibody-coated electron microscope grids. *J. Clin. Microbiol.* **12**, 101.

22   Richmond S. J., Dunn S. M., Caul E. O., Ashley C. R. and Clarke S. K. R. (1979) An outbreak of gastroenteritis in young children caused by adenoviruses. *Lancet* **i**, 1178.

23   Rodger S. M. and Holmes I. H. (1979) Comparison of the genomes of simian, bovine and human rotaviruses by gel electrophoresis and the detection of genomic variation among bovine isolates. *J. Virol.* **30**, 839.

24   Saif L. J., Bohl E. H., Theil K. W., Cross R. F. and House J. A. (1980) Rotavirus-like, calicivirus-like, and 23-nm virus-like particles associated with diarrhoea in young pigs. *J. Clin. Microbiol.* **12**, 105.

25   Snodgrass D. R., Ferguson Anne, Allan Frances, Angus K. W. and Mitchell B. (1979) Small intestinal morphology and epithelial cell kinetics in lamb rotavirus infections. *Gastroenterology* **76**, 477.

26 Taylor P. R., Merson M. H., Black R. E., Mizanur Rahman A. S. M., Yunus M. D., Alim A. R. M. and Yolken R. H (1980) Oral rehydration therapy for treatment of rotavirus diarrhoea in a rural treatment center in Bangladesh. *Arch. Dis. Child.* **55**, 376.

27 Thouless M. E., Bryden A. S. and Flewett T. H. (1978) Serotypes of human rotavirus. *Lancet* **i**, 39.

28 Whitelaw A., Davies H. and Perry J. (1977) Electron microscopy of fatal adenovirus gastroenteritis. *Lancet* **i**, 361.

29 Woode G. N., Bridger J. C., Jones J. M., Flewett T. H., Bryden A. S., Davies H. A. and White G. B. B. (1976) Morphological and antigenic relationships between viruses (rotaviruses) from acute gastroenteritis of children, calves, piglets, mice and foals. *Infect. Immun.* **14**, 804.

30 Woode G. N. and Crouch C. F. (1978) Naturally occurring and experimentally induced rotaviral infections in domestic and laboratory animals. *J. Am. Vet. Med. Assoc.* **173**, 522.

31 Wyatt R. G., James W. D., Bohl E. H., Theil K. W., Saif L. J., Kalica A. R., Greenberg H. B., Kapikian A. Z. and Chanock R. M. (1980) Human rotavirus type 2: cultivation in vitro. *Science* **207**, 189.

32 Yolken R. H. and Stoppa P. S. (1979) Non-specific false positive reactions in rotavirus ELISA tests. *J. Clin. Microbiol.* **10**, 703.

33 Sato K., Inaba, Y., Shinozaki T., Fujii R. and Matumoto M. (1981) Isolation of human rotavirus in cell cultures. *Arch. Virol.* **69**, 155.

34 Urasawa T., Urasawa S. and Taniguchi K. (1981) Sequential passages of human rotavirus in MA-104 cells. *Microbiol. Immunol.* **25**, 1025.

NOTE ADDED IN PROOF

It has recently been shown that human rotaviruses can be isolated in tissue cultures of cynomologous kidney, African green monkey kidney, MA104 cells or LLC-MK2 cells.

Cells from an early passage number of MA104 cells give better results than from some later passages. It is necessary to digest the inoculum (20% suspension of faeces in buffer pH 8) with crystalline trypsin 20 μg/ml for 1 hour at 37°. The inoculum is then allowed to adsorb for 1 hour at 37° to the tissue culture, which must first be carefully washed to remove the serum of the growth medium. Cells are then maintained in a medium consisting of Eagles' minimal essential medium with added glutamine and crystalline trypsin at 2–5 μg/ml and rolled at 37°. With each cell line and each batch of trypsin in it, it is necessary to try different dilutions of trypsin in the maintenance medium. The trick really is to use the highest concentration in the maintenance medium that the cells will stand without rounding up and coming off the glass. Subcultures are made every 5–6 days, the inoculum being trypsinized (20 μg/ml) each time. After the virus has been adapted to the tissue culture a cytopathic effect appears, which when first seen may not appear on the next passage; but thereafter reappears and is consistently present on further subculture.

Most adapted strains can be made to give plaques under agarose if trypsin is included in the medium.[33,34]

9 The challenge of childhood gastroenteritis

M. Gracey

Introduction	187
The extent of childhood gastroenteritis	188
Infections and infestations	190
Enterotoxigenic bacteria	191
Viruses	191
Parasites	192
Intestinal microecology	192
Effects of upper gut contamination on intestinal function	194
The gastrointestinal mucosa	197
Altered gastrointestinal function	198
Environmental factors	198
Approaches to control and prevention	201
References	205

INTRODUCTION

The first hours and days of life form a critical period in which the human host and, in particular, the gastrointestinal tract adjust to an abrupt change from a sterile intrauterine environment to a potentially hostile one, rich in a vast array of microbes. Healthy babies brought into postnatal life in favourable circumstances respond rapidly to this change and the contents of the alimentary tract soon acquire microbial populations which are normally controlled within strict limits. Pathogenic microorganisms are normally suppressed by complex protective mechanisms but these may be overwhelmed by large numbers of a particularly virulent organism or be ineffective in disease states associated with disorders of immune function or gastrointestinal motility. In the so-called developing countries, the common combination of childhood malnutrition and gross environmental contamination, particularly of water by faecal organisms, swamps these normal controlling influences and is associated with the well-known prevalence of gastroenteritis in those regions.

THE EXTENT OF CHILDHOOD GASTROENTERITIS

The World Health Organization lists 'enteritis' and 'diarrhoeal diseases' as the leading two causes of death in infants and children up to the age of 5 years in developing countries.[91] However there are few reliable statistics. Some carefully performed studies of age-specific diarrhoea attack rates from Guatemala, India and Indonesia (Table 9.1) give an indication of the importance of gastroenteritis in children in developing countries.[24] These figures show that diarrhoeal illnesses

Table 9.1 Age-specific diarrhoea attack rates (%) (Elliott and Knight)[24]

Age	Guatemala	India	Indonesia
0–5 months	47	146	99 (up to 1 year)
6–11 months	110	196	
1 year	120	167	
2 years	106	137	163 (1–4 years)
3 years	56	73	
4–6 years	21		40
7–14 years	8		16
15+ years	5		13

are commonest in the second and third years of life when there are more attacks of diarrhoea recorded than individuals in each age group; the excess over 100% is, of course, due to some children suffering more than one diarrhoeal episode each year. The frequency of attacks decreases with advancing age and is slightly less in infancy, depending on local circumstances such as breast-feeding practices.

As the number of children in each age category in the developing parts of the world is known, an estimate can be made of the numbers of diarrhoeal disease episodes and related deaths. In 1975 there were approximately 500 million such episodes in children under 5 in Asia, Africa and Latin America (see Table 9.2)

Table 9.2 Estimates of attacks of diarrhoea in Asia, Africa and Latin America, 1975[24]

Age (years)	Population (millions)	Case rate (%)	Diarrhoeal episodes (millions)
0–1	97.5	100	97.5
1–2	95.5	140	133.7
2–3	93.6	125	117.0
3–4	91.7	80	73.4
4–5	89.9	40	35.9
Total	468.2		457.5

which may have caused 15–20 million deaths in that year. Others have made somewhat different estimates. The studies by Mata *et al.*[93] in Guatemala suggest there may be 2000 million diarrhoeal episodes in children under 5, annually, in developing countries. A more recent review by Barua[92] of 25 published reports of prospective, community-based studies of more than 1 year's duration suggest 760–1000 million episodes each year with about 5 million deaths.

Our own studies done in Aboriginal communities throughout Western Australia,[2] show that this high prevalence of childhood gastroenteritis is not confined to children in developing countries but occurs in socioeconomically disadvantaged sections of otherwise affluent and healthy communities (Table 9.3).

Table 9.3 Age-specific admission rates/1000/year for gastroenteritis for Aboriginal and non-Aboriginal infants and children in Western Australia, 1971–78

Infants		Children aged 1–4 years	
Aboriginal	Non-Aboriginal	Aboriginal	Non-Aboriginal
802	38	202	13

Although Aborigines made up only 3.7% of Western Australia's population under 5 years in 1976 (the last census year), they accounted for 42% of admissions for gastroenteritis and had 58% of the bed occupancy for that disease. The age-specific admission rate for gastroenteritis was over 800/1000/year, or 80% per year, for Aboriginal infants but for non-Aboriginal infants was less than one-twentieth of this (see Fig. 9.1); in the tropical Kimberley region of the state the age-

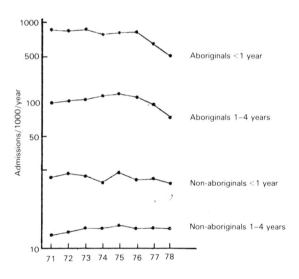

Fig. 9.1 Age-specific admission rates for childhood gastroenteritis in Western Australia, 1971–78 (from Berry and Gracey[2] with permission of The Editor, *Medical Journal of Australia*)

specific admission rate for Aboriginal infants exceeded 1000/1000/year, i.e. > 100%, reminiscent of the figures quoted earlier for developing countries. It is likely that childhood gastroenteritis is a serious problem in urban slums in western cities but its extent is unknown.

Gastroenteritis has an important influence on nutritional status because it suppresses appetite, and because of the widespread practice of withholding food from children with diarrhoeal and vomiting illnesses. The work of Gordon and his colleagues[28] clearly showed that there is a higher prevalence of diarrhoea in malnourished children who are known to have impaired resistance to infection.

These interrelating effects of undernutrition and diarrhoeal disease reflect the well-known synergism of nutrition and infection[73] and, globally, constitute the major health problem facing the majority of the world's children.

INFECTIONS AND INFESTATIONS

In childhood gastroenteritis, most reports from temperate regions used to indicate a low diagnostic yield from faecal cultures,[16] although in developing countries enteric pathogens were reported more frequently.[74] The major pathogenetic mechanisms involved in the production of diarrhoea by these agents are summarized in Table 9.4. A wider range of enteric pathogens is now recog-

Table 9.4 Major mechanisms of pathogenesis of bacterial diarrhoeas

Pathogen	Main effect on intestinal mucosa	Pathogenesis	Main site of action
Vibrio cholerae Enterotoxigenic *E. coli* (ETEC) Other toxigenic bacteria	Adherence	Fluid and electrolyte secretion induced by effect of toxins on cyclic nucleotides	Small intestine
Shigella Other *E. coli*	Penetration and proliferation within enterocytes	Inflammation and histological damage	Small intestine then large intestine
Salmonella	Penetration into the submucosa	Inflammatory infiltration in lamina propria	Small and large intestine

nized. Of these 'newer' agents *Campylobacter jejuni* seems to be particularly important in children,[49] but carriage may occur without diarrhoea, as was found in a prospective study in Aboriginal communities in the north of Western Australia.[3] In one remote, inland settlement *C. jejuni* was prevalent in both the winter, dry season (23%) and in the monsoonal, wet summer season (15%).

In a coastal, tropical community it was not isolated from 82 specimens tested throughout the year. Interestingly, *C. jejuni* was isolated from fresh faecal samples from two out of five randomly selected dogs in the infected community while dogs were banned from the other, campylobacter-free community. In 1979 *C. jejuni* was found in 137 out of 2905 (4.7%) stool specimens submitted to the Western Australian State Health Laboratory Services. In a study in Soweto, South Africa,[7] *C. jejuni* was found in 16% of children without diarrhoea. Thus symptomless carriage of *C. jejuni* is probably not uncommon in children in communities where standards of living and hygiene are low. The role of campylobacter infections in children on a wider scale can only be delineated after adequate, prospective, epidemiological investigations in well studied communities in different localities.

Enterotoxigenic bacteria

Vibrio cholerae and some strains of *E. coli* cause diarrhoea by elaborating toxins which interfere with intestinal fluid and electrolyte transport. These and other enterotoxigenic bacteria produce either a heat-labile toxin (LT), which resembles cholera toxin (CT), or a heat-stable toxin (ST) or both. Development of reliable methods for identification of enterotoxin producers, such as the ELISA assay for LT and the suckling-mouse test for ST, will allow epidemiological studies which will help document the importance of these agents in childhood gastroenteritis in developing countries.

Viruses

Rotaviruses in childhood gastroenteritis were first reported by Bishop *et al.*[4,5] The pathogenesis of viral gastroenteritis is described in Chapter 8; the enterocytes lining the apical parts of the small intestinal villi are damaged[75] with resulting impaired net absorption of fluid, electrolytes and nutrients.

The contribution of rotavirus enteritis to childhood diarrhoeal disease in developing countries is not yet known but may be considerable. For example, Soenarto and her colleagues working in Yogyakarta, central Java, found rotavirus particles in 38% of infants and children with acute diarrhoea in a prospective, year-long study.[78] They found rotaviruses in 11% of 'control' children admitted to hospital for other reasons. There appeared to be little seasonal variation but some increase in the rate of isolation in November and December, the start of the wet monsoonal period. Rotavirus infections were commonest in children aged 6 to 24 months. In temperate or colder climates, rotavirus enteritis is well recognized to have a 'winter peak'; this is shown clearly in Fig. 9.2 which illustrates the monthly

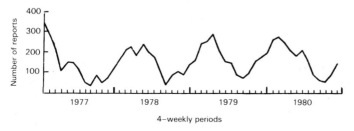

4—weekly periods

Fig. 9.2 Analysis by age, of the 6077 reports received in the three years 1977–79, shows that while 90% of the patients were aged ≤4 years, 688 (11%) of the total were neonates, 48 (0.8%) were aged ≥65 years and 567 (9.3%) reports related to all ages between 5–64 years. (From Communicable Disease Report no. CD8 80/49, published with permission of the Editor, Communicable Disease Surveillance Centre, London)

rotavirus reports over a 4 year period to the Communicable Disease Surveillance Centre at Colindale, London. Analysis of 8011 reports of rotavirus infections received by CDSC since the beginning of 1977 showed an annual peak usually starting in the fourth quarter and reaching a maximum between February and April the following year (Fig. 9.2). The total number of reports increased each year (annual totals: 1804, 1998, 2275, 1934 in weeks 1–48).

Serological tests are now available for accurate and rapid identification of rotavirus infections including an ELISA (enzyme-linked immunosorbent) assay which is being applied in prospective epidemiological surveys of childhood gastroenteritis in developing countries.

Parasites

Parasitic infestations are also important causes of acute and chronic childhood diarrhoea with important regional variations in patterns of infestation. In Aboriginal communities, for example, *Giardia lamblia* infestation from unhygienic living conditions is a common problem.[30] Hookworm infestation is very important in the tropics, particularly in coastal regions and is a significant cause of gastrointestinal blood loss and anaemia, which may be profound. Other parasitic infestations, such as strongyloidiasis and amoebiasis, are important in some regions (see Chapter 10).

INTESTINAL MICROECOLOGY

There are several interrelated factors that control the upper intestinal microflora and normally keep the luminal bacterial populations below 10^4 microorganisms/ ml in the fasting state.[15,27] In 1958 Smythe[76] suggested that the upper intestinal microflora might be disturbed in children with malnutrition; he found coliform bacteria in the gastric contents of 11 of 33 patients in South Africa. In 1965 Dammin[18] reported that malnourished children who died of diarrhoeal illnesses in Guatemala had very large numbers of bacteria in their jejunal contents while malnourished children without diarrhoea had a normal, sparse bacterial flora. Unfortunately, these studies were done some hours after the children had died so the possibility remained that the large numbers of bacteria isolated may have been caused by their proliferation within the intestinal lumen after death and, therefore, were not a true representation of the situation *in vivo*.

In 1972, separate studies from Western Australia[38] and Guatemala[57] of upper gut aspirates, showed that abnormally large numbers of bacteria were present in the upper intestinal contents of malnourished children *in vivo*; in the Guatemalan study most children had 10^7 to 10^8 bacteria/ml. Such numbers occur in the so-called 'contaminated small bowel syndrome'.[29,31] Similar findings were reported from the Gambia, West Africa,[41,69] indicating that bacterial contamination of the upper intestine is an important feature of childhood gastroenteritis.

In a study of malnourished children in Indonesia, Gracey *et al.*[39] found a marked increased of bacteria and *Candida* sp. in aspirates of upper intestinal juice (see Table 9.5).

In a joint study of 27 well-nourished white Australian children and 57 malnourished children (30 Australian Aborigines and 27 Indonesians), a significantly higher rate of isolation of *Candida* sp. was recorded in gastric and intestinal aspirates from the malnourished group[40] (Table 9.6).

Table 9.5 Bacterial contamination of the upper intestine in 20 Indonesian children with malnutrition and diarrhoea (with permission of the Editor, *Am. J. Clin. Nutr.*[39])

Organism	No. of isolations $> 10^4/ml$	Range $\log_{10}$ organisms/ml
Staphylococcus aureus	8	0–7.8
Coagulase-negative Staphylococci	9	0–7.0
Haemophilus influenzae	0	—
Corynebacterium sp.	0	0–3.9
Candida sp.	8	0–6.3
Escherichia coli	7	0–8.0
Klebsiella sp.	3	0–8.9
Pseudomonas sp.	5	0–8.6
Salmonella paratyphi	2	0–4.4
Shigella sp.	1	4.1
Other enterobacteria	8	0–8.7
Aerobic lactobacilli	4	0–5.7
Streptococcus faecalis	0	0–3.5
α-haemolytic *Streptococci*	4	0–6.1
β-haemolytic *Streptococci*	0	—
Other *Streptococci*	9	0–8.0
Anaerobes	6	0–8.0
Total flora	18	0–9.1

Table 9.6 Gastric and small intestinal colony counts of *Candida* sp. in well-nourished white Australian and malnourished Aboriginal Australian and Indonesian children (with permission of the Editor, *Am. J. Clin. Nutr.*[40]). (Results expressed as *Candida* sp./ml as the $\log_{10}$ of the mean viable colony count/ml)

Subjects	Gastric Mean colony count	P	Small intestinal Mean colony count	P
White Australians (27)	0.8		1.6	
Australian Aborigines (30)	2.8	<0.0005	3.1	<0.025
Indonesians (27)	2.0	<0.025	3.5*	<0.01

* 26 studies.

All these findings in malnourished children, some with diarrhoeal illnesses, still leave unanswered the important question of whether the upper intestinal microflora in well-nourished children from favourable circumstances but living in countries where most children are poor, are different from those found in well-nourished children from favourable circumstances in industrialized, western countries from where most of the reports of the 'normal' flora come. Until this question is answered it can be said that most published reports suggest strongly that the upper intestinal microflora is significantly abnormal in childhood malnutrition. If this is so, it raises important questions about its clinical relevance, its pathogenesis and its possible control.

EFFECTS OF UPPER GUT CONTAMINATION ON INTESTINAL FUNCTION

In the so-called 'contaminated small bowel syndrome' or CSBS,[29,31] high bacterial counts in upper intestinal contents have been linked causally with a wide spectrum of clinical consequences, some of which are mentioned in Chapter 14. In brief, it has been established that profuse bacterial overgrowth in the proximal small intestine can cause steatorrhoea, malabsorption of carbohydrate, hypoproteinaemia, vitamin B_{12} deficiency and its associated macrocytic anaemia, and iron deficiency. Several pathogenetic mechanisms are involved. For example, steatorrhoea is associated with bacterial degradation of bile salts and the reduction of the intraluminal concentration of conjugated bile salts to below the critical micellar concentration needed for efficient micellar solubilization prior to intestinal fat absorption.[80] The simultaneous production of abnormally high levels of deconjugated bile salts also has other important effects on intestinal digestion and absorption. For example, impaired carbohydrate absorption has been related to the harmful effects of deconjugated bile salts on the metabolically-dependent, active transport processes in the enterocytes lining the intestinal epithelium which, although virtually normal from a histological viewpoint, shows extensive ultrastructural distortion.[1,33,52]

The pathogenesis of the mucosal lesion consequent on upper gut bacterial contamination is uncertain. It is not due to direct bacterial invasion and until recently the toxic effects of unconjugated bile salts were thought to be causative.[29,33,52] This seemed to be supported by work in experimental animals when similar mucosal lesions were obtained by feeding deconjugated bile salts.[37] However, the role of bile salts has recently been questioned and other mechanisms have been proposed. These include toxins, alcohol, and short chain fatty acids produced by bacteria and injurious to the intestinal mucosa.[26] Jonas *et al.*[47,48] have demonstrated the presence of a bacterial protease in intestinal secretions in experimental intestinal stasis; this enzyme, perhaps a bacterial elastase, releases disaccharidases from the brush border. This and other mechanisms may operate simultaneously to cause the mucosal lesion. The cause of other absorptive defects in this syndrome may be bacterial binding of the vitamin B_{12}-intrinsic-factor complex so that the vitamin is inaccessible to the human host,[72] and conversion of vitamin B_{12} into physiologically inactive analogues, cobamides which causes significant loss of vitamin B_{12} to the host.[9] The cause of hypoproteinaemia is unclear; gastrointestinal loss of protein[45] and bacterial degradation and deamination have been suggested[46] while inhibitory effects of deconjugated bile salts on intestinal amino acid transport may also contribute.[13] The effect of upper intestinal bacterial contamination on other aspects of intestinal function such as water and electrolyte fluxes, has been less intensively studied but defects in jejunal transport of water, sodium and potassium have been shown in animals and humans *in vitro* and *in vivo*.[25,60,61] These are probably relevant to the clinical features of the CSBS and may assume another very important dimension in malnourished children with diarrhoea because of our emerging new knowledge of the role of bacterial enterotoxins in the pathogenesis of watery diarrhoeas.

Although many of the organisms in Table 9.5, such as *Klebsiella* and *Pseudomonas*, would not generally be considered to be enteropathogenic, some strains have been shown, by perfusion of rat jejunum *in vivo*, to interfere with intestinal carbohydrate absorption when pure bacterial broths were perfused through the small intestine (Table 9.7).

Table 9.7 Effect of enteric microorganisms on intestinal monosaccharide absorption *in vivo* (Gracey *et al.* 1975) (reproduced with permission of the Editor, *Am. J. Clin. Nutr.*[94]

Organism	Absorption (μ mole arbutin/cm/h)	P
Controls (8)	0.46 ± 0.13 (S.D.)	
Gram-positive cocci		
Staphylococcus saprophyticus (8)	0.46 ± 0.11	NS
Staphylococcus pyogenes (12)	0.36 ± 0.13	<0.05
Streptococcus viridans (12)	0.30 ± 0.14	<0.0125
Streptococcus faecalis (7)	0.32 ± 0.06	<0.0125
Gram-positive rod		
Lactobacillus (11)	0.36 ± 0.08	<0.05
Enterobacteriaciae		
Non-pathogenic *E. coli* (11)	0.36 ± 0.11	<0.05
E. coli O55 (9)	0.29 ± 0.08	<0.0025
E. coli O111 (9)	0.34 ± 0.07	<0.025
E. coli O142 (7)	0.35 ± 0.11	<0.05
Salmonella paratyphi B (20)	0.42 ± 0.16	NS
Shigella (7)	0.50 ± 0.16	NS
Proteus (8)	0.42 ± 0.08	NS
Klebsiella (8)	0.28 ± 0.10	<0.005
Gram-negative rod		
Pseudomonas (10)	0.32 ± 0.06	<0.005
Candida sp.		
C. albicans (7)	0.33 ± 0.12	<0.05
C. tropicalis (20)	0.38 ± 0.17	NS
C. parapsilosis (8)	0.29 ± 0.11	<0.01

Also in this model impaired intestinal fluid and electrolyte absorption was associated with gross upper intestinal microbial contamination.[81] Using cell-free filtrates of microorganisms isolated from the upper intestinal secretions of malnourished Indonesian children, a decreased net movement out of the intestinal lumen, or actual secretion of water, sodium or potassium into the intestinal lumen, was found with culture filtrates of single isolates of *Staphylococcus epidermidis*, *Escherichia coli* O55, *Escherichia coli* B7A (isolated from an adult),

Shigella sonnei, Klebsiella pneumoniae, Candida albicans and *Candida tropicalis* (see Tables 9.8 and 9.9).

Apart from the well-known enterotoxigenic bacteria, *Vibrio cholerae* and *Escherichia coli*, other reports suggest that a wide range of other microorganisms

Table 9.8 Effect of cell-free culture filtrates on net jejunal fluid flux *in vivo* (from Thelen *et al.*,[81] with permission of the Editor, *J. Med. Microbiol.*)

Organism	*n*	Mean net water flux (ml/cm/h)	Significance
Controls	10	0.041	
Gram-positive cocci			
Staphylococcus epidermidis	12	0.007	*
Streptococcus faecalis	12	0.049	NS
Enterobacteriaceae			
Non-pathogenic *E. coli*	6	0.051	NS
E. coli O55	9	−0.047†	*
E. coli B7A	12	0.023	*
Salmonella paratyphi B	12	0.042	NS
Shigella sonnei	12	0.020	*
Klebsiella pneumoniae	11	0.001	*
Candida species			
C. albicans	11	0.022	*
C. tropicalis	11	0.019	*

* $P < 0.05$. † The negative value indicates net secretion of fluid *into* the intestinal lumen.

Table 9.9 Effect of cell-free culture filtrates on net intestinal flux of sodium and potassium *in vivo* (from Thelen *et al.*,[81] with permission of the Editor, *J. Med. Microbiol.*)

Organism	Mean net ion flux (μ moles/cm/h)			
	Sodium	*P*	Potassium	*P*
Controls	6.16		0.29	
Gram-positive cocci				
Staphylococcus epidermidis	2.41	*	0.01	*
Streptococcus faecalis	7.27	ns	0.20	ns
Enterobacteriaceae				
Non-pathogenic *E. coli*	6.45	ns	0.18	ns
E. coli O55	−5.23	*	−0.33	*
E. coli B7A	2.73	*	−0.06	*
Salmonella paratyphi B	5.44	ns	0.12	ns
Shigella sonnei	5.89	ns	0.11	ns
Klebsiella pneumoniae	−0.34	*	−0.13	*
Candida species				
C. albicans	3.12	*	0.05	*
C. tropicalis	0.41	*	−0.13	*

* $P < 0.05$. The negative values indicate net ion transfer *into* the intestinal lumen.

can have enterotoxigenic properties, including *Shigella flexneri* and *Shigella sonnei*,[51] *Klebsiella* spp. and *Enterobacter* spp.,[53] *Clostridium perfringens*,[20] *Citrobacter* spp., *Proteus* spp., *Aeromonas* spp.,[14] and *Pseudomonas* spp.[86]

The association of *A. hydrophila* with acute diarrhoea[17,83] is discussed in Chapter 5.

A study has been reported of 103 strains of *A. hydrophila*[14] all isolated from faeces except four from water, two from blood, one from an inflamed appendix and one from a wound abscess. Forty-three of the strains came from Western Australia, 51 from South Australia, 6 from India and 3 from Bangladesh. Of the 103 strains 79 produced a heat-labile enterotoxin, as shown by the suckling-mouse test. Rat jejunal perfusion was performed with 50 strains, 12 of which were suckling-mouse negative. The results were in agreement in all instances indicating the relevance of the perfusion method to the intestinal effects of LT and the reliability of the suckling-mouse test for detection of enterotoxigenic strains of *Aeromonas* sp. Enterotoxic activity correlated in general with haemolysin and cytotoxin production, but 6% of strains would have been incorrectly classified by the haemolysin assay without the suckling-mouse test, and 12% by the cytotoxin assay alone. Haemolysin and cytotoxin were not invariably present in the same strain, and thus the three tests may identify separate toxins. It should soon be possible to establish whether *Aeromonas* sp. are important enteric pathogens.

THE GASTROINTESTINAL MUCOSA

There are significant differences in the histological appearances of the small intestinal mucosa in healthy subjects in temperate regions compared with those living in the tropics.[79] Viteri and Schneider[85] showed that the upper intestinal mucosa of fetuses in Central America is indistinguishable from that seen in fetuses elsewhere but by 3 months of age the villi are noticeably broader, shorter and blunted. They attributed this difference to environmental contamination. Apparently these differences persist through childhood to adult life. In children with malnutrition the abnormalities are quite marked with gross thinning of the gut wall, severe flattening and broadening of the villi, extensive inflammatory infiltration of the lamina propria and alteration in the shape of the enterocytes from columnar to cuboidal or squamous.[70] These changes, which have been reported from many parts of the world, are accompanied by very extensive ultra-structural damage to the mucosal epithelial cells.[56] As mentioned later, they have important effects on intestinal digestion and absorption.

The gastric mucosa is also affected. A recent study of malnourished Indonesian children showed that most subjects had chronic gastritis and reduced levels of resting gastric acid secretion. All the subjects investigated had markedly impaired gastric acid secretion following stimulation by the secretagogue, pentagastrin.[34] Secretion of hydrochloric acid by the gastric mucosa is one of the normal factors controlling the upper intestinal microflora and the loss of this mechanism in malnutrition could contribute to bacterial contamination of upper intestinal secretions in malnourished children.

ALTERED GASTROINTESTINAL FUNCTION

The brush border of the small intestinal mucosa is normally rich in digestive enzymes, such as the disaccharidases which hydrolyse disaccharides to their component monosaccharides before absorption. It is not surprising, therefore, that the extensive and sometimes severe histological damage to the mucosa which occurs in protein-energy malnutrition (PEM) is accompanied by a reduction in the activities of these digestive enzymes. This is of considerable clinical importance because secondary lactose intolerance occurs in about a quarter of patients in most reported series.[8,30,89] This causes an osmotic form of diarrhoea which is often profuse and may be life-threatening; bacterial consumption of un-digested and unabsorbed carbohydrate contributes a fermentative element to the diarrhoea which is characteristically frothy and the stools acidic. The presence of reducing substances in the stools can be detected by using the simple Clinitest method which can be used at the bedside or under field conditions.[50] Secondary lactose intolerance should respond promptly to a lactose-free diet by a rapid improvement in the nature of the stools and improved weight gain.[10]

In malnourished children the clinical situation is often not so straightforward; lactose-free formulae are often unavailable or prohibitively expensive in developing countries and it is unwise to cease breast-feeding for a usually self-limiting illness because of the potentially serious longterm effects of removal of breast milk from the child, including its well-known anti-infective properties. Late-onset hypolactasia is also prevalent in some ethnic groups, such as Chinese and Thais, and has to be taken into account in organizing nutritional rehabilitation programmes. In some developing countries, including Thailand, feeding-formulae of low lactose content are being produced from local ingredients including soy beans.

A particularly severe form of carbohydrate malabsorption, temporary mono-saccharide malabsorption,[11] may occur in severe malnutrition. This disorder may be fatal if unrecognized or inadequately managed. It is accompanied by severe dehydration and metabolic acidosis.[55] Malabsorption of other nutrients also occurs. Increased nitrogen losses are associated with impaired protein as-similation and bacterial degradation within the gut lumen.[43] Steatorrhoea may be due to impaired micelle formation and depletion of the bile salt pool[71] or related to decreased intra-luminal lipolysis from depression of exocrine pancreatic secretion[6] or defective β-lipoprotein production for the transport of fat into lymph. The metabolic effects of severe malnutrition are extensive and include fatty infiltration of the liver which may be extreme and even fatal.[87] Lesser degrees of hepatic dysfunction leading to altered sterol metabolism, including bile salt conjugation, could be another factor contributing to malabsorption of fat in malnutrition.

ENVIRONMENTAL FACTORS

The human gastrointestinal tract is constantly exposed to environmental influences — nutritional, microbial and antigenic — which may result in gastro-intestinal disorders. The combination of altered gastrointestinal physiology and vast microbial challenge probably accounts for a significant proportion of diarrhoeal diseases, particularly in children in developing countries. The uniqueness of the gastrointestinal tract in its close contact with the external environment is reflected in the types and numbers of microorganisms inhabiting the upper small intestine.[19] As mentioned earlier, gross bacterial contamination of the upper gut is found in malnourished children. Despite these associations, and despite the obvious widespread faecal pollution of living conditions in the poorest parts of the world, little quantitative evidence is available to relate diarrhoeal disease to environmental pollution, particularly of food and water supplies. We found a startling degree of faecal pollution of surface waters from the Ciliwung River and its adjoining canals in Jakarta (see Table 9.10). Fifteen of the 20

Table 9.10   Isolations of Enterobacteriaceae from 20 specimens from river waters and canals in Jakarta, Indonesia (from Gracey *et al.*[36] with permission of the Editor, *Trans. R. Soc. Trop. Med. Hyg.*)

Samples tested	20
Samples positive	20
E. coli	15
Klebsiella pneumoniae	7
Citrobacter freundii	4
E. cloacae	5
E. agglomerans	7
Salmonella spp.	10
Shigella sp.	1

Mean population of Enterobacteriaceae = 1.6×10^6/dl (range = 1.3×10^5 to 7.9×10^6/dl).

specimens tested grew *E. coli*; *Klebsiella* were isolated from seven and *Citrobacter* from four. *Salmonella* sp. were grown from almost half the water samples examined and from most of the aquatic sediments collected. Altogether, there were 14 serotypes and 37 isolations of *Salmonella* (see Table 9.11). Not surprisingly, this was associated with a high carrier rate of *Salmonella* spp., especially *S. oranienburg*, in symptomless adults and children living in that city; 39 out of 464 or 8.4%. This is in contrast to a carrier rate of only 0.6% in adults seeking employment as meat workers and food handlers in Perth. High rates of isolation of *Salmonella* (6–9%) have also been found in surveys of Aborigines living in unhygienic conditions in remote, tropical parts of Western Australia.[35]

Rowland and his colleagues working in West Africa, clearly related the risk of endemic childhood diarrhoeal disease to contaminated food and water supplies.[69] They showed that microbiological contamination of weaning foods was a common finding with organisms such as *E. coli*, *B. cereus*, *Staphylococcus aureus* and *Clostridia* and, although their attention was focused on commercial baby milks and feeding bottles, traditional weaning foods were also often contam-inated.[67] In studies of remote Aboriginal communities in Western Australia high

Table 9.11 Isolation of *Salmonella* serotypes from surface waters and sediments in Jakarta (from Gracey *et al.*[36] with permission of the Editor, *Trans. R. Soc. Trop. Med. Hyg.*)

| | Salmonella isolations | | |
	Waters	Sediments	Total
S. agona	1	1	2
S. anatum	1	0	1
S. bleadon	0	1	1
S. derby	2	0	2
S. emek	1	0	1
S. heidelberg	0	2	2
S. javiana	1	1	2
S. kentucky	1	0	1
S. lexington	3	3	6
S. london	2	0	2
S. oranienburg	2	6	8
S. paratyphi B	1	0	1
S. senftenberg	3	3	6
S. weltevreden	1	1	2
Total isolations	19	18	37
Samples tested	21	19	40
Samples positive	10	12	22

counts of coliforms have been found which are a recognized index of water quality;[23] the water was stored unhygienically in open metal containers, and was often also contaminated by Gram-positive micro-organisms and yeasts. Tomkins *et al.*[82] found coliform contamination of all water sources examined in a rural community in northern Nigeria where gastroenteritis is common but bacterial counts were significantly less in 'protected water' from deep wells with a high, surrounding parapet. However, coliform counts were even higher in food samples and they suggested that contamination of food and food vessels may be just as important as contaminated water in the causation of diarrhoeal disease.

In some regions seasonal factors are important in determining the incidence of gastroenteritis. For example, in West Africa the number and duration of attacks per child per month are much higher in the wet season than in the dry season;[68,88] although this seasonal effect appears to be unimportant in Guatemala.[58] There is certainly a marked seasonal peak of childhood gastroenteritis in young Aborigines in the north of Western Australia in the first 3 months of the year, which coincides with the summer monsoon or 'wet' season (see Fig. 9.3). Interestingly, the main peak of gastroenteritis in the temperate southern part of the state, including Perth, is in the middle of the year, our winter, when most rainfall occurs.

This reported contamination of the environment by potentially pathogenic microorganisms has some similarities to the environment in which cholera and other serious infectious diseases used to thrive in now industrialized parts of the world, such as London, where these diseases are now largely things of the past.[89] The starkness of conditions in eighteenth century London was clearly chronicled by Tobias Smollett in 1771 who said: 'If I would drink water, I must quaff the

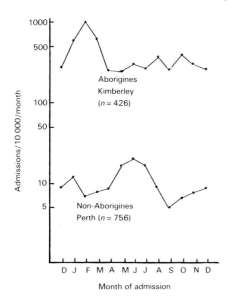

Fig. 9.3 Seasonal incidence of childhood gastroenteritis in Western Australia (0–4 years, 1976). (Note that the scale on the ordinate axis is logarithmic)

maukish contents of an open aqueduct, exposed to all manner of defilement; or swallow that which comes from the river Thames, impregnated with all the filth of London and Westminster — human excreta is the least offensive part of the concrete, ...' This was decades before John Snow's classic epidemiological studies of cholera in central London which clearly traced the source of an epidemic of cholera deaths to tainted water in the Broad Street pump.[77]

APPROACHES TO CONTROL AND PREVENTION

The 'malnutrition-gastroenteritis complex' thrives in children in the poorer parts of the world where poverty, ignorance, overcrowding, undernutrition and poor hygiene are widespread. Eventual eradication of acute diarrhoeal diseases of children has been recognized by the World Health Assembly as central to its goal of 'Health for all by the year 2000'. This has led to the World Health Organization adopting a global, multidisciplinary programme for the control of acute diarrhoeal disease.

The immediate objective of this programme is reduction of deaths caused by diarrhoea and associated malnutrition by the widespread implementation of oral rehydration therapy and the use of appropriate feeding practices during and after diarrhoea.[62] Other approaches to be adopted to support this programme include improved health and nutrition of mothers, better water supplies, sanitation, health education, epidemiological surveillance and control of outbreaks of disease and immunization programmes. The longterm objective of eradication of diarrhoeal disease, or at least its minimization to the extent that is now experienced in industrialized countries, will have to await substantial improvements in overall living standards for children growing up in developing countries.

Meanwhile, short-term solutions must be sought to help alleviate the problem. One of these is oral rehydration therapy (ORT). In the toxigenic diarrhoeas, although adenylate-cyclase-stimulated elevation of intracellular, intestinal cyclic CMP causes net luminal secretion of fluid and electrolytes, the independent sodium-coupled glucose and water absorption mechanisms remain intact. This is the basis for the rationale of ORT which is an effective means of treatment of dehydrated infants with sugar/electrolyte solutions. When used under supervision this is a useful, inexpensive and technologically appropriate approach to the treatment of dehydration from diarrhoea in developing countries.[64] The historical development and physiological basis of ORT has been the subject of an excellent review.[42]

The World Health Organization advocates the use of a single formulation (see Table 9.12) which it claims can be used successfully in all but the most severe

Table 9.12 WHO/UNICEF recommended formulation for oral rehydration therapy

Ingredient	g/l	Ionic concentration (mmol/l)
NaCl	3.5	Na 90
NaHCO$_3$	2.5	K 20
KCl	1.5	HCO$_3$ 30
Glucose	20	Glucose 111
Osmolality 331		

cases of dehydration.[62] However, this unified approach to the treatment of dehydration from diarrhoea is meeting some resistance, particularly from paediatricians who have expressed reservations about the sodium content of the formula which is greater than that generally recommended for treatment of childhood diarrhoea. The recommended formula is designed for treatment of all types of infectious diarrhoeas in all ages and especially in developing countries where hypernatraemia is exceedingly uncommon in childhood gastroenteritis. There is still some dispute about whether sucrose can be used in place of glucose, although its availability and cheapness outweigh the somewhat academic arguments about its minor physiological disadvantages. Another more serious problem about ORT is the variability of the solute concentrations and osmolalities when 'made up' by mothers under field conditions.[54]

The inherent risks of giving oral fluids with potentially dangerous concentrations of sodium and potassium when not under adequate supervision should discourage the 'pinch and scoop' and household methods of making up the solutions and should lead to more desirable, measured aids, such as the double-ended spoon, applicable to field conditions in different places (see. Fig. 9.4).

Workers at the International Centre for Diarrhoeal Disease Research in Bangladesh have shown that chlorpromazine significantly reduces fluid losses in adults with cholera.[66] A recent study suggests that aspirin, and perhaps other salicylates, might be useful in reducing intestinal fluid losses in malnourished children with acute gastroenteritis. Burke *et al.*[12] gave soluble aspirin in

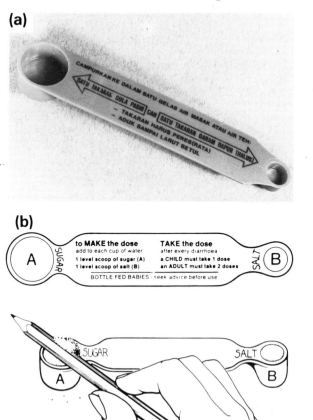

Fig. 9.4 (a) The double-ended blue spoon used in Indonesia to make up oral rehydration solutions. (b) How to add the correct amounts of sugar and salt (from Morley and Woodland[63])

therapeutic doses (25mg/kg/day) in a double blind clinical trial. Stool volume decreased significantly in the patients treated with aspirin, the mean difference in daily stool volume being approximately 100 ml. The mechanism of action of this drug is not known but is currently under investigation in clinical trials in India and Bangladesh. Salicylates have also been shown to have a beneficial, but unexplained, influence on traveller's diarrhoea.[21,22] Further studies are needed before salicylates and other antisecretory drugs can be recommended for treatment in childhood gastroenteritis. In particular, care must be taken to see that known side-effects such as vomiting, acidosis, and gastrointestinal bleeding do not occur.[32,59]

Another strategy being pursued is immunization against the infectious diarrhoeas.[65] The existence of immunological cross-reactivity between cholera toxin (CT) and heat-labile toxin (LT) of *E. coli* suggests that artificial immunity could be induced against a number of toxigenic bacteria. For example, immunization of experimental animals against CT has been shown to protect the small intestine against the secretory effects of *Aeromonas hydrophila* enterotoxin.[44]

Development of cross-reactive immunity in especially vulnerable groups of infants and young children where the microbiological patterns of prevalence of gastroenteritis are known, would seem to be a feasible short-term strategy to pursue. However, there are many technical difficulties to be overcome, such as determination of optimal dosages and routes of administration. The inevitability that childhood gastroenteritis will persist as a major problem in developing countries, in the foreseeable future, should encourage further research into these and other short-term solutions to help relieve this immense problem.

ACKNOWLEDGEMENTS

This work was supported by the TVW Telethon Foundation, Perth, the Wellcome Trust, London, and the National Health and Medical Research Council (Australia).

REFERENCES

1 Ament M. E., Shimoda, S. S., Saunders D. R. and Rubin C. E. (1972) Pathogenesis of steatorrhea in three cases of small intestinal stasis syndrome. *Gastroenterology* **63**, 728.
2 Berry R. J. and Gracey M. (1981) Diarrhoeal disease in Aboriginal and non-Aboriginal infants and Children in Western Australia. *Med. J. Aust.* **1**, 479.
3 Berry R. J., Gracey M. and Bamford V. W. (1981) *Campylabacter jejuni* carriers in Australian Aboriginal Communities. *Med. J. Aust.* **1**, 381.
4 Bishop R. F., Davidson G. P., Holmes I. H. and Ruck B. J. (1973) Virus particles in epithelial cells of duodenal mucosa from children with acute non-bacterial gastroenteritis. *Lancet* **ii**, 1281.
5 Bishop R. F., Davidson G. P., Holmes I. H. and Ruck B. J. (1974) Detection of a new virus by electron microscopy of faecal extracts from children with acute gastroenteritis. *Lancet* **i**, 149.
6 Blackburn W. R. and Vinijchaikul K. (1969) The pancreas in kwashiorkor. An electron microscopic study. *Lab. Invest.* **20**, 305.
7 Bokkenheuser V. D., Richardson N. J., Bryner J. H., Roux D. J., Schutte A. B., Koornhof H. J., Freiman I. and Hartman E. (1979) Detection of enteric campylobacteriosis in children. *J. Clin. Microbiol.* **9**, 227.
8 Bowie M. D., Brinkman G. L. and Hansen J. D. L. (1965) Acquired disaccharide intolerance in malnutrition. *J. Pediatr.* **66**, 1083
9 Brandt L. J., Bernstein L. H. and Wagle A. (1977) Production of vitamin B_{12} analogues in patients with small-bowel bacterial overgrowth. *Ann. Int. Med.* **87**, 546
10 Burke V. and Anderson C. M. (1965) The relationship of dietary lactose to refractory diarrhoea in infancy. *Aust. Paediatr. J.* **1**, 147.
11 Burke V. and Danks D. M. (1966) Monosaccharide malabsorption in young infants. *Lancet* **i**, 1177.
12 Burke V., Gracey M., Suharyono and Sunoto (1980) Reduction by aspirin of intestinal fluid-loss in acute childhood gastroenteritis. *Lancet* **i**, 1329.

13 Burke V., Gracey M., Thomas J. and Malajczuk A. (1975) Inhibition of intestinal amino acid absorption by unconjugated bile salt *in vivo*. *Aust. N.Z. J. Med.* **5**, 430.

14 Burke V., Robinson J., Berry R. J. and Gracey M. (1981) Detection of enterotoxins of *Aeromonas hydrophila* by a suckling-mouse test. *J. Med. Microbiol.* **14**, 401.

15 Challacombe D. N., Richardson J. M. and Anderson C. M. (1974) Bacterial microflora of the upper gastrointestinal tract in infants without diarrhoea. *Arch. Dis. Childh.* **49**, 264.

16 Cramblett H. G., Azimi P. and Haynes R. E. (1971) The etiology of infectious diarrhea in infancy with special reference to enteropathogenic *E. coli*. *Ann. N.Y. Acad. Sci.* **176**, 80.

17 Cumberbatch N., Gurwith M. J., Langston C., Sack R. B. and Brunton J. L. (1979) Cytotoxic enterotoxin produced by *Aeromonas hydrophila*: Relationship of toxigenic isolates to diarrhoeal disease. *Infect. Immun.* **23**, 829.

18 Dammin G. J. (1965) Pathogenesis of acute clinical diarrheal disease. *Fed. Proc.* **24**, 35.

19 Dickman M. D., Chappelka A. R. and Schaedler R. W. (1976) The microbial ecology of the upper small bowel. *Am. J. Gastroenterol.* **56**, 71.

20 Duncan C. L. and Strong D. H. (1969) Ileal loop fluid accumulation and production of diarrhea in rabbits by cell-free products of *Clostridium perfringens*. *J. Bacteriol.* **100**, 86.

21 DuPont H. L., Sullivan P., Evans D. G., Pickering C. K., Evans D. J., Vollet J. J., Ericsson C. D., Ackerman P. B. and Tjoa W. S. (1980) Prevention of travelers' diarrhea (emporiatric enteritis) prophylactic administration of subsalicylate bismuth. *J. Am. Med. Assoc.* **243**, 237.

22 DuPont H. L., Sullivan P., Pickering L. K., Haynes G. and Ackerman P. B. (1977) Symptomatic treatment of diarrhea with bismuth subsalicylate among students attending a Mexican university. *Gastroenterology* **73**, 715.

23 Dutka B. J. (1973) Coliforms are an index of water quality. *J. Environ. Health* **36**, 39.

24 Elliott K. and Knight E. (1976) Acute diarrhoea in childhood. Ciba Foundation Symposium (42) Elsevier, North Holland.

25 Forth W., Rummel W. and Glasner H. (1966) Zur resorptionhemmenden wirkung von gallensäuren. *Naunyn Schmiedebergs Arch. Pharmacol.* **254**, 364.

26 Giannella R. A., Rout W. R. and Toskes P. P. (1974) Jejunal brush border injury and impaired sugar and amino acid uptake in the blind loop syndrome. *Gastroenterology* **67**, 965.

27 Gorbach S. L., Plaut A. F., Nahas L. Weinstein L., Spanknabel G. and Levitan R. (1967) Studies of intestinal microflora. II. Microorganisms of the small intestine and their relations to oral and fecal flora. *Gastroenterology* **53**, 856.

28 Gordon J. E., Chitkara I. D. and Wyon J. B. (1963) Weanling diarrhea. *Am. J. Med. Sci.* **245**, 129/345−161/377.

29 Gracey M. (1971) Intestinal absorption in the 'contaminated small-bowel syndrome'. *Gut* **12**, 403.

30 Gracey M. (1973) Enteric disease in young Australian Aborigines. *Aust. N.Z. J. Med.* **3**, 576.

31 Gracey M. (1979) The contaminated small bowel syndrome: pathogenesis, diagnosis and treatment. *Am. J. Clin. Nutr.* **32**, 234.

32 Gracey M. and Burke V. (1980) Aspirin or loperamide for childhood gastroenteritis. *Med. J. Aust.* **2**, 634.

33 Gracey M., Burke V., Oshin A., Barker J. and Glasgow E. F. (1971) Bacteria, bile salts and intestinal monosaccharide malabsorption. *Gut* **12**, 683.

34 Gracey M., Cullity G. J., Suharjono and Sunoto (1977) The stomach in malnutrition. *Arch. Dis. Childh.* **52**, 325.

35 Gracey M., Iveson J. B., Sunoto and Suharyono (1980) Human salmonella carriers in a tropical urban environment. *Trans. R. Soc. Trop. Med. Hyg.* **74**, 479.

36 Gracey M., Ostergaard P., Adnan S. W. and Iveson J. B. (1979) Faecal pollution of surface waters in Jakarta. *Trans. R. Soc. Trop. Med. Hyg.* **73**, 306.

37 Gracey M., Papadimitriou J., Burke V., Thomas J. and Bower G. (1973) Effects on small-intestinal function and structure induced by feeding a deconjugated bile salt. *Gut* **14**, 519.

38   Gracey M. and Stone D. E. (1972) Small intestinal microflora in Australian Aboriginal children with chronic diarrhoea. *Aust. N.Z. J. Med.* **3**, 215.

39   Gracey M., Stone D. E., Suharjono and Sunoto (1973) Microbial contamination of the gut: another feature of malnutrition. *Am. J. Clin. Nutr.* **26**, 1170.

40   Gracey M., Stone D. E., Suharjono and Sunoto (1974) Isolation of *Candida* species form the gastrointestinal tract in malnourished children. *Am. J. Clin. Nutr.* **27**, 345.

41   Heyworth B. and Brown J. (1975) Jejunal microflora in malnourished Gambian children. *Arch. Dis. Childh.* **50**, 27.

42   Hirschhorn N. (1980) The treatment of acute diarrhea in children. An historical and physiological perspective. *Am. J. Clin. Nutr.* **33**, 637.

43   Holemans K. and Lambrechts A. (1955) Nitrogen metabolism and fat absorption in malnutrition and in kwashiorkor. *J. Nutr.* **56**, 477.

44   James C., Dibley M., Burke V., Robinson J. and Gracey M. (1982) Immunological cross-reactivity of enterotoxins of Aeromonas hydrophila and cholera toxin. *Clin. Exp. Immunol.* **46**, 34.

45   Jeejeebhoy K. N. and Coghill N. F. (1961) The measurement of gastrointestinal protein loss by a new method. *Gut* **2**, 123.

46   Jones E. A., Graigie A., Tavill A. S., Franglen G., and Rosenoer V. M. (1968) Protein metabolism in the intestinal stagnant loop syndrome. *Gut* **9**, 466.

47   Jonas A. and Forstner G. (1979) The effect of biliary diversion on mucosal enzyme activity and brush border glycoprotein degradation in rats with self filling blind loops. *Eur. J. Clin. Invest.* **9**, 167.

48   Jonas A., Krishnan C. and Forstner G. (1978) Pathogenesis of mucosal injury in the blind loop syndrome. *Gastroenterology* **75**, 791.

49   Karmali M. A. and Fleming P. C. (1979) *Campylobacter* enteritis in children. *J. Pediatr.* **94**, 527.

50   Kerry K. R. and Anderson C. M. (1964) A ward test for sugar in faeces. *Lancet* **ii**, 981.

51   Keusch G. T. and Jacewicz M. (1977) The pathogenesis of *Shigella* diarrhea. VI. Toxin and antitoxin in *Shigella flexneri* and *Shigella sonnei* infections in humans. *J. Infect. Dis.* **135**, 552.

52   King C. E. and Toskes P. P. (1979) Small intestine bacterial overgrowth. *Gastroenterology* **76**, 1035.

53   Klipstein F. A., Holdeman L. V., Corcino J. J. and Moore W. E. C. (1973) Enterotoxigenic bacteria in tropical sprue. *Ann. Int. Med.* **79**, 632.

54   Levine M. M., Hughes T. P., Black R. E., Clements M. L., Matheny S., Siegel A., Cleaves F., Futierrez C., Foote D. P. and Smith W. (1980) Variability of sodium and sucrose levels of simple sugar/salt oral rehydration solutions prepared under optimal and field conditions. *J. Pediatr.* **97**, 324.

55   Lifshitz F., Coello-Ramirez P., Gutierrez-Topete G. and Gutierrez M. L. C. (1970) Monosaccharide intolerance and hypoglycemia in infants with diarrhea. II. Metabolic studies in 23 infants. *J. Pediatr.* **77**, 604.

56   Martins Campos J. V., Fagundes Neto U., Patricio F. R. S., Wehba J., Carvalho A. A. and Shiner M. (1979) Jejunal mucosa in marasmic children. Clinical, pathological and fine structure evaluation of the effect of protein-energy malnutrition and environmental contamination. *Am. J. Clin. Nutr.* **32**, 1575.

57   Mata L. J., Jiminez F., Cordon M., Rosales R., Prera E., Schneider R. E. and Viteri F. E. (1972a) Gastrointestinal flora of children with protein-calorie malnutrition. *Am. J. Clin. Nutr.* **25**, 1118.

58   Mata L. J., Urrutia J. J., Albertazzi C., Pellecer O. and Arellano E. (1972b) Influence of recurrent infections on nutrition and growth of children in Guatemala. *Am. J. Clin. Nutr.* **25**, 1267.

59   Medical Journal of Australia (1980) Aspirin for childhood gastroenteritis. *Med. J. Aust.* **2**, 358.

60   Mekhjian H. S. and Phillips S. F. (1970) Perfusion of the canine colon with unconjugated bile acids. Effect on water and electrolyte transport, morphology and bile acid absorption. *Gastroenterology* **59**, 120.

61 Mekhjian H. S., Phillips S. F. and Hofmann A. F. (1968) Conjugated bile salts block water and electrolyte transport by the human colon. *Gastroenterology* **54**, 1256.

62 Merson M. H. and Sterky G. (1980) The WHO programme for diarrhoeal diseases control (CDD): The value of oral rehydration therapy. In Abstracts of Symposia and Colloquia, XVI International Congress of Pediatrics, Barcelona, p.434.

63 Morley D. and Woodland M. (1979) *See how they grow — monitoring child growth for appropriate health care in developing countries.* Macmillan, London.

64 Nalin D. R., Levine M. M., Mata L., de Cespedes C., Vargas W., Lizano C., Loria A. R., Simhon A. and Mohs E. (1978) Comparison of sucrose with glucose in oral therapy of infant diarrhoea. *Lancet* **ii**, 277.

65 Pierce N. F. and Gowans J. L. (1975) Cellular kinetics of the intestinal immune response to cholera toxoid in rats. *J. Exp. Med.* **142**, 1550.

66 Rabbani G. H., Greenough W. B. III, Holmgren J. and Lönnroth I. (1979) Chlorpromazine reduces fluid-loss in cholera. *Lancet* **i**, 410.

67 Rowland M. G. M., Barrell R. A. E. and Whitehead R. G. (1978) Bacterial contamination in traditional Gambian weaning foods. *Lancet* **i**, 136.

68 Rowland M. G. M., Cole T. J. and Whitehead R. G. (1977) A quantitative study into the role of infection in determining nutritional status in Gambian village children. *Br. J. Nutr.* **37**, 441.

69 Rowland M. G. M. and McCollum J. P. K. (1977) Malnutrition and gastroenteritis in the Gambia. *Trans. R. Soc. Trop. Med. Hyg.* **71**, 199.

70 Schneider R. E. and Viteri F. (1972) Morphological aspects of the duodenojejunal mucosa in protein-calorie malnourished children and during recovery. *Am. J. Clin. Nutr.* **25**, 1092.

71 Schneider R. E. and Viteri F. (1974) Luminal events of lipid absorption in protein-calorie malnourished children, relationship with nutritional recovery and diarrhea. I. Capacity of the duodenal content to achieve micellar solubilization of lipids. *Am. J. Clin. Nutr.* **27**, 777.

72 Schjönsby H., Drasar B. S., Tabaqchali S. and Booth C. C. (1973) Uptake of vitamin B_{12} by intestinal bacteria in the stagnant loop syndrome. *Scand. J. Gastroenterol.* **8**, 41.

73 Scrimshaw N. S., Taylor C. E. and Gordon J. E. (1968) Interactions of Nutrition and Infection. World Health Organization Monograph Series, Number 57, World Health Organization, Geneva.

74 Sebodo T., Soetarjo Sadjimin T., Soenarto Y. and Sanborn W. T. (1978) Study on the etiology of diarrhea. *Trop. Paediatr. Environ. Child Health* **24**, 107.

75 Shepherd R. W., Butler D. G., Outz E., Gall D. G. and Hamilton J. R. (1979) The mucosal lesion in viral enteritis. Extent and dynamics of the epithelial response to virus invasion in transmissible gastroenteritis of piglets. *Gastroenterology* **76**, 770.

76 Smythe P. M. (1958) Changes in Intestinal Bacterial flora and role of Infection in Kwashiorkor. *Lancet* **ii**, 724.

77 Snow J. (1849) On the pathology and mode of communication of the cholera. *Lond. Med. Gaz.* **44**, 730, 745, 923.

78 Soenarto Y., Sebodo T., Ridho R., Alrasjid H., Rohde J. E., Bugg H. C., Barnes G. L. and Bishop R. F. (1981) Acute diarrhoea and rotavirus infection in newborn babies and children in Yogyakarta, Indonesia, from June 1978 to June 1979. *J. Clin. Microbiol.* **14**, 123.

79 Sprinz H., Scribhibhadh R., Gangarosa B. J., Benyajati C., Kundel D. and Halstead S. (1962) Biopsy of small bowel in Thai people with special reference to recovery from Asiatic cholera and to an intestinal malabsorption syndrome. *Am. J. Clin. Pathol.* **38**, 43.

80 Tabaqchali S., Hatzioannou J. and Booth C. C. (1968) Bile salt deconjugation and steatorrhoea in patients with the stagnant loop syndrome. *Lancet* **ii**, 12.

81 Thelen P., Burke V. and Gracey M. (1978) Effects of intestinal micro-organisms on fluid and electrolyte transport in the rat. *J. Med. Microbiol.* **11**, 463.

82 Tomkins A. M., Drasar B. S., Bradley A. K. and Williamson W. A. (1978) Water supply and nutritional status in rural northern Nigeria. *Trans. R. Soc. Trop. Med. Hyg.* **72**, 239.

83 Trust T. J. and Chipman D. C. (1979) Clinical involvement of *Aeromonas hydrophila. Can. Med. Assoc. J.* **120**, 942.

84   Ulshen M. H. and Rollo J. L. (1980) Pathogenesis of *Escherichia coli* gastroenteritis in man
     — another mechanism. *N. Eng. J. Med.* **302**, 99.
85   Viteri F. and Schneider R. E. (1974) Gastrointestinal alterations in protein-calorie
     malnutrition. *Med. Clin. North Am.* **58**, 1487.
86   Wadstrom T., Aust-Kettis A., Habte D., Holmgren J., Meeuwisse G., Mollby R. and
     Söderlind O. (1976) Enterotoxin-producing bacteria and parasites in stools of Ethiopian
     children with diarrhoeal disease. *Arch. Dis. Childh.* **51**, 865.
87   Waterlow J. C. (1975) Amount and rate of disappearance of liver fat in malnourished infants
     in Jamaica. *Am. J. Clin. Nutr.* **28**, 1330.
88   Waterlow J. C. (1981) Observations on the suckling's dilemma — a personal view. *J. Hum.
     Nutr.* **35**, 85.
89   Wharton B. (1975) Gastroenterological problems of children in developing countries in
     Paediatric Gastroenterology ed. C. M. Anderson and V. Burke, Blackwell, Oxford.
90   Wharton B. A., Howells G. and Phillips I. (1968) Diarrhoea in kwashiorkor. *Br. Med. J.* **4**,
     608.
91   World Health Organization (1976) New trends and approaches in the delivery of maternal
     and child care in health services. WHO Technical Report series No. 600, Geneva.
92   Barua D. (1981) Diarrhoea as a global problem and the WHO programme for its control. In:
     Acute Enteric Infections in Children. New Prospects for Treatment and Prevention pp.1–6,
     Eds T. Holme, J. Holmgren, M. H. Merson and R. Mollby, Elsevier/North-Holland
     Biomedical Press, Amsterdam.
93   Mata L., Kronmal R. A. and Villegas H. (1980) Diarrhoeal diseases: a leading world health
     problem. In: *Cholera and Related Diarrhoeas: Molecular Aspects of a Global Health
     Problem*, p.1–14. Eds O. Ouchterlony and J. Holmgren, S. Karger, Basle.
94   Gracey M., Burke V., Thomas J. A. and Stone D. E. (1975) Effects of microorganisms
     isolated from the upper gut of malnourished children on intestinal sugar absorption *in vivo*.
     Am. J. Clin. Nutr. **26**, 841.

10 Amoebic dysentery, intestinal protozoa and helminths

D. Grove

Introduction	209
Protozoal infections	212
Amoebiasis	212
Giardiasis	216
Helminthic infections	218
Nematode infections	219
Enterobiasis	219
Trichuriasis	223
Ascariasis	224
Hookworm infection	226
Strongyloidiasis	227
Trematodes infections	229
Schistosomiasis *mansoni*	229
Schistosomiasis *japonicum*	233
Cestode infections	234
Taeniasis *saginata*	234
Taeniasis *solium*	237
References	238

INTRODUCTION

Parasitic infections of the gastrointestinal tract are spread widely throughout the world. The prevalence and intensity of these infections is greatest, however, in persons living in the developing countries of the tropics. Indeed, millions of people in these regions harbour multiple infections. It has been estimated that *Entamoeba histolytica* may be found in 500 million people and perhaps 250 million people are infected with *Giardia lamblia*. Helminth infections are even more prevalent. One thousand million people have *Ascaris* infections, several hundred million people have hookworm, *Trichuris*, *Enterobius* or schistosome infections, and tens of millions are infected with *Strongyloides*, *Clonorchis* and *Taenia*.

Many people with parasitic infections are asymptomatic or have only minor symptoms, but the effects in others may be devastating. Since such large numbers of people are infected with gastrointestinal parasites, the contribution of these

TROPHOZOITES   CYSTS

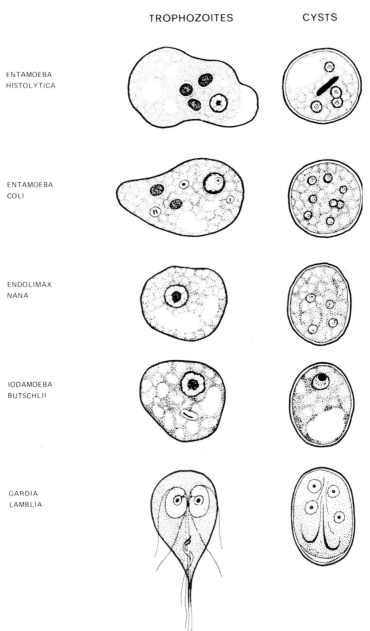

ENTAMOEBA
HISTOLYTICA

ENTAMOEBA
COLI

ENDOLIMAX
NANA

IODAMOEBA
BUTSCHLII

GARDIA
LAMBLIA

Fig. 10.1   Trophozoites and cysts of intestinal protozoa

organisms to human misery is almost incalculable. This chapter reviews the important protozoal infections, amoebiasis and giardiasis. It then discusses the major nematode infections (enterobiasis, trichuriasis, ascariasis, hookworm

WORMS

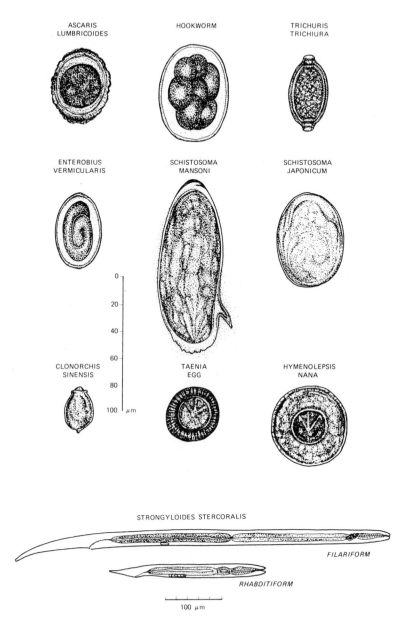

Fig. 10.2 Helminth eggs and *Strongyloides* larvae in the faeces

infection and strongyloidiasis), trematode infections (schistosomiasis) and cestode infections (taeniasis). The appearances of parasites commonly found in the faeces are illustrated in Figs 10.1 and 10.2.

PROTOZOAL INFECTIONS

Protozoa infecting the gastrointestinal tract are able to live and reproduce in the bowel, thus they behave biologically rather like gut bacteria. Representatives of amoebae (Sarcodina), flagellates (Mastigophora) and ciliates (Ciliata) can infect humans. Most of the protozoa found in the gastrointestinal tract dwell in the lumen, although *Entamoeba histolytica* and *Balantidum coli* have the capacity to invade the tissues. The forms found in the bowel are trophozites, while those which are passed in the faeces are encysted in order to withstand the rigours of the environment and facilitate transmission to other individuals.

When a protozoan is found in the faeces, the first question which must be asked is whether the organism is a commensal or a pathogen. If the parasite is a potential pathogen, then it is necessary to decide whether the parasite is likely to be causing disease in that patient. This can only be done by taking into account the clinical manifestations in that person. Protozoa found in the gastrointestinal tract which are either nonpathogenic or of only limited significance are listed in Table 10.1.

Table 10.1 Protozoal infections of minor importance

Parasite	Clinical features	Drug of choice
Balantidium coli	Usually nil Diarrhoea	Tetracycline
Chilomastix mesnili	Nonpathogenic	Unnecessary
Dientamoeba fragilis	Usually nil ? diarrhoea	Tetracycline
Endolimax nana	Nonpathogenic	Unnecessary
Entamoeba coli	Nonpathogenic	Unnecessary
Entamoeba hartmanni	Nonpathogenic	Unnecessary
Entamoeba polecki	Nonpathogenic	Unnecessary
Enteromonas hominis	Nonpathogenic	Unnecessary
Iodamoeba butschlii	Nonpathogenic	Unnecessary
Isopora species	Usually nil Diarrhoea	Usually self-limited
Trichomonas hominis	Nonpathogenic	Unnecessary

Note: most infections occur worldwide.

AMOEBIASIS

TAXONOMY AND PATHOGENICITY

Controversy has surrounded the parasitic amoebae of humans for most of the twentieth century. An inaccurate description of the reproduction of *E. histolytica* and *E. coli* caused years of confusion. This was compounded by those who promulgated the doctrine that *E. histolytica* is always a pathogen. It is only in recent times that this dispute has been resolved; most investigators now agree that this parasite, although a potential pathogen, is usually a commensal inhabitant of the gastrointestinal tract.[3]

Nevertheless, problems still remain. Morphologically similar or identical forms of *E. histolytica* have been subclassified in several ways. Firstly, organisms have been categorized on the basis of size. Cysts have been divided into 'large race' with a diameter $>10\,\mu m$ and 'small race' with a diameter of $\leqslant 10\,\mu m$. Argument still continues as to whether the latter form merits designation as a separate species, *E. hartmanni*. Such taxonomic niceties do not matter for the clinician, however, as it is only the large forms which are likely to be pathogenic and require intervention. Secondly, *E. histolytica* has been classified on the basis of growth characteristics. Classical strains grow best at 37° C, whereas atypical, 'Laredo-type' strains grow well at both 37° C and at room temperature (25° C). Some authors consider the latter strains to be a separate species, as yet unnamed. 'Laredo-type' strains are less likely to be pathogenic than are classical strains. Thirdly, *E. histolytica* strains have been demarcated recently by the presence or absence of an enzyme, phosphoglucomutase.[23] This enzyme is present in organisms obtained from patients with clinical amoebiasis, but not in amoebae isolated from asymptomatic carriers. Finally, there are other types of amoebae which are similar morphologically to *E. histolytica* but are nonpathogenic for man; they include *E. polecki*, *E. moshkovskii* and *E. invadens* in pigs, sewage, and snakes, respectively.

MORPHOLOGY AND LIFE CYCLE

There are three different stages in the life cycle of *E. histolytica*. Motile trophozoites range in size up to $50\,\mu m$ in 'diameter'. There is a single nucleus with a delicate membrane, finely beaded peripheral chromatin and a small central endosome. The cytoplasm of the large race form may contain ingested red cells. Precysts are formed when food particles are digested or extruded; the parasite shrinks, becomes more spherical in shape, and secretes a cell wall. Cysts are non-motile, spherical and smaller in size than trophozoites, usually being $< 20\,\mu m$ in diameter. Depending upon the degree of maturation, they contain one, two or four nuclei, which resemble those seen in trophozoites. In young cysts chromatoid bodies with rounded ends may be seen in the cytoplasm.

All three stages of the organism may be found in the faeces of infected persons; trophozoites predominate in diarrhoeic stools and cysts are found in formed material. Trophozoites are not infective if ingested as they are destroyed by gastric secretions. The cysts are resistant, however, and excyst in the small intestine; the released trophozoites divide by binary fission.

EPIDEMIOLOGY

E. histolytica is found throughout the world; the prevalence is inversely proportional to environmental sanitation and personal hygienic practices.[12] Consequently, the prevalence of infection in some developing countries in the tropics approaches 50% but is only 1% in many industrialized countries. High prevalence rates are probably the result of constant reinfection. The organism is transmitted primarily via cysts present in contaminated water and food, particularly fresh vegetables. Cysts are viable for several days in water at 30° C; they are killed by hyperchlorination, but not by the usual municipal chlorination methods. The organism may also be transmitted venereally, especially in homosexuals.

PATHOGENESIS

Invasive amoebiasis is common in tropical regions while significant disease is rare in temperate zones. The factors which determine virulence are ill-understood. There may be a spectrum of pathogenicity among the various strains of *E. histolytica*,[3] although it has been claimed that any strain can become invasive under the right conditions.[10,30] It is probable that amoebae are only pathogenic in the presence of intestinal bacteria.[32] Avirulent organisms live in the intestinal lumen while virulent trophozoites invade host tissues by discharging enzymes which destroy cells. Primary lesions begin as minute erosions which enlarge by lateral necrosis producing flask-shaped ulcers up to 2 cm across. Lesions may involve the whole of the large bowel. There is little inflammatory reaction until secondary bacterial infection supervenes. During invasion of the submucosa, amoebae may enter blood vessels and be carried to other parts of the body, particularly the liver.

CLINICAL FEATURES

The majority of patients have asymptomatic amoebic infections. In symptomatic patients, there is a wide range in the modes of presentation and in the severity of the clinical manifestations.[1] The onset is usually gradual over several weeks with the appearance of abdominal discomfort, which may become painful and colicky, and frequent, loose, watery stools containing variable amounts of blood and mucus. Some patients have few constitutional symptoms while others are prostrated. Examination frequently reveals lower abdominal tenderness. The liver may be slightly enlarged and tender; this is nonspecific and does not indicate hepatic amoebiasis. In severe cases, patients look ill, are febrile and dehydrated. Weight loss is common. Sigmoidoscopy commonly reveals ulcers in the rectal mucosa. There may be pinpoint erosions or well-developed ulcers up to 2 cm in diameter with a punched-out appearance, a whitish-yellow base and a narrow rim of swollen mucosa. Symptoms and signs often subside spontaneously after a few weeks or months, but relapses are frequent.

A number of complications may supervene. Amoebic colitis may become fulminant. Peritonitis may result from acute perforation or slow leakage. Intestinal obstruction may follow the formation of an amoebic stricture or amoeboma. Occasionally, an ulcer may haemorrhage severely. In some patients, a chronic, irritative bowel syndrome may persist for several weeks to months after treatment, even though amoebae can no longer be found; this usually subsides spontaneously.

Extraintestinal spread may occur whether or not amoebic dysentery is present. A number of organs may be affected; the liver is most frequently involved but the lungs, pericardium, brain and skin may occasionally be invaded. These conditions have been well reviewed.[2,16]

LABORATORY DIAGNOSIS

Microscopy

A definitive diagnosis of amoebiasis depends upon finding *E. histolytica* in the stools or in scrapings of rectal mucosa. Unfortunately, errors of omission or commission in the laboratory are not uncommon. Failure to find organisms may result from incorrect handling of specimens or inexperience of laboratory personnel.[14] Trophozoites may lyse if left standing at room temperature. A number of substances may interfere with stool examinations; these include prior administration of antibiotics, antiprotozoal agents, radiological contrast media, antidiarrhoeal preparations containing bismuth or kaolin, and finally tap water, which lyses trophozoites. At the other extreme, false positive identifications may be made, usually by mistaking white cells (which may ingest red cells) for parasites.[20]

Ideally, specimens should be examined within 1 hour of collection; this allows identification of motile, haematophagous trophozoites in saline preparations. In addition, faeces should be preserved in 10% formalin (for cysts) and in polyvinyl alcohol (for trophozoites) in order to permit confirmation of the diagnosis and to provide a permanent record. Slides prepared from this material may be stained with iron haematoxylin or Wheatley's trichrome at leisure.

Serology

Serological tests are a useful aid in invasive amoebiasis. They are positive in $\leqslant 95\%$ of patients with extraintestinal amoebiasis and in 80–90% of those with amoebic dysentery, but are of little value in asymptomatic cyst-passers. Some assays, such as the indirect haemagglutination and latex agglutination tests remain positive for months or years after treatment, whereas precipitin reactions like the gel diffusion and cellulose acetate precipitin tests are usually positive only when there is active disease.[22]

TREATMENT

Opinions differ as to which persons with amoebic infection should be treated and which drugs should be used.[17.19] Whether or not patients with asymptomatic infections should be treated is much debated. A compromise view is that persons living in endemic areas should not be treated as rapid reinfection is so common, but that the organisms should be eradicated from patients in industrialized countries. A luminal amoebicide which kills cysts, such as diloxanide furoate, should be given 5 mg/kg t.d.s. orally for 10 days. *E. hartmanni* does not need to be treated.

Patients with symptomatic amoebic dysentery should be treated with a tissue amoebicide. In recent years, metronidazole 10 mg/kg t.d.s. orally for 5 days has been most frequently prescribed; this regimen is effective in more than 90% of patients.[1] Recent studies have suggested that tinidazole given in a daily dose of 30 mg/kg for 3 days has less side-effects and is more effective in both amoebic dysentery and in amoebic liver abscess.[5] This regimen will probably become the treatment of choice. Since both metronidazole and tinidazole are inactive against cysts, therapy with those drugs should be followed by a course of diloxanide furoate.

CONTROL

Wherever possible, the source of infection should be determined and organisms eradicated. This is not feasible in most developing countries, however, and prevention depends upon interruption of transmission. Faecal contamination of food and water should be avoided. If the source of food and water is uncertain, the only sure way of killing amoebae is by boiling water and thorough cooking of vegetables, while fresh vegetables such as lettuce should be avoided.

GIARDIASIS

TAXONOMY

The nomenclature of the organism causing giardiasis is unresolved. The human parasite has been given a number of names including, *Giardia lamblia*, *Giardia intestinalis*, *Lamblia intestinalis* and *Giardia duodenalis.*[25.26]

MORPHOLOGY AND LIFE CYCLE

Giardia lamblia is a flagellate protozoan. The trophozoites are 9×15 μm in size; the dorsal surface is convex and the flattened ventral surface has a large sucking disc. The organisms have two nuclei, a crescent-shaped parabasal body, two central axostyles and four pairs of flagella. They multiply by binary fission and are found attached to the epithelium of the upper small intestine. Some parasites encyst in the gut lumen. The ovoid cysts, 7×11 μm in size and with four nuclei, are passed in the faeces. When cysts are ingested, trophozoites excyst in the upper small intestine.

EPIDEMIOLOGY

Human infections are found throughout the world but are more common in the tropics where prevalence rates may reach 30%. In most areas, the infection is endemic and is related to poor standards of hygiene; the parasite is spread from hand and food contaminated with infected faeces to mouth. In such communities, the prevalence and severity of symptoms is greatest in children. In recent years, water-borne epidemics of giardiasis have been recognized, particularly in temperate areas such as the USA.[40] *G. lamblia* may also be transmitted venereally, particularly among homosexuals.[27]

In endemic areas, humans are the major reservoir of infection. The recognition of water-borne epidemics in areas where there is faecal pollution of animal but not human origin has raised the possibility that animal *Giardia species* may infect man. Cysts do not survive desiccation but remain viable in water for up to 4 days at 37° C and for several months at 8° C. They are killed by boiling but freeze-thawing is unreliable; they are resistant to chlorination.

PATHOGENESIS

It is uncertain whether the pathological and clinical manifestations of infection result from mechanical obstruction by trophozoites lining the small bowel mucosa, mechanical irritation with functional enzyme deficiencies, or bacterial overgrowth.[48] In some patients, the sheer multitude of trophozoites lining the small bowel may impair absorption. Scanning electron microscopical studies have shown that the sucking discs by which the trophozoites adhere to the mucosa cause considerable irritation to the microvilli. This may be associated with functional deficiencies of disaccharidase, peptide hydrolase and enteropeptidase activity. In some *Giardia* infections, there may be overgrowth of bacteria in the small bowel lumen which may exacerbate malabsorption. Other suggestions include competition by *Giardia* with the host for nutrients, and the production of toxins by the organisms.

Different geographical strains of *Giardia* may vary in their pathogenicity. Large inocula of cysts may facilitate infection as do a number of host factors. Hypochlorhydria and achlorhydria have been shown to enhance infection. Since adults in endemic areas have low intensities of infection and little symptomatic disease, it seems likely that there is some acquired resistance to this infection.[18] Studies in Colorado have shown that short-term residents had higher attack rates than did longterm inhabitants. Similar observations have been made in animal models. For example, mice acquired resistance to reinfection with *G. muris*. On the other hand, hypothymic mice with impaired cell-mediated immunity were unable to eliminate the infection. The importance of immune responses is indicated by the marked association between symptomatic giardiasis and hypo-gammaglobulinaemia in humans. It is possible that the immunodeficient individual is at no greater risk than the immunocompetent person of acquiring giardiasis, but should he do so, then he is more likely to have a symptomatic illness. Patients with selective IgA deficiency do not appear to be more prone to giardiasis.

CLINICAL FEATURES

Many infected persons are asymptomatic, particularly in endemic areas. The acute illness is most marked in those exposed to the organism for the first time. After an incubation period of 1–3 weeks, there is frequently a sudden onset of explosive, watery diarrhoea, abdominal distension and discomfort, flatulence, nausea and anorexia. After a week or so, the symptoms resolve spontaneously or subside into a low-grade, chronic infection with diarrhoea, weight loss and debility which may last for several months. The stools may be greasy and some patients with heavy infections develop a malabsorption syndrome.

LABORATORY DIAGNOSIS

Parasites can usually be found in the stools, although examination of different specimens of faeces may need to be repeated.[48] When *Giardia* cannot be found in the faeces in patients in whom the diagnosis is strongly suspected, the organisms may sometimes be identified in duodenal fluid obtained with the string test.[7] Serology is of little use in the diagnosis of giardiasis.

TREATMENT

Symptomatic persons must be treated as should infected persons in nonendemic areas. It is pointless treating asymptomatic, infected people in endemic areas as reinfection is common. The usual regimen has been to administer metronidazole 5 mg/kg t.d.s. orally for 5 or 10 days; infection is eradicated in up to 90% of patients. Recent studies have shown that tinidazole is more effective and has less side-effects;[5] it is given in a dose of 30 mg/kg orally each day for 2 days.

CONTROL

In endemic areas, only foods which have been cooked or peeled should be eaten. Water should be boiled.

HELMINTHIC INFECTIONS

The biological behaviour of helminths is quite different from protozoa. With the important exception of *S. stercoralis*, worms are not able to replicate within the human host. This has major implications for pathogenesis, clinical manifestations and treatment. In gastrointestinal helminth infections, the prime determinant of whether infection causes ill-health is the number of worms. Since worms are unable to multiply and there is relatively little development of immunity to reinfection, the worm burden is proportional to both the intensity and duration of exposure to infective forms. Thus, the severity of schistosomiasis depends upon the worm burden and this can be correlated with the number of eggs excreted in the faeces. Similarly, the degree of iron deficiency anaemia in hookworm infection is proportional to the blood loss, which in turn reflects the worm burden. Consequently, it is important to quantify the intensity of infection as well as to assess the patient for evidence of the presence and severity of disease. Even so, it is often difficult to be certain whether symptoms and signs are due to a given worm, as concurrent infections with other gastrointestinal pathogens are frequent. When all of these factors are taken into account, rational therapy may be instituted. In most instances, asymptomatic patients with small worm burdens do not require treatment but patients with heavy intensities of infection or evidence of disease need to be treated. Furthermore, since low intensities of infection are unlikely to lead to disease, it is unnecessary to eradicate all the worms; a marked reduction in worm burden is sufficient.

NEMATODE INFECTIONS

Nematodes are roundworms; they are cylindrical in shape, unsegmented, have a body cavity and gut, and are either male or female. Intestinal roundworms are the most important helminth infections of man; more than 1000 million people are infected with one or more of these parasites. The life cycles of the major pathogens are relatively simple as there are no intermediate hosts. *Enterobius vermicularis* and *Trichuris trichiura* are acquired by ingestion of eggs; they develop directly into adult worms in the gut, the former usually lying free in the lumen and the latter being partly attached to the intestinal mucosa. Infection with *Ascaris lumbricoides* also occurs after ingestion of eggs, but larvae liberated in the intestinal lumen invade the tissues and pass via the bloodstream to the lungs before returning to the gastrointestinal tract where they mature. Hookworms and *Strongyloides stercoralis* have a similar migration, but infection occurs when larvae penetrate the intact skin rather than after ingestion of eggs. Eosinophilic and IgE responses develop only when parasites are in direct contact with the tissues. With the exception of strongyloidiasis, immunological tests have little place in the diagnosis of these infections. These five species will be discussed in some detail. Nematode infections of lesser importance are summarized in Table 10.2.

Enterobiasis

LIFE CYCLE

When eggs of *E. vermicularis* are ingested, larvae hatch in the upper intestine and

Table 10.2 Nematode infections of minor importance

Parasite	Geographical distribution	Mode of acquisition	Location in host	Clinical features	Drug of choice
Angiostrongylus costaricensis	Central America	Ingestion of contaminated vegetables	Mesenteric vessels	Abdominal pain, abdominal mass, fever	Nil satisfactory
Anisakis species	Worldwide	Ingestion of infected, raw salt-water fish	Intraluminal or invasion of stomach or intestinal mucosa	Variable	Nil satisfactory
Capillaria philippinenis	Philippines, Thailand	Ingestion of infected, raw, freshwater fish	Partly embedded in SI mucosa	Abdominal pain, diarrhoea, malabsorption	Mebendazole
Trichostrongylus species	Predominantly Asia	Ingestion of contaminated food	Heads embedded in SI mucosa	Usually nil	Bephenium hydroxynapthhoate

SI, small intestine.

migrate to the region of the caecum where they mature, copulate, and may temporarily attach to the intestinal mucosa. Between 3 and 6 weeks after infection, the white, thread-like, 1 cm long, gravid females move down the bowel and pass out of the anus at night; each worm deposits approximately 10 000 eggs, 25×55 µm in size, on the peri-anal skin then dies. The eggs embryonate and are infective within a few hours of deposition.

EPIDEMIOLOGY

The worm is found in both tropical and temperate areas where up to 20% of the population may be infected. There is no predilection for specific socioeconomic conditions, but infections are commonly clustered in families and institutions. Man is the only reservoir of infection and children are more frequently infected. Autoinfection occurs when eggs are transferred from anus to mouth by fingers; this is enhanced by pruritis ani. Eggs remain viable for up to 3 weeks and may be transferred from person to person by contaminated clothing, bedding or dust.

PATHOGENESIS

There is little host response to adult worms and eosinophil and IgE levels are normal. Resistance does not develop and reinfections are common. Pruritis ani may be related to an immunological reaction, but this is unproven. In women, parasites may sometimes migrate through the vagina and uterus to the Fallopian tubes or, less frequently, the peritoneal cavity, or via the urethra to the bladder. Rarely, worms may invade the appendix and produce a granulomatous reaction.

CLINICAL FEATURES

Most patients are asymptomatic.[11,47] A small proportion of patients complain of nocturnal pruritis ani and consequent insomnia.

LABORATORY DIAGNOSIS

Adult worms may be seen with the naked eye, particularly when the peri-anal region is inspected at night. Eggs are rarely seen in conventional stool examinations. They are best recovered using a sticky cellophane tape which is pressed repeatedly on the peri-anal skin on arising in the morning. It is then placed, adhesive side down, onto a drop of toluene (which clears the tape) on a microscope slide and scanned under low power.

Table 10.3 Anthelmintics for intestinal nematode infections

	E. vermicularis	T. trichiura	A. lumbricoides	Hookworms	S. stercoralis
Bephenium hydroxynaphthoate	—	—	(5 g once)	5 g once	—
Levamisole	—	—	2.5 mg/kg once	(2.5 mg/kg 3 days)	—
Mebendazole	100 mg once	100 mg b.d. 3 days	100 mg b.d. 3 days	100 mg b.d. 3 days	—
Piperazine citrate	50 mg/kg 7 days	—	50 mg/kg 2 days	—	—
Pyrantel embonate	10 mg/kg once	—	10 mg/kg once	10 mg/kg† 1–3 days	—
Thiabendazole	25 mg/kg b.d.* 1 day	—	(25 mg/kg 2 days)	(25 mg/kg b.d. 3 days)	25 mg/kg b.d. 3 days
Viprynium embonate	5 mg/kg once	—	—	—	—

( ), Partial activity, not drug of choice. *Unpleasant side effects. †Once for *Ancyclostoma duodenale*, 3 days for *Necator americanus*.

TREATMENT

A large number of drugs are effective (Table 10.3). Mebendazole in single dose of 100 mg for all ages is perhaps the drug of choice.[28] It may be necessary to repeat the course in 2–3 weeks. Since the infection frequently occurs in families, it is reasonable to treat all other members of the family. While sanitary measures alone do not eradicate infection,[37] they may be used in conjunction with specific anthelmintic therapy as this may reduce the chances of reinfection. Children should be showered in the morning and their finger nails cut, clothing and bedding boiled, and the rooms thoroughly vacuumed.

CONTROL

It is difficult to prevent reinfection, particularly from extrafamilial sources.[24] Treatment must be reinstituted if symptoms return and eggs are found.

Trichuriasis

LIFE CYCLE

When eggs of *T. trichiura* are ingested, larvae hatch in the small intestine. Mature worms, 3–5 cm long and with a whip-like anterior 60% and fleshy posterior 40%, attach to the large intestinal mucosa by the head and begin producing eggs 1–3 months after infection. Adult worms probably live for several years and each female produces 5000 eggs, $25 \times 50 \, \mu m$ in size, per day. After excretion in the faeces, embryonic development takes place over the next 2–4 weeks in a warm, shady, humid environment; the egg is then infective.

EPIDEMIOLOGY

The worm is found in warm, moist areas of the world where it may infect up to 100% of the population. It is most common in poor, rural areas where sanitary conditions are lacking. Man is the principal reservoir. Infection is acquired by ingestion of contaminated food, water or soil.

PATHOGENESIS

Resistance to reinfection probably does not develop. Light infections produce little reaction in the bowel but massive infections may lead to inflammation and mucosal necrosis. Opinions differ as to whether a blood eosinophilia is found. It is controversial whether blood loss occurs, but one group of investigators estimated that adult worms suck 0.005 ml of blood/worm/day from the mucosa;[21] anaemia is very unlikely as a result of trichuriasis.

224   *D. Grove*

CLINICAL FEATURES

The vast majority of infected persons are asymptomatic. In heavy infections, diarrhoea, abdominal pain and rectal prolapse due to mucosal oedema may appear.

LABORATORY DIAGNOSIS

Eggs are readily seen on a simple faecal smear as *Trichuris* has a high egg output (200 eggs/g faeces/female worm). Occasionally, adult worms may be seen on proctoscopy or sigmoidoscopy.

TREATMENT

Anthelmintic therapy is only required in symptomatic patients or persons with heavy infections ($\geqslant$30,000 eggs/g faeces $\equiv$ 300 worms). Mebendazole is the most effective drug[39] (Table 10.3). Trichuriasis can only be controlled with improved environmental sanitation.

Ascariasis

LIFE CYCLE

When eggs of *A. lumbricoides* are ingested, larvae hatch in the small intestine then penetrate the mucosa and pass via the bloodstream to the lungs where they enter the alveolar spaces and ascend the airways. They are then swallowed and within 1–2 weeks of infection return to the intestines where they mature. The adult worms, 15–35 cm long, live in the gut lumen, especially in the jejunum. Egg production begins two months after infection. Adult worms live for up to 12 months and each female produces 200 000 ova, $40 \times 60\ \mu m$ in size, per day. Under warm, shady, moist conditions, eggs become infective 2–3 weeks after excretion in the faeces.

EPIDEMIOLOGY

Ascariasis occurs widely throughout the tropics and subtropics. It has been estimated that more than 1000 million people are infected. Man is the only reservoir of infection. Infection is prevalent in areas where sanitation is poor and human faeces are used as fertilizer. The eggs are highly resistant to heat and desiccation and may survive for months to years in the soil. Transmission is continuous throughout the year in moist climates, but embryogenesis occurs only during the rainy season in drier regions. Infection is acquired by ingestion of contaminated food and soil. It is found in all age groups, but more commonly in children.

PATHOGENESIS

The pathological responses to migratory larvae are speculative; it is probable that there is usually little reaction, but sometimes granulomas may develop around larvae in the lungs producing ascaris pneumonia. Adult worms in the intestines rarely cause pathological changes. *Ascaris* infections may contribute to malnutrition by inhibiting protein absorption[42] but this is probably significant only in areas where food intake is deficient.[9] Resistance to reinfection is absent or incomplete.

CLINICAL FEATURES

Although larval migration through the lungs may be associated with pulmonary infiltrates with eosinophilia, this is uncommon; only four cases were found in 13 000 patients in Colombia.[41] For uncertain reasons, it is a more frequent event in some areas such as Saudi Arabia where transmission is seasonal.

Most persons with small adult worm loads are either asymptomatic or have ill-defined abdominal discomfort. Occasionally, a bolus of worms may cause intestinal obstruction; this usually happens in young children.[8] Obstructive jaundice has rarely resulted from worms ascending the biliary tree. Ascarids have been found in a number of aberrant sites, but such events occur in only a very small proportion of infected persons.

LABORATORY DIAGNOSIS

Since *A. lumbricoides* has a high egg output (5000 eggs/g faeces/female worm), ova are readily seen in a simple faecal smear. Occasionally, adult worms are passed spontaneously.

TREATMENT

All patients with intestinal ascariasis should be treated. A number of effective drugs are available, but in uncomplicated patients, mebendazole is probably the drug of choice (Table 10.3). In early intestinal obstruction thought to be due to ascariasis, a trial of conservative treatment is warranted. Piperazine should be used as it narcotizes the worm. It is administered as a syrup through a nasogastric tube, 150 mg/kg initially, followed by several doses of 50 mg/kg at 12–hourly intervals. This regimen may also be useful in biliary obstruction. Advanced obstruction requires surgical intervention.

CONTROL

Ascariasis can be controlled by improved environmental sanitation with the installation of waste disposal systems and by not using human faeces as fertilizer for vegetable gardens. Unfortunately, these ideals are unlikely to be met in most endemic areas where economic conditions are poor. Where facilities are available, health education measures need to be improved. Even in rich countries like the USA, ascariasis is endemic in some areas. Repeated mass administration of anthelmintics has been used with success in some areas but not in others.[4]

Hookworm infection

Humans are infected commonly with either *Ancylostoma duodenale* or *Necator americanus*, but a dog hookworm, *Ancylostoma ceylanicum* sometimes reaches maturity.[6] Since the eggs of *N. americanus* and *A. duodenale* are indistinguishable, infections are usually classified as hookworm rather than necatoriasis or ancylostomiasis.

LIFE CYCLE

Infective (filariform) larvae penetrate intact skin and pass via the bloodstream to the lungs where they enter the alveolar spaces and ascend the airways. They are then swallowed and mature in the small intestine. The white, cylindrical adult worms, about 1 cm long, attach to the small intestinal mucosa by the mouth and may live for several years. Egg deposition usually begins 4–6 weeks after skin penetration. The average output of eggs, 40×60 μm in size, by adult females is 10–20 000 per day. The ova are deposited in the faeces on the ground and under warm, moist conditions, they hatch larvae which moult twice over the next 1–2 weeks and become infective filariform larvae.

The cycle just described is the usual one, but variations may occur with *A. duodenale*. This parasite may also be acquired by oral ingestion[29] and possibly by transmammary transmission.[6] Furthermore, in some circumstances, it may have a dormant period with maturity being delayed some months.[6]

EPIDEMIOLOGY

Hookworms are widespread in warm regions of the world and infect hundreds of millions of people. Man is the reservoir of infection. Infection is prevalent where sanitation is poor and people walk barefoot. Maximal development of larvae occurs in well-aerated, moist, shaded soil with temperatures between 23° and 33° C.

PATHOGENESIS

A mild inflammatory reaction develops around the site of attachment of worms to the intestinal mucosa. The average daily blood loss is 0.03 ml/worm for *N. americanus* and 0.2 ml/worm for *A. duodenale*. Whether or not hookworm disease results from hookworm infection depends upon the worm burden (which determines blood loss) and nutritional status (which determines the ability to replace lost blood). For example, in Venezuela, only egg counts of >2000/ml faeces in women and children and >5000/ml faeces in men were associated with anaemia.[36] Significant immunity to hookworm probably does not develop.

CLINICAL FEATURES

Skin penetration by larvae may cause a pruritic, papulovesicular rash, particularly in repeated infections. Migration of larvae through the lungs is usually asymptomatic, but occasionally pulmonary infiltrates with eosinophilia may occur. The majority of persons with light worm loads are asymptomatic. The major manifestations of hookworm disease are iron deficiency anaemia and hypoalbuminaemia with their attendant symptoms and signs.

LABORATORY DIAGNOSIS

Eggs can be readily detected in simple faecal smears when the concentration is above 1000/g faeces, *N. americanus* has an egg output of approximately 50 ova/g faeces/female worm. The intensity of infections must be quantitated.

TREATMENT

Light infections in asymptomatic persons need no treatment. Patients with symptoms or women and children with egg counts of >1000/g faeces and men with levels of >2000/g faeces should be treated with one of the anthelmintics indicated in Table 10.3. Iron should be replaced and when anaemia is very severe, blood transfusion may be necessary.

Control measures are similar to those described for ascariasis.

Strongyloidiasis

LIFE CYCLE

The life cycle of *Strongyloides stercoralis* is complex. The infection is acquired in the same way as hookworm with infective larvae penetrating the skin, passing via the bloodstream to the lungs and then to the small intestine where they mature.

Males are rarely found, but female worms burrow into the mucosa and release eggs which rapidly develop into first-stage (rhabditiform) larvae, 250 μm long which first appear in the stools 3–4 weeks after infection. These larvae may then enter either a free-living or parasitic cycle. In the free-living cycle, larvae develop either directly into infective (filariform) larvae or into free-living adults which in turn produce large numbers of filariform larvae, 500 μm long. In the parasitic cycle, autoinfection occurs, i.e. rhabditiform larvae develop into infective larvae within the human host and penetrate the intestinal mucosa or the perianal skin and undergo the usual migration. It is this ability, extremely unusual among worms, of replicating within man that accounts for persistence of infection for up to 40 years.

EPIDEMIOLOGY

S. stercoralis is widespread in warm, moist regions of the world, but it is also found in some temperate areas. Man is the reservoir of infection and tens or hundreds of millions of people are infected. Environmental conditions conducive to the spread of hookworm also favour transmission of strongyloidiasis.

PATHOGENESIS

A mild inflammatory reaction may be seen around adult worms in the intestinal mucosa. Complete immunity does not develop as infection persists for many years. However, the infection is contained as the prime manifestations are usually limited to the skin and the gastrointestinal tract. If a person with strongyloidiasis should become immunosuppressed as a result of the administration of cortico-steroids, irradiation, malnutrition, lepromatous leprosy, lymphoma or leu-kaemia, then hyperinfection occurs with rapid multiplication and dissemination of worms throughout the body, often with concomitant septicaemia, resulting in death.[38]

CLINICAL FEATURES

Many patients are asymptomatic but others have cutaneous or gastrointestinal complaints.[13] Larva currens is pathognomonic; transient urticarial eruptions migrate in a serpiginous fashion at speeds of up to 10 cm/hour. More commonly, crops of stationary weals appear, particularly on the buttock and around the waist; they last 1–2 days and recur at irregular intervals. Weight loss may develop and patients may complain of diarrhoea, pruritis ani, indigestion and lower abdominal pain. In more severe infections, malabsorption or protein-losing enteropathy may develop. Although pulmonary infiltrates with eosinophilia have been described, they are probably uncommon. In disseminated strongyloidiasis, severe abdominal pain, intestinal obstruction, Gram-negative septicaemia, pneumonitis, and meningitis may supervene.

LABORATORY DIAGNOSIS

The definitive diagnosis depends upon finding larvae in faeces or duodenal fluid, but this may be extremely difficult as the parasite load is usually low. Duodenal fluid may be obtained with an Enterotest capsule.[7] The most reliable technique however, is repeated examination of fresh samples of faeces.[13]

TREATMENT

All persons infected with *S. stercoralis* should be treated with the aim of eradicating the infection. The drug of choice is thiabendazole, 25 mg/kg b.d. for 3 days. Unfortunately, this regimen is not always effective in achieving eradication. Control measures are similar to those described for ascariasis.

TREMATODES INFECTIONS

Trematodes, or flukes, are distinguished from other worms by their shape, which is often leaf-like, the lack of segmentation, the absence of a body cavity and an incomplete gut. All of the species parasitic in man have an alternation of generations in which sexual reproduction of adult worms in the human is followed by asexual multiplication of the larval stages in a molluscan intermediate host. Human parasites may be divided into two groups: (a) the schistosomes which are more cylindrical in shape, have separate sexes, and dwell in blood vessels and (b) the rest which are leaf-like, hermaphroditic and live in the gut, liver or lung. The schistosomes are of major importance with more than 200 million people around the globe being infected. The two species infecting the gastrointestinal system, *Schistosoma mansoni* and *S. japonicum*, will be discussed in some detail. Infection with intestinal and liver flukes are usually diagnosed by finding eggs in the faeces or duodenal fluid. These organisms are of less importance on a worldwide scale, and the salient features are summarized in Table 10.4.

Schistosomiasis *mansoni*

LIFE CYCLE

Fork-tailed larvae known as cercariae rapidly penetrate the intact skin when a person comes into contact with infected water. They lose their tails in the process and the resultant schistosomula migrate through the lungs to the portal vessels where they mature. Adult worms, 1–2 cm long, mate to form worm pairs in which the cylindrical female worm lies in a canal formed by the folded margins of the male. They migrate backwards to the small venules of the gut where they may live for 5–10 years. Approximately 6 weeks after infection, egg production begins; most eggs pass through the intestinal mucosa and are excreted in the faeces, but a

Table 10.4 Trematode infections of minor importance

Parasite	Geographical distribution	Mode of acquisition	Location in host	Clinical features	Drug of choice
Clonorchis sinensis	East Asia	Ingestion of infected, raw freshwater fish	Bile ducts	Usually nil	Nil satisfactory
Dicrocoelium dendriticum	Worldwide	? Ingestion of parasitized ants	Bile ducts	Usually nil	Nil satisfactory
Echinostoma ilocanum	Asia	Ingestion of infected, raw snails and clams	Attached to SI mucosa	Usually nil	Nil satisfactory
Fasciola species	Worldwide	Ingestion of contaminated vegetation	Liver parenchyma or bile ducts	Nil hepatitis	Nil satisfactory
Fasciolopsis	Asia	Ingestion of contaminated fruit and vegetables	Attached to SI mucosa	Usually nil	Hexylresorcinol
Gastrodiscoides hominis	Asia	?	Attached to LI mucosa	Usually nil	Nil satisfactory
Heterophyes heterophyes	North Africa Asia	Ingestion of infected, raw fish	Attached to SI mucosa	Usually nil	Hexylresorcinol
Metagonimus yokogawi	Predominantly East Asia	Ingestion of infected, raw freshwater fish	Attached to SI mucosa	Usually nil	Hexylresorcinol
Opisthorchis species	Europe Asia	Ingestion of infected, raw freshwater fish	Bile ducts	Usually nil	Nil satisfactory
Schistosoma intercalatum	West and Central Africa	Contact with infected water	Mesenteric vessels	Usually nil	Niridazole

SI, small intestine. LI, large intestine.

proportion of them embolize to the liver. The oval-shaped eggs are approximately 60×160 μm wide and have a characteristic sharp lateral spine. If faeces are deposited in fresh water, the eggs hatch and release motile larvae called miracidia which penetrate the bodies of snails. Within each snail, the miracidium forms a sporocyst in which asexual multiplication occurs; 3–4 weeks later, large numbers of cercariae are released into the water.

EPIDEMIOLOGY

S. mansoni is endemic in many countries in Africa, the Middle East and Central and South America. In many areas the prevalence of infection is increasing, particularly in association with irrigation projects.

The transmission of schistosomiasis depends upon the presence of water, suitable intermediate hosts, various environmental factors and the social habits of the population. Man is the only significant reservoir of infection. *S. mansoni* will only develop in snails of the genus *Biomphalaria*. They are found principally in still, shallow areas of ponds and waterways with appropriate vegetation, abundance of organic material, and little pollution. Schistosomiasis can only occur in areas with inadequate sewerage where people defaecate near streams. The intensity of infection in a person is related to the degree of water contact, much of which is determined by the availability of piped water sources and social customs.

PATHOGENESIS

The main factors affecting the severity of disease are the parasite load and the host response.[43] The number of adult worms, and hence the number of eggs within the body, are limited by the number of cercariae which penetrate the skin and mature. The numbers of eggs in the faeces generally reflect the worm burden. The most important pathological consequence of infection is involvement of the liver. Lesions are due, not so much to the egg itself, but to the host reaction to those eggs. Cell-mediated immune processes lead to granuloma formation which may ultimately result in fibrosis. If granulomas around eggs trapped in the pre-sinusoidal venules of the liver cause sufficient obstruction to blood flow, portal hypertension develops with splenomegaly and oesophageal varices.[45] The roles of immune processes in modulating these events and providing resistance to reinfection are controversial and are subjects of intensive investigation.

CLINICAL FEATURES

Acute schistosomiasis

This is occasionally seen in people who come in contact with water only sporadic-ally. A pruritic, maculopapular rash may develop where cercariae penetrate the skin; it is more commonly seen in reinfections. One to two months after infection, there may be a gradual onset of fever and malaise. Urticaria may occur. Nausea and vomiting are common and heavy infections may produce diarrhoea or dysentery. Upper abdominal discomfort may be prominent and hepatospleno-megaly may be palpable. These features usually subside within several weeks or months.

Chronic schistosomiasis

The vast majority of infected persons have low to moderate worm burdens and are asymptomatic. Death occurs in only a small proportion of those with sympto-matic infection. Patients may complain of fatigue, abdominal pain and diarrhoea, but these symptoms are often difficult to disentangle from concurrent infections with other gastrointestinal organisms. Intestinal polyps are seen in Egyptian patients. The most definite signs are hepatomegaly and splenomegaly. The spleen may reach massive dimensions and is firm; anaemia, leucopenia and thrombo-cytopenia may result from hypersplenism. Rupture of oesophageal varices may lead to haematemesis and melaena. Liver function is usually not significantly impaired until the terminal stages when ascites and jaundice may be found. Although gastrointestinal and hepatic features usually predominate, eggs may be carried via collateral vessels to the lungs and produce cor pulmonale.

LABORATORY DIAGNOSIS

A definitive diagnosis of schistosomiasis mansoni can only be made by finding eggs in the faeces or in a biopsy specimen, usually from the rectum. Since the severity of disease is related to intensity of infection, it is essential to quantitate the number of eggs per gram of faeces. Rectal biopsies are taken through the proctoscope with a sharp curette; tissue samples are compressed between two glass slides and examined for eggs at low magnification. A number of immuno-logical diagnostic techniques, including skin tests and antibody assays, have been described, but they are usually of little assistance as they provide no quantitative data on the intensity of infection.

TREATMENT

Since antischistosomal agents have significant toxicity, specific treatment is only indicated when patients are symptomatic or have moderately heavy worm burdens, i.e. more than 100 eggs/g faeces. Furthermore, since schistosomes cannot multiply in man, it is not necessary to aim for eradication of parasites, but simply a marked reduction in worm burden. This can be achieved with smaller doses of drug and thus less toxicity. A number of drugs are available, but oxam-niquine has become the drug of choice.[33] It is given orally as a single dose of 15 mg/kg. The most common side-effects are dizziness and somnolence, but occasional hallucinations and convulsions may be experienced.

CONTROL

Schistosomiasis is a disease of poor communities. The most satisfactory way of controlling infection is by interrupting transmission by the installation of safe water supplies and efficient sewage disposal systems. Unfortunately, this is unlikely to be possible in most developing nations. Attempts have been made, therefore, to influence the prevalence and intensity of infection by health education, snail control by environmental, biological and chemical means, and by mass treatment with schistosomicides.[15] Perhaps the most promising approach is targeted mass treatment in which patients with heavy infections in a community are identified and treated.[46]

Schistosomiasis *japonica*

S. japonicum is found in eastern Asia, particularly China, the Philippines and Indonesia. Although the life cycle of this organism is similar to that of *S. mansoni* there are a number of important biological, epidemiological and clinical differences between the two infections.

EPIDEMIOLOGY

S. japonicum has a large animal reservoir as well as occurring in man; it is found in water buffalo, cattle, pigs, dogs and rodents. It is transmitted by snails of the genus *Oncomelania* which live in the mud of irrigation ditches, rice fields and marshes.

PATHOGENESIS

S. japonicum produces 10 times more eggs per worm pair than does *S. mansoni*. When antibodies first appear and large amounts of antigen are present in heavy primary infections, acute schistosomiasis develops, probably as a result of immune complexes producing a serum sickness-like syndrome. *S. japonicum* eggs tend to be laid in large aggregates rather than singly, and have a much greater tendency to calcify. The mechanism of granuloma development around them is uncertain, but may be related to immune complex deposition rather than cell-mediated immunity.[44]

CLINICAL FEATURES

Acute schistosomiasis (Katayama fever)

This is similar to that seen in schistosomiasis mansoni but probably occurs more commonly.

Chronic schistosomiasis

As in schistosomiasis mansoni, most patients have low or moderate worm burdens and are asymptomatic. Severe hepatosplenic disease with portal hypertension, ascites and varices may develop. Cor pulmonale may occur but does not seem to be as frequent as in schistosomiasis mansoni. Cerebral schistosomiasis has been estimated to occur in 2–4% of the infected population. Worms migrate to the brain and deposit masses of eggs in the cortical venules; eggs may be absent from the faeces. The most frequent sign is Jacksonian epilepsy, but signs of a space-occupying lesion or generalized encephalopathy may occasionally be found. The laboratory diagnosis is made in the same way as in schistosomiasis mansoni.

TREATMENT

S. japonicum is more resistant to treatment than the other major human schistosomes. Niridazole is the drug of choice at present.[44] Reduction in numbers rather than eradication of worms should be aimed for. The drug is given orally in divided doses of 25 mg/kg per day for 7 days. Toxic effects include nausea, vomiting, dizziness and insomnia. Psychotic reactions may occur in persons with hepatosplenic disease. A new agent, praziquantel, may be more effective, and is currently under investigation.

CONTROL

The same problems apply as in schistosomiasis mansoni, but control of schistosomiasis japonica is made even more difficult by the presence of an animal reservoir of infection.

CESTODE INFECTIONS

Cestodes, or tapeworms, are distinguished from other worms by their tape-like appearance, segmentation, absence of both gut and body cavity, and their bisexual nature. Man is the definitive host of a number of species which have different life cycles, but only *Taenia saginata* and *T. solium* will be discussed in detail. Human cestode infections of lesser importance are summarized in Table 10.5.

Taeniasis *saginata*

LIFE CYCLE

Adult tapeworms may live for years in the small intestine of man. The small head,

Table 10.5 Cestode infections of minor importance

Parasite	Geographical distribution	Mode of acquisition	Location in host	Clinical features	Drug of choice
Diphyllobothrium latum	Europe North America	Ingestion of infected, raw freshwater fish	Head attached to SI mucosa	Usually nil pernicious anaemia	Niclosamide
Dipylidium caninum	Worldwide	Ingestion of parasitized dog and cat fleas	Head attached to SI mucosa	Usually nil	Niclosamide
Hymenolepis diminuta	Worldwide	Ingestion of parasitized insects in grain, cereals	Head attached to SI mucosa	Usually nil	Niclosamide
Hymenolepis nana	Worldwide	Ingestion of eggs from soiled fingers, fomites	Head attached to SI mucosa	Usually nil	Niclosamide

SI, small intestine.

or scolex, 1–2 mm in diameter, is attached to the mucosal surface. Behind this comes the strobila which includes a neck 5–10 mm long, then a ribbon-like series of immature, mature and finally, gravid proglottids or segments. The whole worm may be up to 10 m long. The gravid proglottids, 6×20 mm in size, break off and are passed in the faeces, together with free, yellow-brown eggs 35 μm in diameter. The eggs are deposited on the ground and ingested by cattle. In the animal's intestine, the larva (called an oncosphere) hatches, penetrates the mucosa and spreads throughout the tissues and develops into a fluid-filled sac, less than 10 cm in size, called a cysticercus, which contains a single head. Ingestion of tissues containing cysts with viable scolices by man allows development of the larval stage into an adult over 3 months and completion of the life cycle.

EPIDEMIOLOGY

T. saginata is spread widely throughout the world but is most prevalent in East Africa, the Middle East and Central and South America. Adult worms develop only in man and the infection is acquired when poorly cooked meat of diseased cattle is ingested. Transmission can only occur, however, when there is also contamination of grazing lands with human faeces.

PATHOGENESIS

Adult tapeworms in the intestinal lumen cause little host reaction and immunity does not develop. Although it might seem that tapeworms utilize significant quantities of nutrients, calculations have suggested that the total amount of worm produced and lost in faeces each year is only 1 kg.[35]

CLINICAL FEATURES

The most obvious sign of taeniasis is the spontaneous passage of white, motile proglottids, or segments of worm even up to a metre in length, an experience which may be most frightening to the patient.[31] Most patients are otherwise asymptomatic, but there may be mild abdominal pain.

LABORATORY DIAGNOSIS

Taeniasis is confirmed by finding either the characteristic eggs in the stools, or the recovery of gravid proglottids. The eggs of *T. saginata* cannot be distinguished from those of *T. solium*. The definitive diagnosis of taeniasis saginata is made by inspecting the proglottids; the characteristic feature is 15 to 20 lateral uterine branches.

TREATMENT

Niclosamide is the drug of choice; adults and children more than 6 years of age are given 2 g of tablets which are chewed thoroughly in a single dose after a light meal. Nearly 90% of patients are cured on the first treatment with passage of a degenerate worm (the scolex is destroyed). The major side-effects are nausea and abdominal cramps. Failure of treatment can be followed by a second dose.

CONTROL

A number of measures can be taken to control taeniasis including proper cooking of meat, freezing at $-10°$ C for 2 weeks, inspection of meat at abattoirs, and prevention of human faecal contamination of grazing lands.

Taeniasis *solium*

LIFE CYCLE

T. solium has a life cycle similar to that described for *T. saginata*. Man is the only definitive host, but pigs are the major intermediate host. The most important difference, however, is the capacity of eggs ingested by man to behave like those in the intestines of swine, i.e. to penetrate the gut mucosa and migrate through the body where they develop into cysticerci cellulosae. The sites of predilection are the subcutaneous tissues, brain, eyes, muscle, heart, liver, lungs and peritoneum.

EPIDEMIOLOGY

T. solium occurs in many countries; it is most prevalent in parts of Asia, Central and South America, Africa and Europe, uncommon in North America, and unknown in Australasia. Adult worms develop when partly cooked, infected pork containing cysticerci is eaten. Human cysticercosis is acquired in several ways: (a) ingestion of food and water contaminated with human faeces containing eggs (most common), (b) autoinfection from anus to mouth by a person with an adult tapeworm and (c) reversed peristalsis and internal autoinfection in a person with an adult tapeworm (least common).

PATHOGENESIS

The pathogenesis of illness due to adult worms is similar to that described for taeniasis saginata. In human cysticercosis, cysticerci mature within 3 months and the cysts, up to 1 cm in diameter, may remain viable for 3–5 years, when they degenerate and evoke an inflammatory reaction followed by calcification. It is uncertain whether immunity develops in human cysticercosis.

CLINICAL FEATURES

Adult worms have the same manifestations as do those of *T. saginata.* Cysticercosis may be asymptomatic or produce variable symptoms and signs, depending upon the numbers and locations of cysticerci. Epilepsy is probably the most common problem, but features of a space-occupying lesion or raised intracranial pressure may be present. Occasionally, mass lesions may appear in other sites.

LABORATORY DIAGNOSIS

Taeniasis is confirmed by finding eggs and gravid proglottids in the stools. The proglottids of *T. solium* have 7–12 lateral uterine branches. The diagnosis of cysticercosis is more difficult, particularly in the early stages. There may be an eosinophilia and elevated serum IgE level. Serology may be useful.[34] A CAT scan may demonstrate numerous space-occupying lesions. Occasionally, a cysticercus may be biopsied. Finally, plain X-rays may demonstrate calcific lesions in advanced cysticercosis.

TREATMENT

Adult worms are eliminated with niclosamide. Many authorities recommend purging several hours later to prevent reversed peristalsis and the possibility of cysticercosis. The therapy of cysticercosis is largely palliative; epilepsy should be controlled with anticonvulsants. Public health measures to control infection are the same as those described under taeniasis saginata.

REFERENCES

1 Adams E. B. and Macleod I. N. (1977) Invasive Amebiasis. I. Amebic dysentery and its complications. *Med. (Baltimore)* **56**, 315.
2 Adams E. B. and Macleod I. N. (1977) Invasive amebiasis. II. Amebic liver abscess and its complications. *Med. (Baltimore)* **56**, 325.
3 Albach R. A. and Booden T. (1978) *Amoeba. Parasitic Protozoa*, vol. 2, p.455, Ed. J. P. Kreier, Academic Press, New York.
4 Arfaa F., Sahba G. H., Farahmandian I. and Jalali H. (1977) Evaluation of the effect of different methods of control of soil-transmitted helminths in Khuzestan, Southwest Iran. *Am. J. Trop. Med. Hyg.* **26**, 230.

5   Baksji J. S., Ghiara J. M. and Nanivadekar A. S. (1978) How does tinidazole compare with metronidazole? A summary report of Indian trials in amoebiasis and giardiasis. *Drugs* (Suppl. 1) **15**, 33.

6   Banwell J. G. and Schad G. A. (1978) Hookworm. *Clin. Gastroenterol.* **7**, 129.

7   Beal C. B., Viens P. and Grant R. G. (1970) A new technique for sampling duodenal contents: demonstration of upper small bowel pathogens. *Am. J. Trop. Med. Hyg.* **19**, 349.

8   Blumenthal D. S. and Schultz M. G. (1975) Incidence of intestinal obstruction in childen infected with *Ascaris lumbricoides*. *Am. J. Trop. Med. Hyg.* **24**, 801.

9   Blumenthal D. S. and Schultz M. G. (1976) Effects of *Ascaris* infection on nutritional status in children. *Am. J. Trop. Med. Hyg.* **25**, 682.

10 Bos H. J. and Hage A. J. (1975) Virulence of bacteria-associated, Crithidia-associated, and axenic *Entamoeba histolytica*: experimental hamster liver infections with strains from patients and carriers. *Zeitschr. Parasit.* **47**, 79.

11 Cram E. B. (1943) Studies on oxyuriasis. XXVIII. Summary and conclusions. *Am. J. Trop. Dis. Child.* **65**, 46.

12 Elsdon-Dew R. (1968) The epidemiology of amoebiasis. *Adv. Parasit.* **6**, 1.

13 Grove D. I. (1980) Strongyloidiasis in Allied ex-prisoners of war in Southeast Asia. *Br. Med. J.* **280**, 598.

14 Healy G. R. (1971) Laboratory diagnosis of amebiasis. *Bull. N.Y. Acad. Med.* **47**, 478.

15 Jordan P. (1977) Schistosomiasis — research to control. *Am. J. Trop. Med. Hyg.* **26**, 877.

16 Juniper K. (1978) Amoebiasis. *Clin. Gastroenterol.* **7**, 3.

17 Kean B. H. (1976) The treatment of amebiasis. A recurrent agony. *J. Am. Med. Assoc.* **235**, 501.

18 Knight R. (1978) Giardiasis, isosporiasis and balantidiasis. *Clin. Gastroenterol.* **7**, 31.

19 Krogstad D. J., Spencer H. C. and Healy G. R. (1978) Current concepts in parasitology: amebiasis. *N. Eng. J. Med.* **298**, 262.

20 Krogstad D. J., Spencer H. C., Healy G. R., Gleason N. N., Sexton D. J. and Herron C. A. (1978) Amebiasis: epidemiologic studies in the United States, 1971–1974. *Ann. Int. Med.* **88**, 89.

21 Layrisse M., Aparcedo L., Martinez-Torres C. and Roche M. (1967) Blood loss due to infection with *Trichuris trichiura*. *Am. J. Trop. Med. Hyg.* **16**, 613.

22 Leading Article (1978) Misdiagnosis of amoebiasis. *Br. Med. J.* **211**, 379.

23 Leading Article (1979) Pathogenic *Entamoeba histolytica*. *Lancet* **i**, 303.

24 Matsen J. M. and Turner J. A. (1969) Reinfection in enterobiasis (pinworm infection). *Am. J. Dis. Child.* **118**, 576.

25 Meyer E. A. and Jarroll E. L. (1980) Giadiasis. *Am. J. Epid.* **111**, 1.

26 Meyer E. A. and Radulescu S. (1979) *Giardia* and giardiasis. *Adv. Parasit.* **17**, 1.

27 Meyers J. D., Kuharic H. A. and Holmes K. K. (1977) *Giardia lamblia* infection in homosexual men. *Br. J. Ven. Dis.* **53**, 54.

28 Miller M. J., Krupp I. M., Little M. D. and Santos C. (1974) Mebendazole. An effective anthelmintic for trichuriasis and enterobiasis. *J. Am. Med. Assoc.* **230**, 1412.

29 Mizuno T. and Yanagisawa R. (1963) Studies on the infection route of hookworms with reference to experimental infection in human hosts with larvae of *Ancylostoma duodenale* and *Necator americanus*. *Jpn. J. Hyg.* **13**, 311.

30 Neal R. A. (1971) Pathogenesis of amebiasis. *Bull. N.Y. Acad. Med.* **47**, 462.

31 Pawlowski Z. and Schultz M. G. (1972) Taeniasis and cysticercosis (*Taenia saginata*). *Adv. Parasit.* **10**, 269.

32 Phillips B. P., Wolfe P. A. and Rees C. W. (1955) Studies on the ameba-bacteria relationship in amebiasis: comparative results of the intracecal inoculations of germfree mono-contaminated and conventional guinea pigs with *Entamoeba histolytica*. *Am. J. Trop. Med. Hyg.* **4**, 675.

33 Prata A. (1978) Schistosomiasis mansoni. *Clin. Gastenterol.* **7**, 49.

34 Proctor E. M., Powell S. J. and Elsdon-Dew R. (1966) The serological diagnosis of cysticercosis. *Ann. Trop. Med. Parasit.* **60**, 146.

35 Rees G. (1967) Pathogenesis of adult cestodes. *Helminth Abst.* **36**, 1.

36 Roche M. and Layrisse M. (1966) The nature and cause of hookworm anaemia. *Am. J. Trop. Med. Hyg.* **15**, 1030.

37 Sawitz W., D'Antoni J. S., Rhude K. and Lob S. (1940) Studies on the epidemiology of oxyuriasis. *South Med. J.* **33**, 913.

38 Scowden E. B., Schaffner W. and Stone W. J. (1978) Overwhelming strongyloidiasis; an unappreciated opportunistic infection. *Med. (Baltimore)* **57**, 527.

39 Scragg J. N. and Proctor E. M. (1977) Mebendazole in the treatment of severe, symptomatic trichuriasis in children. *Am. J. Trop. Med. Hyg.* **26**, 198.

40 Shaw P. K., Brodsky R. E., Lyman D. O., Wood B. T., Hibler C. P., Healy G. R. *et al.* (1977) A community-wide outbreak of giardiasis with evidence of transmission by a municipal water supply. *Ann. Int. Med.* **87**, 426.

41 Spillman R. K. Pulmonary ascariasis in tropical communities. *Am. J. Trop. Med. Hyg.* **24**, 791.

42 Triparthy K., Gonzales F., Lotero H. and Bolanos O. (1971) Effects of *Ascaris* infection on human nutrition. *Am. J. Trop. Med. Hyg.* **20**, 212.

43 Warren K. S. (1973) Regulation of prevalence and intensity of schistosomiasis in man: imunology or ecology? *J. Infect. Dis.* **127**, 595.

44 Warren K. S. (1978) Schistosomiasis japonica. *Clin. Gastroenterol.* **7**, 77.

45 Warren K. S. (1978) The pathology, pathobiology and pathogenesis of schistosomiasis. *Nature* **273**, 609.

46 Warren K. S., Arap Siongok T. K., Ouma J. H. and Houser H. B. (1978) Hycanthone dose-response in *Schistosoma mansoni* infection in Kenya. *Lancet* **i**, 352.

47 Weller T. H. and Sorenson C. W. (1941) Enterobiasis: its incidence and symptomatology in a group of 505 children. *N. Eng. J. Med.* **224**, 174.

48 Wolfe M. S. (1978) Giardiasis. *N. Eng. J. Med.* **298**, 319.

11 *Yersinia* infections including mesenteric adenitis, and gastrointestinal tuberculosis

C. S. Goodwin

Introduction   241
Yersinia infections   242
  Causative organisms   242
  Epidemiology   242
  Pathogenesis   243
  Clinical features   244
  Laboratory diagnosis   245
  Antibiotic treatment   246
  Control   246
Gastrointestinal tuberculosis   247
  Clinical features and epidemiology   247
  Laboratory diagnosis   247
  Epidemiology   248
  Antimicrobial treatment   248
  Control   248
References   249

INTRODUCTION

In recent years there has been increasing interest in human disease due to *Yersinia enterocolitica* and *Yersinia pseudotuberculosis*, and the former have been found in cow's milk and goat's milk;[32,65] the incidence of infection with these organisms may be underestimated. Although *Y. pseudotuberculosis* is probably only a rare cause of gastroenteritis,[22] both organisms can be causes of mesenteric adenitis, which can be misdiagnosed as acute appendicitis.[29,69] *Y. enterocolitica* is an important cause of diarrhoea in children in some countries. *Mycobacterium tuberculosis* infection of the gut is very rare in developed countries but gastrointestinal tuberculosis is an important aspect of a disease which is all too common in developing countries. Among immigrants to the United Kingdom and among Asian refugees who enter developed countries tuberculosis is frequently found, and so gastrointestinal tuberculosis should be borne in mind by the discerning physician.

YERSINIA INFECTIONS

Causative organisms

Yersinia enterocolitica and *Y. pseudotuberculosis* are Gram-negative bacilli, which are characteristically motile at 22° C but not at 37° C. However, the demonstration of motility can depend on media; some strains are mobile at both temperatures and some at neither temperature.[18]

The organisms were previously included in the genus Pasteurella.[56] In 1939 *Y. enterocolitica* was described and named *Bacterium enterocoliticum*.[50] *Y. enterocolitica* was probably the organism referred to in 1961 as *Pasteurella pseudotuberculosis* type B.[20] It was not until after 1964 that enteritis due to *Y. enterocolitica* was recognized as being a common disease around the world.[9,21,41,67,68] In 1949 Hassig[28] reported two cases of septicaemia caused by an organism called *Pasteurella pseudotuberculosis* type X. *Y. pseudotuberculosis* was isolated from mesenteric lymph nodes in 1954,[36] and was shown to be the probable cause of symptoms in children diagnosed as suffering from acute appendicitis.[40]

There are biochemical differences between the two species, for example in contrast to *Y. enterocolitica*, *Y. pseudotuberculosis* does not have ornithine decarboxylase, fails to ferment sucrose and is lysed by specific *Y. pseudotuberculosis* bacteriophage.[35] *Y. pseudotuberculosis* is recognized as having at least six serological subtypes of which type II is antigenically related to group B *Salmonella*, and type IV to *Salmonella* groups D and H. The bacteriology of *Y. enterocolitica* has been described by Bottone[9] and Keusch,[35] but there has been considerable argument as to whether biochemically atypical strains should be assigned new names such as *Y. intermedia*,[10] *Y. frederiksenii*[60] and *Y. kristensenii*.[5] On the basis of somatic O antigens 34 serogroups have been described for *Y. enterocolitica*. The O antigens are found in all the four species just mentioned; for example O:16 can occur in all these species.[52] The commonest serogroup is O:3,[14,52] and this has been found in both *Y. enterocolitica* and *Y. intermedia*.[52] Most human illness has been caused by serogroups O:3, O:5, O:8 and O:9.[35] *Yersinia* sp. may be phage-typed.[52]

Epidemiology

Y. enterocolitica and *Y. pseudotuberculosis* have been found in a wide range of animals, including dogs and cats,[2] in rodents and foxes,[33] in monkeys,[12] in pigs,[58] and in goat's milk[32] and cow's milk.[65] Birds and small rodents may become chronic faecal carriers of *Y. enterocolitica*,[52] and of *Y. pseudotuberculosis*.[43] Both organisms have been isolated from water,[52] and from oysters but the serogroups from these sources are often different from those encountered in man. Human serogroups of *Y. enterocolitica*, including serogroup O:3, have been isolated from pigs.[9,58] In patients with yersiniosis a history of pork ingestion or direct contact with a pig or pigkeeper may often be obtained. It has been considered that pigs should be regarded as the main source of human enteric yersiniosis.[58] Both species have been isolated from deer in the USA; *Y. enterocolitica* O:8 was isolated from water infected with deer faeces and the same serogroup was isolated from a man with septicaemia who had been hunting in that area.[34] In the Camargue in France, three strains of *Y. enterocolitica* were isolated from the coypu, but the serogroups seemed different from those in humans.[4]

In a study in the USA of 4448 human, animal and environmental samples 339 isolates of *Yersinia* species were identified; serogroups implicated in human disease were recovered from both human and non-human sources.[52] In Alsace, France, of 75 raw cow's milk samples 81.4% yielded *Y. enterocolitica*, but most of the serogroups were those not found commonly in humans.[65] In New South Wales, Australia, 35 of 274 samples (12.8%) of raw goat's milk were found to contain *Y. enterocolitica*.[32] Most of the goat's milk in New South Wales is marketed raw and much is consumed by infants and other people with allergy to cow's milk. The serogroups from goat's milk were not the same as those commonly isolated from humans, but there remains the suspicion that some animal isolates may cause mesenteric adenitis especially in infants without any laboratory specimen yielding the organism.

The modes of transmission to humans have not been clearly elucidated. However the organism can be spread by direct or indirect human transmission, especially among children. One outbreak of gastroenteritis due to *Y. enterocolitica* involved 222 children, and was due to contaminated chocolate milk.[7] In some parts of the world the value of looking routinely for *Y. enterocolitica* in faeces is minimal. In Adelaide in South Australia only 3 out of 3298 faecal specimens were found to yield the organism, and one of these patients had acquired the infection overseas.[57]

Pathogenesis

Yersinia species can invade many tissues of the body, producing clinical features described in the next section; *Yersinia* sp. are entero-invasive in the gut. However *Y. enterocolitica* have also been found to elaborate a heat-stable enterotoxin which activates guanylate cyclase, as does the heat-stable toxin of *E. coli*, with resulting alterations of intestinal ion transport and diarrhoea.[45,46] In an animal model of *Y. enterocolitica* infection, the gerbil, virulent strains of the organisms possessed a plasmid which also enabled these strains to detach tissue culture cells from glass surfaces.[45] This plasmid has also been found in *Y. pseudotuberculosis*.[26] However, strains that had lost this plasmid, although they were avirulent for gerbils, could still invade tissue culture cells. *Y. enterocolitica* have V and W antigens which are similar to those of *Y. pestis*.[15] An enterotoxin-negative strain of *Y. enterocolitica* O:3 was capable of producing diarrhoea in mice,[49] which throws doubt on the significance of the enterotoxin. The production of diarrhoea in mice has been correlated with the ability to autoagglutinate at 35° C in a tissue culture medium.[49] The enterotoxin has not been detected in species that caused diarrhoea in rabbits.

Clinical features

Y. enterocolitica, and very occasionally *Y. pseudotuberculosis*[22,36] cause mild or severe diarrhoea, nearly always with abdominal pain and fever. Both organisms can cause mesenteric adenitis,[9,22,29,40] and widespread symptoms throughout the body (see below). Some patients may have diarrhoea for many months and may appear to be suffering from Crohn's disease,[48] or ulcerative colitis. It is important to distinguish yersinia ileitis from these other conditions. With both organisms the diarrhoea may be accompanied by faecal leucocytosis and occasionally by blood. Vomiting is usually not a prominent symptom in adults, but occurs more commonly in children.[37] Two-thirds of infections with *Y. enterocolitica* apparently occur in children. Because *Yersinia* can cause terminal ileitis, the pain and tenderness may be localized to the right iliac fossa.[38,50] A comparison of the clinical aspects of acute abdominal disease due to these organisms has been made by Bottone,[9] and is shown in Table 11.1.

Table 11.1 Comparison of clinical and laboratory aspects of acute abdominal disease due to *Y. enterocolitica* and *Y. pseudotuberculosis* (after Bottone 1977[9])

Feature	*Y. enterocolitica*	*Y. pseudotuberculosis*
Age	Usually children (enteritis) and young adults; 60% incidence under 7 years of age; predilection for males.	Usually children and young adults (2–24 years), especially males; low incidence among 5–12 year olds.
Fever	Usually present for more than 2 weeks (38–40° C).	Usually present early in course; lasts for less than 2 weeks (38–40° C).
Antibody titres acute	Low or absent.	Usually present at time of abdominal symptoms; parallels course of disease; titres of 80–12 800 recorded.
Convalescent	High titres (80–20 480 recorded) may persist for several years; highest in patients with arthritis or erythema nodosum.	Titre disappears rapidly during convalescence (1–4 months if uncomplicated).
Common serogroups	3,8,9; antibody response poor to other serogroups; Serogroup 9 cross-reacts with *Brucella* sp.	Specific for Serotypes I,III,V; Types II and IV cross-react with *Salmonella* groups B,D; Serotype I causes 90% of human infections; Type IV rarely isolated from man.
Stool culture	Usually positive within 2 weeks after onset of disease, especially in patients with symptoms necessitating appendectomy (i.e. terminal ileitis, mesenteric adenitis).	Seldom positive.

Mesenteric adenitis, which usually occurs in children, is characterized by a central dull abdominal pain, usually continuous, but distinct from the sharp colicky pain that usually develops in appendicitis. Palpation of the abdomen may show direct or rebound tenderness. Yersinial adenitis may be accompanied by high fever.[38] However, other causes of mesenteric adenitis may be enteroviruses, and with these there may be a history of upper respiratory tract infection in the patient or a near relative, and the pulse rate will not rise steadily as it usually does in appendicitis. In Scandinavia in a series of 964 patients with symptoms of appendicitis 581 underwent appendicectomy and 383 did not; 3.8% of those operated on, and 5.6% of the others yielded *Y. enterocolitica* in their stools. Only one of 974 controls yielded the microorganism.[42] In the USA one study of 808 children with abdominal pain showed that *Y. enterocolitica* were isolated from 15 children (1.9%) including five who had appendicectomies; only one of the latter had pathologically confirmed acute appendicitis, and *Y. enterocolitica* was cultured from three of the remaining four appendices.[69]

THE GENERALIZED SYMPTOMS OF YERSINIA INFECTION

Polyarthritis with or without associated erythema nodosum is increasingly being associated with *Yersinia* infection.[1,39] Occasionally severe septicaemic forms of infection occur especially in patients with underlying diseases.[6] In Sweden, of 75 patients with infection due to *Y. enterocolitica* 58 had gastroenteritis but 17 had no gastrointestinal symptoms; erythema nodosum occurred in 24 patients.[3] Ten patients had arthritis. Diagnosis was based on the culture of *Y. enterocolitica* (usually type O:3) from stools or by serological evidence of specific antibody.[3] In Finland from 1971–73 60 patients were hospitalized for infections due to *Y. enterocolitica* O-types 3 and 9, and for infections due to *Y. pseudotuberculosis* serotype 1. All the patients were older than 15 years.[38] *Y. enterocolitica* has been recovered from the blood of an infant with sepsis and fever but with few gastrointestinal symptoms.[13] In New York, of a series of five children aged from 5 weeks to 6½ years old with infection due to *Y. enterocolitica,* four had a primary enteric illness while the fifth had associated ocular and joint involvement.[47] In the aged, debilitated, or immunosuppressed patients a typhoid-like septicaemia may be caused by both species.[9] A wide range of other symptoms including meningitis, myocarditis, panophthalmitis, haemolytic anaemia, Reiter's disease and abscesses of the liver and spleen may occur.[9]

Laboratory diagnosis

On routine laboratory media *Y. enterocolitica* may produce a similar biochemical result to *E. coli,* and thus be discarded, and *Y. pseudotuberculosis* may be assumed to be *Proteus* sp. because it fails to ferment lactose and is urease-positive.[35] Cold temperature (4–7° C) enrichment procedures[44,61] are of unquestionable value for the recovery of *Y. enterocolitica* from faeces, although holding periods of a month or more are required to allow Yersinia species to multiply at the low temperature while other vegetative organisms do not multiply. A discussion of different media has been made by Vidon and Delmas,[65] who reported that isolation of *Y. enterocolitica* from raw milk is achieved most frequently by incubation in selective broth at 4° C for 1 month, followed by transfer to another selective medium at 28° C for 48 hours, followed by subculture to a solid medium containing ampicillin. A more rapid method of isolating *Y. enterocolitica* from faeces has been described using a medium containing cellobiose and arginine and lysine, with incubation at 25° C. After 40 hours incubation at 25° C characteristic colonies could be recognized.[21] The ELISA antibody technique has been utilized to diagnose *Y. enterocolitica* infection in children in Sweden. In 286 children with acute diarrhoea two patients had large rises to serotype O:3.[64] Diarrhoea due to *Y. enterocolitica* can usually be diagnosed by culture of the organism during the first 2 weeks of the disease, but *Y. pseudotuberculosis* is rarely cultured from the faeces and diagnosis must be made by serological methods.

Antibiotic treatment

Antibiotics are not indicated for the acute gastroenteritis caused by *Y. enterocolitica* which is usually self-limiting. Other forms of illness due to *Yersinia* should be treated with antibiotics according to the clinical state, and guided by sensitivity tests. Arthritis due to *Y. enterocolitica* in southern Sweden was treated successfully with tetracycline.[39] Isolates of *Y. enterocolitica* are usually highly susceptible *in vitro* to tetracyclines and the aminoglycosides, and to the sulphonamides and cotrimoxazole. Isolates are also highly susceptible to cefotaxime, and moderately susceptible to cefoperazone and cefamandole. Resistance to ampicillin is not infrequent.[25]

Control

The hazards of raw milk can certainly be overcome by pasteurization and this should obviously be applied to goat's milk as much as to cow's milk. Presumably people who handle animals infected with serogroups that can cause human disease, such as pigs, should be meticulous in washing their hands before eating so that the chain of infection can be broken. Some serogroups may come from dogs and cats, and it is interesting that children seem to be mostly affected by these organisms, and they may have aquired them from domestic animals. Contact with areas contaminated by rodents can also be a cause of acquiring the disease and rodents may presumably contaminate food. The moral of the deer-hunter story should be that water contaminated by deer faeces can be a source of the infection. However, it does seem fortunate that many animal serogroups are apparently not the cause of human disease.

GASTROINTESTINAL TUBERCULOSIS

Clinical features and epidemiology

The clinical features of gastrointestinal tuberculosis are frequently those of intestinal obstruction, vomiting, colicky abdominal pain and constipation. Abdominal pain is a very consistent feature, occurring in 94% of one series of 182 Indian patients[19] but in only 66% of 35 Ceylonese patients.[66] Vomiting may occur without intestinal obstruction.[19] Fever is common,[19,66] but diarrhoea is infrequent. Anorexia and weight loss may be marked features.[54] The ileo-caecal region appears to be a common site of gut tuberculosis.[17,66]

In a patient with pulmonary tuberculosis intestinal bleeding may indicate intestinal tuberculosis.[53] In developed countries gut tuberculosis may be wrongly diagnosed as Crohn's disease.[51] In a series of 21 patients seen in New York during 44 years 90% of the patients had evidence of pulmonary tuberculosis. Surgical exploration was strongly recommended to make a diagnosis. In the years before streptomycin was available the mortality rate was 67%, and after the availability of streptomycin the rate was still 21% in patients receiving appropriate drug therapy. Chemotherapy obviated the necessity of intestinal resection in most patients.[30] Only about 30% of patients with gut tuberculosis have a positive tuberculin reaction.[27] Malabsorption and the stagnant loop syndrome can occur in association with intestinal tuberculosis.[59]

In the Sudan, of 65 patients with abdominal tuberculosis, abdominal pain and a palpable mass were the commonest clinical features. A high erythrocyte sedimentation rate and a positive Mantoux test were relatively infrequent.[23] A complaint of abdominal swelling was given by 83% of patients. Laparotomy was the preferred method of making the diagnosis. In developed countries the value of colonoscopy with biopsies for histological and cultural purposes avoids the need for laparotomy.[11,24]

At Chandigarh, India, of 102 patients, 81 experienced obstructive symptoms, 62 had radiographic evidence of intestinal obstruction and four had bowel perforation.[62] Pulmonary tuberculosis was detected in 28 patients. The commonest sites of bowel involvement were ileo-caecal, the ileum, and the ascending colon. Duodenal lesions were seen in three patients, and in another three patients there was isolated involvement of the appendix. Right hemicolectomy was necessary in 55 of the 74 patients who had surgical exploration. Open peritoneal biopsy, performed after making a small incision in the right iliac fossa, has been found to be a most useful investigation in the diagnosis of abdominal tuberculosis.[19]

On examination abdominal tenderness and a mass may be found; ascites may be present. A 'doughy feel to the abdomen' used to be regarded as typical of tuberculosis of the gut, but this was present in only 6% in one series of 182 patients.[19]

Laboratory diagnosis

Mycobacterium tuberculosis is difficult to culture from faeces.[31] The use of highly selective media containing substances inhibitory to bowel bacteria may yield a higher isolation rate of *M. tuberculosis*. Biopsy specimens obtained by colonoscopy may be less useful than laparotomy specimens. Histological appearances including the demonstration of acid-fast bacilli should be diagnostic. However in one series of 58 patients with gut tuberculosis acid-fast bacilli could be demonstrated in only 19 biopsies,[31] and in another series of 50 cases, acid-fast bacilli were cultured from only 7 biopsies.[55]

Epidemiology

The milk of cows infected with bovine tuberculosis may contain *M. tuberculosis* var. *bovis*, and if milk is drunk raw there is obviously a possibility of acquiring abdominal tuberculosis. However, most reports of gastrointestinal tuberculosis indicate that the human *M. tuberculosis* bacillus is the commonest causative organism.

Antimicrobial treatment

The classical method of treating tuberculosis with three drugs such as isoniazid, ethambutol and streptomycin or rifampicin should be undertaken until the sensitivities of the organism are known. However, it has been reported that medical treatment alone can lead to increased fibrosis,[8] and many patients treated with antibiotics may require hemicolectomy later. However, in one series of 166 patients more than 50% of patients responded to chemotherapy alone.[16] The value of various surgical procedures is discussed by Croker, Record and Wright.[17]

Control

Eradication of bovine tuberculosis is obviously essential to eliminate causes of disease from that source. However, in communities where pulmonary tuberculosis is very common it is apparent that only improvement of the socio-economic status of people will allow them to avoid close contact with people infected with *M. tuberculosis*, and improved nutrition may decrease the likelihood of overt disease.

Several authorities emphasize the need for a high index of suspicion so that the diagnosis can be considered at an early stage after presentation of the first clinical symptoms.[51]

REFERENCES

1 Ahvonen P., Sievers K. and Aho K. (1969) Arthritis associated with *Yersinia enterocolitica* infection. *Acta Rheumatol. Scand.* **15**, 232.
2 Ahvonen P., Thal E. and Vasenius H. (1973) Occurrence of *Yersinia enterocolitica* in animals in Finland and Sweden. In: *Contributions to Microbiology and Immunology*, vol. 2, p. 135, Ed. S. Winblad, Karger, Basel.
3 Arvastson B., Damgaard K. and Winblad S. (1971) Clinical Symptoms of Infection with *Yersinia enterocolitica. Scand. J. Infect. Dis.* **3**, 37.
4 Baylet R., Rollin P. E. and Rollin D. (1980) Isolement de *Yersinia enterocolitica* chez le ragondin *Myocastor coypu* (Kerr) en Camargue. (Isolation of *Yersinia enterocolitica* from *Myocastor coypu* (Kerr) in the Camargue). *Bull. Soc. de Pathol. Exotique* **73**, 35.
5 Bercovier H., Ursing J., Brenner D. J., Steigerwalt A. G., Fanning G. R., Carter G. P. and Mollaret H. H. (1980) *Yersinia kristensenii* a new species of Enterobacteriaceae composed of sucrose-negative strains (formerly called atypical *Yersinia enterocolitica*-like). *Curr. Microbiol.* **4**, 219.
6 Bissett M. L. (1976) *Yersinia enterocolitica* Isolates from Humans in California, 1968–1975. *J. Clin. Microbiol.* **4**, 137.
7 Black R. E., Jackson R. J., Medvesky M., Shayegani M., Feeley J. C., Macleod K. I. E. and Wakelee A. M. (1978) Epidemic *Yersinia enterocolitica* infection due to contaminated chocolate milk. *N. Engl. J. Med.* **298**, 76.
8 Bondurant R. E. and Reid D. (1975) Ileocaecal tuberculosis. *Am. J. Gastroenterol.* **63**, 58.
9 Bottone E. J. (1977) *Yersinia enterocolitica*: a panoramic view of a charismatic microorganism. *Crit. Rev. Microbiol.* **5**, 211.
10 Brenner D. J., Bercovier H., Ursing J., Alonso J. M., Steigerwalt A. G., Fanning G. R., Carter G. P. and Mollaret H. H. (1980) *Yersinia intermedia* a new species of Enterobacteriaceae composed of rhamnose-positive, melibiose-positive, raffinose-positive strains (formerly called *Yersinia enterocolitica* or *Yersinia enterocolitica*-like). *Curr. Microbiol.* **4**, 207.
11 Bretholz A. and Knoblauch M. (1979) Colonic tuberculosis. *Gastroenterology* **77**, 606.
12 Buhles J. R. W. C., Vanderlip J. E., Russell S. W. and Alexander N. L. (1981) *Yersinia pseudotuberculosis* infection: Study of an Epizootic in Squirrel Monkeys. *J. Clin. Microbiol.* **13**, 519.
13 Caplan L. M. (1978) *Yersinia enterocolitica* Septicaemia. *Am. J. Clin. Pathol.* **69**, 189.
14 Caprioli T., Drapeau A. J., and Kasatiya S. (1978) *Yersinia enterocolitica*: Serotypes and Biotypes Isolated from Humans and the Environment in Quebec, Canada. *J. Clin. Microbiol.* **8**, 7.
15 Carter P. B., Zahorchak R. J. and Brubaker R. R. (1980) Plague virulence antigens from *Yersinia enterocolitica. Infec. Immun.* **28**, 638.
16 Chuttani H. K. (1970) Intestinal tuberculosis. In: *Modern Trends in Gastro-Enterology* vol. 4, p. 309, Eds I. W. Card and B. Creamer, Butterworths, London.
17 Croker J., Record C. O. and Wright J. T. (1978) Ileo-caecal tuberculosis in immigrants. *Postgrad. Med. J.* **54**, 410.
18 D'Amato R. F. (1981) Influence of Media on Temperature-Dependent Motility Test for *Yersinia enterocolitica. J. Clin. Microbiol.* **14**, 347.
19 Das P., and Shukla H. S. (1976) Clinical diagnosis of abdominal tuberculosis. *Brit. J. Surg.* **63**, 941.
20 Dickinson A. B. and Mocquot G. (1961) Studies on the bacterial flora of the alimentary tract of pigs. *I. Enterobacteriaceae* and other Gram-negative bacteria. *J. Appl. Bacteriol.* **24**, 252.
21 Dudley M. V. and Shotts E. B. Jr (1979) Medium for Isolation of *Yersinia enterocolitica. J. Clin. Microbiol.* **10**, 180.
22 El-Maraghi N. R. H. and Mair N. S. (1979) Histopathology of enteric infection with *Yersinia pseudotuberculosis. Am. J. Clin. Path.* **71**, 631.

23 El Masri S. H., Boulos P. and Mallick M. O. A. (1977) Abdominal tuberculosis in Sudanese patients. *East Afr. Med. J.* **54**, 319.

24 Franklin G. O., Mohapatra M. and Perrillo R. P. (1979) Colonic tuberculosis diagnosed by colonoscopic biopsy. *Gastroenterology* **76**, 362.

25 Gaspar M. C. and Soriano F. (1981) Susceptibility of *Yersinia enterocolitica* to eight β-lactam antibiotics and clavulanic acid. *J. Antimicrob. Chemother.* **8**, 161.

26 Gemski P., Lazere J. R., Casey T. and Wohlhieter J. A. (1980) Presence of a virulence-associated plasmid in *Yersinia pseudotuberculosis. Infect. Immun.* **28**, 1044.

27 Grange J. M. (1980) *Mycobacterial Diseases*, p. 76, Arnold, London.

28 Hassig A., Karrer J. and Pusterla F. (1949) Über Pseudotuberculose beim Menschen. *Schweiz. Med. Wochenschr.* **79**, 971.

29 Henshall T. C. (1963) Pasteurella pseudotuberculosis mesenteric adenitis. *N.Z. Med. J.* **62**, 462.

30 Homan W. P., Grafe W. R. and Dineen P. (1977) A 44-Year Experience with Tuberculous enterocolitis. *World J. Surg.* **1**, 245.

31 Hoon J. R., Dockerty M. D. and Pemberton J. de J. (1950) Collective review: ileocaecal tuberculosis including comparison of this disease with non-specific regional enterocolitis and non-caseous tuberculated enterocolitis. *Surg. Gynae. & Obstet,* **60**, 417.

32 Hughes D. and Jensen N. (1981) *Yersinia enterocolitica* in raw goat's milk. *Appl. Environ. Microbiol.* **41**, 309.

33 Kapperud G. (1977) *Yersinia enterocolitica* and Yersinia like microbes isolated from mammals and water in Norway and Denmark. *Acta Path. Microbiol. Scand. Sect. B* **85**, 129.

34 Keet E. E. (1974) *Yersinia enterocolitica* septicemia. Source of infection and incubation period idenitfied. *N.Y. State J. Med.* **74**, 2226.

35 Keusch G. T. (1981) Yersinia enteritis. In: *Medical Microbiology and Infectious Diseases*, p. 1063 vol. 2, Ed. A. I. Braude, Saunders, Philadelphia.

36 Knapp von W. and Masshoff W. (1954) Zur Ätiologie der abszedierenden Retikulozytaren Lymphadenitis. *Dtsch Med. Wochenschr.* **79**, 1266.

37 Kohl S., Jacobson J.. A. and Nahmias A. (1976) *Yersinia enterocolitica* infection in children. *J. Pediatr.* **89**, 77.

38 Leino R. and Kalliomaki J. L. (1974) Yersiniosis as an Internal Disease. *Ann. Int. Med.* **81**, 458.

39 Marsal L., Winblad S. and Wollheim F. A. (1981) *Yersinia enterocolitica* arthritis in southern Sweden: a four-year follow-up study. *Br. Med. J.* **283**, 101.

40 Masshoff W. (1953) Eine neuartige Form der mesenterialen Lymphadenitis. *Dtsch. Med. Wochenschr.* **78**, 532.

41 Mollaret H. H. (1971) L'infection humaine à 'Yersinia enterocolitica' en 1970, à la lumière de 642 cas reçents. Aspects cliniques et perspectives épidémiologiques. *Pathol. biol. (Paris)* **19**, 189.

42 Nilehn B. (1969) Studies on *Yersinia enterocolitica* with special reference to bacterial diagnosis and occurrence in human acute enteric disease. *Acta Path. Microbiol. Scand.* **206**, (Suppl), 1.

43 Obwolo M. J. (1976) A review of yersiniosis (*Yersinia pseudotuberculosis*) infection. *Vet. Bull.* **46**, 167.

44 Pai C. H., Sorger S., Lafleur L., Lackman L. and Marks M. I. (1979) Efficacy of cold enrichment techniques for recovery of *Yersinia enterocolitica* from human stools. *J. Clin. Microbiol.* **9**, 712.

45 Portnoy D. A., Moseley S. L. and Falkow S. (1981) Characterization of Plasmids and Plasmid-Associated Determinants of *Yersinia enterocolitica* Pathogenesis. *Infect. Immun.* **31**, 775.

46 Rao M. C., Guandalini S., Laird W. J., Field M. (1979) Effects of heat-stable enterotoxin *Yersinia enterocolitica* on ion transport and cyclic guanosine $3',5'$-monophosphate metabolism in rabbit ileum. *Infect. Immun.* **26**, 875.

47 Rodriguez W. J., Controni G., Cohen G. J., Florence B., Khan W. N. and Ross S. (1978) *Yersinia enterocolitica* Enteritis in children. *J. Am. Med. Assoc.* **242**, 1978.

48 Savage A. and Dunlop D. (1976) Terminal iletis due to *Yersinia pseudotuberculosis. Br. Med. J.* **2**, 916.

49 Schiemann D. A. (1981) An enterotoxin-negative strain of *Yersinia enterocolitica* serotype O:3 is capable of producing diarrhea in mice. *Infect. Immun.* **32**, 571.

50 Schleifstein J. and Coleman M. B. (1939) An unidentified microorganism resembling *B. lignieri* and *Past. pseudotuberculosis*, and pathogenic for man. *N.Y. State J. Med.* **39**, 1749.

51 Schulze K., Warner H. A. and Murray D. (1977) Intestinal tuberculosis Experience at a Canadian Teaching Institution. *Am. J. Med.* **63**, 735.

52 Shayegani M., DeForge I., McGlynn D. M. and Root T. (1981) Characteristics of *Yersinia enterocolitica* and related species isolated from human, animal and environmental sources. *J. Clin. Microbiol.* **14**, 304.

53 Sherman H. I., Johnson R. and Brock T. (1978) Massive gastrointestinal bleeding from tuberculosis of the small intestine. *Am. J. Gastroenterol.* **70**, 314.

54 Shukla H. S. and Hughes L. E. (1978) Abdominal tuberculosis in the 1970s: a continuing problem. *Br. J. Surg.* **65**, 403.

55 Singh H. N., Vaidya M. P. and Roy S. K. (1973) The laboratory diagnosis of intestinal tuberculosis: a study of 50 cases. *Aust. N.Z. J. Surg.* **42**, 411.

56 Smith J. E. and Thal E. (1965) A taxonomic study of the genus *Pasteurella* using a numerical technique. *Acta Pathol. Microbiol. Scand.* **64**, 213.

57 Steele T. W. and McDermott S. N. (1979) Enterocolitis due to *Yersinia enterocolitica* in South Australia. *Pathology* **11**, 67.

58 Szita J., Svidro A., Kubinyi M., Nyomarkay I. and Mihalyfi I. (1980) *Yersinia enterocolitica* infection of animals and human contacts. *Acta Microbiol. Acad. Sci. Hung.* **27**, 103.

59 Tandon R. K., Bansal R., Kapur B. M. L. and Shriniwas (1980) A study of malabsorption in intestinal tuberculosis: stagnant loop syndrome. *Am. J. Clin. Nutr.* **33**, 244.

60 Ursing J., Brenner D. J., Bercovier H., Fanning G. R., Steigerwalt A. G., Brault J. and Mollaret H. H. (1980) *Yersinia frederiksenii*: a new species of Enterobacteriaceae composed of rhamnose-positive strains (formerly called a typical *Yersinia enterocolitica* or Yersinia *enterocolitica*-like). *Curr. Microbiol.* **4**, 213.

61 Van Noyen R., Vandepitte J., Wauters G. and Selderslaghs R. (1981) *Yersinia enterocolitica*: its isolation by cold enrichment from patients and healthy subjects. *J. Clin. Pathol.* **34**, 1052.

62 Vaidya M. G. and Sodhi J. S. (1978) Gastrointestinal Tract Tuberculosis: A study of 102 cases including 55 Hemicolectomies. *Clin. Radiol.* **29**, 189.

63 Venables G. S. and Rans P. S. J. B. (1979) Colonic tuberculosis. *Postgrad. Med. J.* **55**, 276.

64 Vesikari T., Granfors K., Maki M. and Gronroos P. (1980) Evaluation of ELISA in the diagnosis of *Yersinia enterocolitica* diarrhoea in children. *Acta Pathol. Microbiol. Scand.* **88B**, 139.

65 Vidon D. J. M. and Delmas C. L. (1981) Incidence of *Yersinia enterocolitica* in raw milk in Eastern France. *Appl. Environ. Microbiol.* **41**, 355.

66 Vyravanathan S. and Jeyarajah R. (1980) Tuberculous peritonitis: a review of thirty-five cases. *Postgrad. Med. J.* **56**, 649.

67 Wauters G. (1970) Contribution à l'étude de *Yersinia enterocolitica* Thèse d'agrégation de l'Enseignement Supérieur, Vander, Brussels.

68 Zen-Yoji H. and Maruyama T. (1972) The first successful isolation and identification of *Yersinia enterocolitica* from human cases in Japan. *Jpn. J. Microbiol.* **16**, 493.

69 Pai C. H. (1982) Infection due to *Yersinia enterocolitica* in children with abdominal pain. *J. Infect. Dis.* **146**, 705.

12 Immunization against gut infections

G. N. Cooper

Introduction	253
Typhoid fever vaccines	254
Cholera vaccines	258
Shigella vaccines	261
Escherichia coli infections	263
The future for immunization against gut pathogens	264
References	266

INTRODUCTION

In the first half of this century many of the claims for success of immunization against a variety of diseases were based on ill-conceived, poorly-designed and badly-controlled studies in animals and man. Today it is clear that, with few exceptions, bacterial vaccines are only moderately effective and some may even be next to useless. This holds true particularly for those designed to provide longterm protection against intestinal infections. Discussion in this chapter is limited for the most part to four major bacterial diseases of the intestine — typhoid fever, cholera, shigellosis and *Escherichia coli* infection.

There are two legitimate purposes for immunization against intestinal infection. The first is for individual protection, for example travellers through high-risk areas. The second is for community control. This approach assumes that herd immunity (expressed when more than 80% of the population is immune) will effectively reduce the incidence of a particular disease in the community, though this has never really been demonstrated for intestinal infections. An ideal vaccine would be inexpensive, devoid of side-reactions, and confer longterm immunity. Unfortunately, none of the present-day vaccines for gut pathogens meets all these criteria and it is therefore important to weigh the advantages and disadvantages of immunization against those of the two alternatives — prevention by hygiene, and chemoprophylaxis.

The age-old advice of avoiding unwashed vegetables or cold collations, drinking only boiled water or bottled beverages and eating only recently-cooked foods can provide excellent protection against the major bacterial intestinal infections, amoebic dysentery, and traveller's diarrhoea. There are, of course,

253

occasions when even the most fastidious individual is unable to maintain this strict control; incidents of typhoid fever, cholera and *E. coli* infection associated with airline foods attest to this fact. For chemoprophylaxis, clioquinol and related hydroxyquinoline drugs are now known to be valueless and, if used continually, potentially dangerous. However, recent studies suggest that single or daily doses of doxycycline or sulphadoxine may be effective in preventing cholera or *E. coli* infection in persons in high risk areas;[7,39] but their use cannot be recommended for longterm prophylaxis and they are not likely to be effective against typhoid fever or amoebic dysentery.

Chemoprophylaxis cannot be contemplated for community control, but the reservoirs and pathways of transmission of intestinal pathogens indicate opportunities for disease control in large populations by methods other than immunization. The dramatic decline in typhoid fever, cholera and severe bacillary dysentery that has occurred over the last five decades or more in many countries has not been due to the immunologist; rather it is linked to improved housing and purer water supplies, better attention to personal hygiene and a variety of utilities and health services designed to interrupt infection pathways, provide rapid diagnosis of cases, identify carriers, and maintain effective epidemiological surveillance.

However, these public services are not cheap. They are therefore unlikely to provide immediate solutions to the problems of highly populated, under-privileged countries. Although the simple expedient of chlorinating well-water has eliminated cholera from villages in the Philippines, it is doubtful whether measures of this nature alone would be similarly effective in densely populated urban areas. The cost-benefits of a control programme can be assessed by mathematical models of the type devised by Cvjetanovic and his colleagues,[6] but the information they yield is only valid if the input data is directly relevant to the community in question.

Immunization for individual protection and community control is simple, cheap and, at the present time, probably the best method available. But each vaccine differs in effectiveness, inherent risks, overall costs, and likelihood of public acceptance.

TYPHOID FEVER VACCINES

The first parenteral typhoid vaccine was developed in 1897 by Almroth Wright; despite a cursory investigation of its protective capacity, this heat-killed preparation of *Salmonella typhi* was used, with only minor modifications, to immunize probably millions of people over the ensuing half-century. Because *S. typhi* is uniquely pathogenic for man, the only methods for assessing the effectiveness of a typhoid vaccine are those involving volunteers or extensive, rigorously controlled, field trials. Such trials were not mounted until 1954, by the World Health Organization in Yugoslavia, British Guyana, Poland and Russia and these were finally assessed between 1962 and 1965.[5] Community control was attempted and therefore high-risk areas were selected for the studies. Almost 1.5 million people were involved and most subjects were school-age children, the group most susceptible to serious disease in high risk areas. The vaccines and

Table 12.1 Effectiveness of various parenteral typhoid vaccines assessed by field trials in Yugoslavia, British Guyana, Poland and USSR

Vaccine type	No. of doses	No. of trials	Duration of trials (y)	Effectiveness[1]	
				Maximal	Minimal
(a) *Whole organisms inactivated by:*					
Acetone	2	3	2–3½	94%	79%
	1	2	2–3½	100%	—
Heat–phenol	2	6	2–6	86%	51%
	1	1	2–3½	78%	—
Alcohol	2	4	2–5	75%	39%
Formalin	2	1	2	90%	—
(b) *Extracted antigens*					
Endotoxoid	2	2	2	61%	0%
'Chemical vaccine'					
+ Adjuvant	2	2	2	68%	59%
	1	3	2	77%	58%
	2	2	2	61%	23%
− Adjuvant	1	1	2	11%	—

[1]Effectiveness = $100(b-a)/b$, where a = incidence rate in immunized group and b = incidence rate in control group.

antigens used in the trial are shown in Table 12.1. Full details of these trials have been reported[16,21,36,43,47] and the most pertinent results are summarized in Table 12.1. The acetone-inactivated vaccine was the most effective, though potency variations might have occurred with vaccines manufactured under different conditions. The heat-phenol-inactivated vaccine was the next most effective but in only one trial was it found to have a protective efficiency of more than 80%. Differences in potency of different preparations of this vaccine may have accounted for the relatively broad range of results (51–86%). The trials also showed that the combined typhoid-paratyphoid vaccines, though having some effect against typhoid fever, had little influence on the incidence of the milder paratyphoid fevers; the use of these vaccines has now been discontinued in many countries. Although the results suggested that a single dose was more effective than two doses, a more detailed trial in Tonga using an acetone-inactivated vaccine showed the superiority of two doses of vaccine spaced by approximately four weeks.[42] In some trials, booster doses given 1 year after the first course were found to be useful in extending the duration of immunity.

These and later trials have led to the conclusion that, *in areas where typhoid fever is prevalent*, parenteral immunization with acetone-inactivated vaccine can be expected to have an efficiency of approximately 80% and that immunity may last for a period of up to 5 years. Epidemiological evidence strongly supports the view that significant natural immunity, acquired through frequent exposure to subinfectious doses of *S. typhi*, exists in most adults living in high-risk areas and, *pari passu* that parenteral immunization may serve as no more than a useful booster to it. There is, however, no evidence that primary immunization produces the same degree of immunity in persons who normally reside in low-risk areas. Volunteers who had not been previously exposed to the organism have been studied; although the acetone and heat-phenol vaccines gave approximately 70% protection against doses of 100 000 organisms ($\equiv$ID25) or less, they were totally ineffective when 100-fold greater doses ($\equiv$ID50) were used.[18] Thus though parenteral immunization may offer protection against water borne outbreaks of typhoid fever — when the dose level would normally be low — it may have little benefit against infections that result from food contamination when prior multiplication to yield large numbers of organisms can be expected. In high-risk areas the individual may only be protected against low doses of *S. typhi*. The advice of one senior U.S. public health administrator is relevant for travellers, 'certainly have typhoid immunization, but when you get there, behave as if you hadn't'.

Despite the success of the field trials, mass immunization campaigns in densely populated, underprivileged countries have not been mounted partly because of the local and systemic reactions to the vaccine, but mainly because the cost of the programme would be prohibitive. Furthermore, it has yet to be established that mass immunization alone will have any effect on the carrier rate of *S. typhi* in these communities; this may be the most important factor in determining the incidence of the disease.

A correlation was found between the effectiveness of various vaccines used in the trials and the levels of H (flagella) antibodies in the sera of different groups of vaccines,[1] but it is doubtful whether this simple serological test can be used as a measure of antityphoid immunity or as a means of assessing the immune status of an immunized population. One quality control test — the active mouse protection test — yielded reasonable correlations with the performance of different vaccines used in the field trials, but as noted by Cvjetanovic and Uemura,[5] '... the results ... tend to differ when performed in different laboratories and even in the same laboratory they often give different results'. However, there is no better test, and thus there is no guarantee that any given batch of vaccine, whatever its method of preparation, will contain a required standard of potency.

Oral immunization has long been considered as an alternative to parenteral injection of vaccines. At the end of the First World War Besredka developed 'bili-vaccination'. Ox-bile capsules plus approximately 1×10^{10} killed *S. typhi*, were given orally for 3 or 4 days, and epidemics of typhoid apparently were arrested.[2] As there were no properly designed tests of its efficiency, it was not accepted by medical scientists in Britain and the USA. In Europe, heat-killed or acetone-inactivated whole organisms have been used for these vaccines. Humoral antibody responses against *S. typhi* are induced and local defence mechanisms may be activated. However, controlled trials in areas of high prevalence have shown that, even with doses of 1×10^{12} organisms the vaccines were ineffective.[3]

Despite the proven efficacy of the parenteral acetone-killed vaccines, there is a continued search for safer, less costly and more effective typhoid vaccines especially oral vaccines. Studies on rodent *Salmonella* infections have clearly established that systemic immunity to the pathogen is essential, that it is cell-mediated and is best induced by exposure to live organisms. This may not hold true for typhoid in man, because systemic experience of *S. typhi* during clinical infection offers no guarantee of immunity to a second infection;[29] moreover in the longterm typhoid carrier the hepatic and splenic macrophages are sites of residence for the organism which must survive apparently in the face of specifically-activated cell-mediated mechanisms. Thus *S. typhi* seems to have become so well adapted to survival in its natural host, that effective systemic immunity to the organism may be difficult to achieve.

The typhoid carrier presents a curious paradox; in these persons the biliary and intestinal tracts often contain large numbers of virulent *S. typhi* yet reinvasion from the intestinal lumen does not occur. Does this imply that specific, local defence mechanisms are the key to typhoid immunity? If so, it might be argued that vaccines should be designed primarily to promote local rather than systemic, immunity. Intestinal antibody (presumed to be of the sIgA class) is highly protective in rodent salmonellosis.[24] In man most attention has been given to live vaccines prepared from mutants of *S. typhi*. It has been argued that provided the mutation leads to loss of virulence without affecting the organism's antigenic characteristics, live organism vaccines may be retained in the intestine for a period sufficient to permit induction of local, possibly general, immunity.

The first generation of oral typhoid vaccines was based on mutants which grow only in the presence of streptomycin (SmD).

One strain (27V) has been tested extensively in chimpanzees and volunteers. When given once weekly over a period of 4–5 weeks, it was found to be safe, stable and retained in the intestine for 2–3 days. Moreover, if the vaccine was given immediately after the organisms were harvested, a high level of protection was found in volunteers challenged with a dose of virulent *S. typhi* equivalent to one ID50. Surprisingly, lyophilized preparations of this vaccine were not protective; this could not be ascribed to loss of viability and as there is no other means of preparing this type of vaccine for distribution on a large scale it is not likely to be considered for routine use.[27] Other SmD mutants have been developed and are currently being evaluated.

A second type of mutant appears more promising. These are described as gal-E mutants and lack the enzyme uridine-5-diphosphate-glucose-4-epimerase which is necessary for complete assembly of the specific polysaccharide side chains of the O-antigens (LPS). Grown in the presence of galactose these mutants develop the complete LPS of smooth strains but, because of accumulation of galactose-1-phosphate and UDP-galactose, they lyse. *In vivo* exogenous galactose would ensure the development of the smooth O-antigen but automatically restrict the organism's capacity to proliferate for any significant period. These mutants were first shown to be highly protective in rodent salmonellosis[12] and one *S. typhi* gal-E mutant vaccine has been tested in volunteers.[14] Five to eight doses of 3^{10}–10^{10} organisms given orally have been used; the mutant survived in the intestine for no more than 3 days yet conferred a high level of protection against subsequent challenge. In all respects it appeared superior to the acetone-killed parenteral vaccine tested under the same conditions. The results of a 3-year field trial in young school children living in a typhoid-endemic area suggest that oral immunization with the vaccine (designated Ty 21a) may be highly successful.

Though the incidence of the disease in nonvaccinated groups was not high (36 cases per 10 000) the vaccine's protective efficacy was found to be 95%.[44] Should further, more extensive trials in other regions substantiate this result, a strong case could be made for its use as a routine typhoid immunoprophylactic.

CHOLERA VACCINES

Parenteral vaccines have been prepared from whole *Vibrio cholerae* organisms, and were first used about 1901. Epidemics were apparently arrested but it is likely that the simultaneous application of simple hygiene relating to faeces disposal and water supply had a far greater effect on the rate at which these epidemics waned. The results of many extensive studies over the past 20 years have, however, clearly demonstrated that currently-available cholera vaccines do not effectively control epidemics, nor do they prevent asymptomatic carriage of the organism. The continued use of cholera vaccines for these purposes is difficult to justify particularly as simple sanitation methods control epidemics, and chemo-prophylaxis can prevent asymptomatic carriage of the organism.

Since 1962 trials have been undertaken to assess the efficacy of routine vaccines, and also some new types. The routine vaccines contained both antigenic types of *V. cholerae*, Ogawa and Inaba, inactivated by heat, phenol or formalin, and were issued either in fluid or freeze-dried forms. The newer test vaccines included monovalent whole organism preparations, bivalent preparations with oil or aluminium hydroxide as adjuvant, and purified lipopolysaccharide preparations. These trials were strictly controlled, involved many thousands of subjects and were conducted in a number of different regions so that vaccine efficacy against the El Tor and classical biotypes and the two major serotypes of *V. cholerae* could be investigated. The results of some of these trials are briefly shown in Table 12.2. From these and from more detailed reports,[33,34] it was concluded that routine vaccines did not have an efficacy of 80%, and could not maintain immunity for 2–3 years, and thus are of little practical value. Their efficacy ranged from 4–72%, and their maximum efficacy lasted for about 3 months then declined. The immunity was of shorter duration in children under 14 years than in adults, but in endemic areas the disease is more common and serious in children. Second or booster doses of the vaccine appeared to increase the duration and level of immunity in young children to some extent. The frequency of side-effects of these vaccines was low and, with rare exceptions, there were very mild local effects.

In one trial a monovalent vaccine was found to provide protection of more than 80% over a period of 3 years against the homologous strain (Inaba). However, a subsequent trial in another region did not confirm this. Monovalent vaccines may increase the chances of antigenic shift of the endemic strains.

Aluminium hydroxide adjuvant seems to enhance the efficacy of vaccines,[38] but not enough to be useful. Oil-based adjuvants have problems of severe local side-reactions.

Table 12.2 Effectiveness of parenteral cholera vaccines assessed by various field trials in endemic areas

Vaccine type	Side reactions*	Range of vaccine effectiveness† (%)	Duration of effective immunity (months)
'Routine' bivalent vaccines			
Freeze dried	±	9–57	0–3 mths
Fluid	±	4–72	0–18 mths
'Monovalent' vaccines	±	11–84	6–36 mths
Lipopolysaccharide	±	43	6
Adjuvant vaccines	±		
Oil based	++++	66	8
Al(OH)$_3$	±	68	14

* ± slight reactions (local or general) in small percentages of vaccinees, ++++ severe local abscesses in some vaccinees. †Effectiveness = $100 (b-a)/b$, where a = incidence rate in immunized group and b = incidence rate in control group.

In Bangladesh cholera occurs more commonly in young children than in adults. Levels of serum vibriocidal antibodies were found to be higher in adults than children.[32] Antibacterial antibodies may indicate immunity, but studies in the field and in volunteer trials showed that disease could occur when vibriocidal titres were high or low and, conversely, did not occur in cholera contacts who had low serum levels of these antibodies. The correlation between vibriocidal titres and vaccine efficacy was poor.[34] At present there is nothing to recommend the use of parenteral cholera vaccines or purified lipopolysaccharides either as a means of public health control in endemic areas or as a reasonable guarantee of protection for individuals against the disease.

Oral immunization with cholera organisms was developed by Besredka. Initial reports of this vaccine were enthusiastic, but were devoid of meaningful statistical data. Since then there have been no extensive field studies designed to assess the true, or potential, value of oral cholera vaccines.

Epidemiological studies and volunteer experiments have suggested that man's resistance to cholera infection is enhanced by intestinal exposure to *Vibrio cholerae*. Whilst this encourages the belief that oral immunization may be a viable approach to the control of cholera, there are very few experimental immunizing agents that can be regarded as strong candidates to replace the present, poorly effective, parenteral vaccines.

During the past 20 years a great deal has been learned of the pathogenic mechanisms of *V. cholerae*; the organism is restricted to the intestinal lumen and disease results only if it attaches to and proliferates on the duodenal mucosa, then releases an enterotoxin which binds to, and directly affects, these cells. Immunity is mediated by antibodies within the lumen or associated with the mucosal surface, preventing the organism's association with the surface or directly interfering with the enterotoxin. Antibacterial and antitoxic antibodies appear in the intestinal secretions and faeces of convalescent cholera cases and it is assumed that if one or both types of antibody are maintained in the intestine, or are rapidly recalled in the face of challenge by the virulent organism, effective immunity will be achieved.

Many experiments in different animal models have established that anti-bacterial antibodies function by interfering, in some way, with the organism's colonization of the intestinal surface. Antibodies of the IgM, IgG and IgA classes are equally effective and no better than F(ab)$_2$ fragments, suggesting that they function by direct interference rather than by exploitation of amplification mechanisms requiring participation of the Fc region of the molecule.[37] Anti-LPS antibodies are protective in the intestine; whether antibodies that react with other components of the *V. cholerae* cell (e.g. flagella[46]) also have protective functions has yet to be evaluated properly. Antitoxic antibodies are also protective in the intestine; in this case only IgG and IgA antibodies appear to have significant toxin-neutralizing activity and the former appears to be far more avid than the latter.[17]

The purely local nature of immunity to cholera has, in recent years, directed some attention to the development of oral immunizing agents designed to induce either antibacterial or antitoxic immunity. A variety of genetic recombinants of *V. cholerae* and other cholera-like organisms, designed to reduce the natural virulence through loss of toxigenicity or modification of surface antigens have been developed and tested in animals and volunteers. Some have provided protection in animals and one mutant has been claimed to maintain copro-antibody production in volunteers for 3 months after two large oral doses;[40] the efficacy of such mutant vaccines against natural or challenge infection has not been properly assessed. One detailed study in volunteers[11] has yielded results that do little to encourage the belief that the present generation of live mutant vaccines are likely to be effective. It was found that the antibacterial antibody content of intestinal secretions was no greater in individuals immunized with a total of ca 8×10^{11} live vaccine organisms than in those given a normal course of a parenteral killed vaccine; curiously, the highest antibody responses were found in the group which received two oral doses of 1×10^{11} phenol-inactivated organisms. Most importantly, in all instances the antibodies in the intestinal secretions disappeared within 4 weeks of the last vaccine dose.

Oral immunization techniques designed to promote local antitoxic immunity have been considered at the experimental level also. In most animals, cholera toxin is highly immunogenic when given intraintestinally; local formation and secretion of antitoxin (primarily of the IgA class) develops rapidly and correlates with the development of immunity to challenge infection.[23] However, two factors mitigate against this approach; firstly the local antitoxin responses are short-lived and second cholera toxoid is poorly immunogenic in the intestine. However, recent studies in dogs have suggested another approach;[35] subcutaneous priming with purified aluminium phosphate precipitated toxoid, followed some weeks later by several intraintestinal doses, conferred longterm protection against challenge infection. Curiously, in these studies immunity could not be directly correlated with residual local or systemic antitoxin nor with rapid recall of local antitoxin, a situation that bears a superficial relationship to the longterm immunity found in volunteers following recovery from cholera infection. As yet there is no information available concerning the efficacy of the subcutaneous plus oral immunizing regime in man.

Doubts concerning the capacity of the intestinal lymphoid tissues to mount prolonged antibody responses to any specific antigen (and thus maintain effective antibody levels in the intestine) have been expressed in Chapter 2; a corollary is that oral immunization techniques that are designed to induce local immunity may have little to offer in diseases such as cholera where it is entirely dependent upon humoral antibodies. However, despite the obvious importance of sIgA antibodies in local intestinal immunity, there is now ample evidence to indicate that intestinal immunity can also be mediated by IgM and IgG antibodies which cross the epithelial surface into mucus associated with it. In the case of antitoxin of the IgG class there is a direct correlation between serum concentration and immunity; this can be attributed to transudation of a small portion of it across the epithelial surface.

In this instance, then, a case can be made for considering parenteral immunizing agents provided they are highly immunogenic and maintain serum antibodies at high levels over a long period. Most attention has been focused on cholera toxoid and though a field trial with a glutaraldehyde-inactivated preparation was not successful,[4] more recent studies with a heat-inactivated, formalin-treated toxoid appear encouraging.[13] Additionally, with elucidation of the structure-function relationships of cholera enterotoxin, an immunizing agent based on the non-toxigenic, highly immunogenic B-subunit has been developed and is currently being assessed.[17] The possibility of combining this material with purified antigens of the *V. cholerae* cell (e.g. LPS) as a means of inducing both antitoxic and antibacterial immunity has been considered at the experimental level[17] and may offer yet another approach to the solution of what is clearly a difficult problem.

SHIGELLA VACCINES

Climate, economic conditions and community standards of hygiene greatly influence the nature of dysentery infections in different communities. In most developing countries *Shigella flexneri* serotypes are endemic, and *S. dysenteriae* type 1 (Shiga's bacillus) has caused major, severe epidemics; in contrast *S. sonnei* exists as the major endemic organism in most industrialized countries but occasional epidemics of *S. flexneri* occur. Moreover, in these countries, institutional shigellosis, usually due to *S. flexneri* and *S. dysenteriae* serotypes, remains an important problem. A strong case can be made for immunization on a wide scale in areas where the disease is highly endemic and also as a means of controlling institutional shigellosis.

Killed oral and parenteral *Shigella* vaccines have been used for many years. The absence of any routine immunization programme can be accounted for by the fact that these vaccines have proved to be ineffective. However, recent studies have clarified the pathogenic mechanisms of the shigellae. It has been suggested that the initially intraluminal production of an enterotoxin in the jejunum causes an early watery diarrhoea and then invasion and multiplication of the organism within the colonic epithelium occurs. Intracellular toxin production may lead to death of these cells leading to the inflammatory responses that are characteristic of the pathology of the disease.[20] The enterotoxin is produced by all virulent strains of *Shigella* and appears to be antigenically identical in all serotypes. Genetic studies have implicated three separate regions of the chromosome of these organisms which all have some role in the attachment and invasive processes that lead to proliferation in the colon; at least one of these regions is associated with somatic antigen formation and thus it is reasonable to believe that immune mechanisms which might protect against invasion are serotype specific.

It has been known for many years that serotype specific antibacterial antibodies appear in the faeces of dysentery convalescents and more recently toxin-neutralizing antibodies have also been found in these persons.[19] It might therefore be assumed that immunity to the disease can be expressed through both types of antibodies and thus immunizing agents which induce one or the other might be protective. Curiously, in contrast to cholera, an aluminium hydroxide-absorbed toxoid prepared from *S. dysenteriae* was found to be devoid of protective activity in rhesus monkey, despite its capacity to induce high serum antitoxin titres.[31] If this result is confirmed, antibacterial immunity must serve as the basis for vaccine development.

Parenteral injections of live or killed *Shigella* induce high anti-LPS antibody titres in sera of laboratory animals, nonhuman primates and human vaccinees; despite this they offer no protection against dysentery infection. Again this contrasts with cholera; the explanations may lie, firstly, in the fact that as *Shigella* organisms pass from cell to cell in the colonic mucosa[15] they may be inaccessible to serum antibodies and, secondly, in that the peculiar environment of the colonic surface may not be conducive to transudation or survival of serum antibodies which may otherwise serve to prevent surface colonization by the organism.

Despite the lack of encouragement from animal infection-immunity studies, significant advances have been made in dysentery vaccine developments over the past 15 years; these derive from quite empirical studies by Mel and his colleagues in Yugoslavian army volunteers who were given oral doses of streptomycin-dependent mutants (SmD) of that country's endemic strains. Subsequent extensive field trials in adults and children established that, provided the vaccine doses were appropriately adjusted for different age groups, these live vaccines caused few side-effects and showed no evidence of reversion to the virulent phenotype. Immunity was found to be serotype specific and usually a protective efficacy of 80% or greater was recorded against the homologous infection.[30] A first course of four oral doses, given at 3-day intervals, containing $c\ 50 \times 10^{10}$ live organisms generally protected for 12 months and revaccination boosted protection to $c.$ 90% in the second year.

Volunteer studies in individuals who were, on serological grounds, thought not to have been previously infected with *Shigella* demonstrated that the SmD vaccines conferred statistically significant protection; however, the protection rates were no more than 50–60%. This finding suggests that the high efficacy of the vaccines reported in the Yugoslavian trials might be attributed to their boosting of pre-existing immunity acquired by natural subclinical infection.[9] Furthermore, studies in a children's institution in the United States revealed that the stability of the live vaccines varied, that a high rate of reversion to streptomycin-independence occurred and that transmission of the vaccine strains to non-immunized individuals could not be prevented.[26] These observations caution against the use of vaccines that are based on one-step mutations as there can be no guarantee that continual, uncontrolled intestinal passage might not lead to selection of virulent strains.

A second approach is favoured, particularly by workers in the United States. It depends upon selection of avirulent mutants followed by hybridization with *E. coli* K12. These mutant-hybrid (MH) vaccines were developed from earlier generations of mutants or hybrids which caused severe reactions, even frank dysentery, in volunteers.[8] Unfortunately, the MH vaccines conferred no protection in volunteers and in one instance reversion to virulence occurred.[25] A third generation of candidate oral vaccines has been developed by hybridization of *E. coli* K12 with *S. flexneri* 2a with the aim of inserting into the recipient's chromosome those genes responsible for expression of the *Shigella* somatic antigens. Though nonreactogenic, this vaccine was not found to protect volunteers against challenge infection.[28]

The development of an effective *Shigella* vaccine therefore seems to be confounded by an obvious paradox. Effective local immunity is likely to develop only when the vaccine colonizes and invades the colonic mucosa, yet these activities are essential components of virulence. Thus the vaccine might unavoidably induce inflammatory responses which are essential features of the pathology of the disease. Until this paradox is resolved or circumvented, it is unlikely that any substantial progress will be made towards the widespread use of oral immunization against bacillary dysentery.

ESCHERICHIA COLI INFECTIONS

Enterotoxigenic *E. coli* (ETEC) strains are known to be responsible for many severe diarrhoeal diseases in young children and infants and also for the common adult syndrome of traveller's diarrhoea. Immunization is not warranted for the latter infection but the severity of infantile diarrhoea in developing nations is of sufficient concern to warrant the use of some effective prophylactic procedure on a wide scale.

The elegant studies on *E. coli* infections in piglets have clearly established that ETEC infection is in practically all respects similar to that of cholera.[41]

However, adhesion has been specifically linked with the presence of plasmid-controlled, antigenically and morphologically distinctive pili that form part of the cell envelope. Vaccines prepared from purified pili promote production of antibodies in serum and in the intestines and these prevent colonization by challenge organisms, thus acting protectively against the disease.

Studies with human ETEC have lagged far behind those concerned with piglet infection. Nonetheless, it is now certain that the pathogenesis of infection in man is similar; however, the two adhesive pilus antigens so far identified (CFA I, CFA II) are different from those of the animal strains.[10] In recent years, most research effort has been concerned with the nature and function of the enterotoxin produced by the human ETEC strains. Two diarrhoeogenic toxins may be produced (singly or together) by these strains. One is heat-stable (ST) and non-antigenic; the other is heat-labile (LT), antigenic and shares common antigenic determinants with *V. cholerae* enterotoxin.[22] This finding has encouraged the belief that a cholera prophylactic that induces antitoxin production might protect against both cholera and ETEC infections. The hypothesis has yet to be substantiated, however.

A recent report of a WHO Scientific Working Group acknowledges the importance of developing an effective means of immunizing against ETEC infection.[45] Whilst live, avirulent strains may be most suitable for oral immunization, the potential value of nonreplicating antigens, e.g. colonization factors (pili), cell wall materials or toxoid cannot be discounted. Further, the Working Group raised the question whether immunization of mothers near term may also be effective in reducing the incidence of neonatal infection through passive immunity acquired by transfer of antibody in milk.

Thus, at the moment, the potential value of immunization against *E. coli* infection is largely a matter of conjecture rather than reality. Furthermore, it is not yet known whether immunization against the enteropathogenic (EPEC) and enteroinvasive (EIEC) strains is warranted. It seems certain that, because of the antigenic diversity that exists between pathogenic *E. coli* strains and the obviously different mechanisms by which they produce disease, the problems of developing satisfactory immunizing agents will prove far more complex than those which have been revealed by more detailed and extensive studies with other, less complicated bacterial diseases of the intestine.

THE FUTURE FOR IMMUNIZATION AGAINST GUT PATHOGENS

With the exception of preformed bacterial toxins in food, bacterial disease is the direct consequence of proliferation of pathogenic organisms on or within the host at a greater rate than can be controlled by the host's natural defence mechanisms. The mechanisms of bacterial pathogenesis are shown in Table 12.3.

If disease is to occur, a pathogenic bacterium must express two, or more, of the primary mechanisms listed. The pathogen may have 'adhesins' which enable it to overcome the normal surface defence mechanisms, and then attach to and flourish at a particular epithelial/mucosal surface. In *E. coli* pili are thought to be adhesins. For some organisms — *V. cholerae, E. coli* — surface proliferation is all that is required but in many diseases, the organisms must invade tissues by means of 'invasins', but little is known of their nature. Recent studies with *Shigella* species have permitted mapping of genes associated with this activity.

Exotoxin production is of paramount importance for *Vibrio cholerae* (see Chapter 5) and enteroxigenic *E. coli* (see Chapter 4). Specific immunological

Table 12.3 Mechanisms of bacterial pathogenesis

Primary mechanisms	Surface colonization	('ADHESINS')
	Invasiveness	('INVASINS')
	Exotoxin production	Acting locally
		Acting peripherally
	Survival and proliferation	('AGGRESSINS')
	in tissues	Extracellular survival
		Intracellular survival
Secondary mechanisms	Cytotoxins	
	Enzymes	

defence depends upon the host mounting responses, humoral or cell-mediated, that are specifically antagonistic to the primary mechanisms used by the pathogen in its attack on the host (Table 12.4).

If active immunization is to be successful, it must ensure that the appropriate protective immune responses are evoked, and more importantly, that they are accompanied by longterm memory which permits their rapid recall on subsequent exposure to the pathogenic organism or its appropriate antigens. In the case of the intestinal diseases, in which the vaccines offer only moderate or poor protection, some or all of the pathogenic mechanisms remain within the obscurity of the terms adhesin, invasin or aggressin; until the nature of these components — once commonly described as the 'protective antigens' — has been identified precisely, it is unlikely that effective vaccines will be developed.

Though nonhuman primates are generally susceptible to the human intestinal pathogens, basic costs of management usually preclude their use in detailed studies. Unfortunately more convenient laboratory animals are naturally resistant to these pathogens and as a result, experimental models of infection which completely mimic the human diseases have been difficult to devise.

For virus infections it is only within recent years that some of the causative organisms — the Norwalk agent and the rotavirus — have been identified and only a few have been propagated *in vitro*. Furthermore, there is insufficient sero-epidemiological data to indicate whether active immunization is likely to be useful in their prevention. Potential rotavirus vaccines are discussed in Chapter 8.

Table 12.4 Defence mechanisms against bacterial pathogenesis

Pathogenic mechanism	Host defence mechanism Humoral	Cell-mediated
Surface colonization (Adhesins)	Interference	—
Invasins	?	?
Exotoxin	Antitoxin	—
Aggressins	Opsonization causing enhanced phagocytosis and digestion	Enhanced intracellular digestion through macrophage activation

REFERENCES

1 Benenson A. S. (1964) Serological responses of man to typhoid vaccines. *Bull. WHO* **30**, 659.
2 Besredka A. (1923–24) Local immunity in infectious diseases. *Trans. R. Soc. Trop. Med. Hyg.* **17**, 346.
3 Chuttani C. S., Prakash K., Gupta P., Grover V. and Kumar A. (1977) Controlled field trial of a high dose oral killed typhoid vaccine in India. *Bull. WHO* **55**, 643.
4 Curlin G., Levine R, Aziz K. M. A., Rahman A. S. M. and Verwey W. F. (1976) Field trial of cholera toxoid. Proc. 11th Joint Conf. U.S. Jap. Coop. Med. Sci. Prog. Symp. on Cholera, p. 314.
5 Cvjetanovic B. and Uemura K. (1965) The present status of field and laboratory studies of typhoid and paratyphoid vaccines with special reference to studies sponsored by World Health Organisation. *Bull. WHO* **32**, 29.
6 Cvjetanovic B., Grab B. and Uemura K. (1970) Epidemiological model of typhoid fever and its use in the planning and evaluation of antityphoid immunization and sanitation programmes. WHO Document WHO/ENT/70.12.
7 Deb B. C., Sen Gupta P. G., De S. P., Sil J., Sikdar S. N. and Pal S. C. (1976) Effect of sulfadoxine on transmission of *Vibrio cholerae* infection among family contacts of cholera patients in Calcutta. *Bull. WHO* **54**, 171.
8 Du Pont H. L., Hornick R. B., Snyder M. J., Libonati J. P., Formal S. B. and Gangarosa E. J. (1972) Immunity in Shigellosis I. Response of man to attenuated strains of Shigella. *J. Infect. Dis.* **125**, 5.
9 Du Pont H. L., Hornick R. B., Snyder M. J., Libonati J. P., Formal S. B. and Gangarosa E. J. (1972) Immunity in Shigellosis II. Protection induced by oral live vaccine or primary infection. *J. Infect. Dis.* **125**, 12.
10 Evans D. G., Evans D. J. Jr and Du Pont H. L. (1977) Virulence factors of enterotoxigenic *Escherichia coli*. *J. Infect. Dis.* **136**, S118.
11 Ganguly R., Clem L. W., Bencic Z., Sinha R., Sakazaki R. and Woldman R. H. (1975) Antibody response in the intestinal secretions of volunteers immunised with various cholera vaccines. *Bull. WHO* **52**, 323.
12 Germanier R. (1972) Immunity in experimental salmonellosis. 3. Comparative immunization with viable and heat-inactivated cells of *Salmonella typhimurium*. *Infect. Immun.* **5**, 792.
13 Germanier R., Furer E., Varallyay S. and Inderbitzen T. M. (1977) Antigenicity of cholera toxoid in humans. *J. Infect. Dis.* **135**, 512.
14 Gilman R. H., Hornick R. B., Woodard W. E., Du Pont H. L., Snyder M. J., Levine M. M. and Libonati J. P. (1977) Evaluation of a UDP-glucose-4-epimeraseless mutant of *Salmonella typhi* as a live oral vaccine. *J. Infect. Dis.* **136**, 717.
15 Hale T. L. and Bonventre P. F. (1977) Shigella infection of Henle intestinal epithelial cells: role of the bacterium. *Infect. Immun.* **24**, 879.
16 Hejfec L. B. (1965) Results of the study of typhoid vaccines in four controlled field trials in the USSR. *Bull. WHO* **32**, 1.
17 Holmgren J. and Svennerholm A. M. (1977) Mechanisms of disease and immunity in cholera: a review. *J. Infect. Dis.* **136**, Suppl: S105.
18 Hornick R. B., Woodward T. E., McCrumb F. R., Snyder M. J., Dawkins A. T., Bulkeley J. T., de la Macorra F. and Corozza F. A. (1967) Typhoid fever vaccine — yes or no? *Med. Clin. Nth America* **51**, 617.
19 Keusch G. T. and Jacewicz M. (1973). Serum enterotoxin-neutralizing antibody in human shigellosis. *Nature* **241**, 31.
20 Keusch G. T. and Jacewicz M. (1977). The pathogenesis of Shigella diarrhoea VI. Toxin and antitoxin in *Shigella flexneri* and *Shigella sonnei* infections in humans. *J. Infect. Dis.* **135**, 552.
21 Khasanov M. I., Kheifets L. B. and Salmin L. V. (1962) A controlled field trial of the typhoid component of polyvalent enteric vaccine (NIISI Polyvaccine). *Bull. WHO* **26**, 371.

22 Klipstein F. A. and Engert R. F. (1977) Immunological interrelationships between cholera toxin and the heat-labile and heat-stable enterotoxins of coliform bacteria. *Infect. Immun.* **18**, 110.

23 Lange S., Hansson H. A., Molin S. O. and Nygren H. (1979) Local cholera immunity in mice: intestinal antitoxin-containing cells and their correlation with protective immunity. *Infect. Immun.* **23**, 743.

24 Levanou Y. and Rossetini S. M. O. (1968). Reagins from orally immunized animals. 1. Nature and protection effect. *Progr. Immunobiol. Standards.* **4**, 347.

25 Levine M. M., Du Pont H. L., Formal S. B., Hornick R. B., Takeuchi A., Gangarosa E. J., Snyder M. J. and Libonati J. P. (1973) Pathogenesis of *Shigella dysenteriae* 1 (Shiga) dysentery. *J. Infect. Dis.* **127**, 261.

26 Levine M. M., Gangarosa E. J., Barrow W. B., Morris G. K., Wells Joy G. and Weiss C. F. (1975) Shigellosis in custodial institutions. IV. *In vivo* stability and transmissibility of oral attenuated streptomycin-dependent Shigella vaccines. *J. Infect. Dis.* **131**, 704.

27 Levine M. M., Du Pont H. L., Hornick R. B., Snyder M. J., Woodward W., Gilman R. H. and Libonati J. P. (1976) Attenuated streptomycin-dependent *Salmonella typhi* oral vaccine: potential deleterious effects of lyophilization. *J. Infect. Dis.* **133**, 424.

28 Levine M. M., Woodward W. E., Formal S. B, Gemski P. Jr, Du Pont H. L., Hornick R. B., and Snyder M. J. (1977) Studies with a new generation of oral attenuated Shigella vaccine: *Escherichia coli* bearing surface antigens of *Shigella flexneri*. *J. Infect. Dis.* **136**, 577.

29 Marmion D. E., Naylor G. R. E. and Steward I. O. (1953) Second attacks of typhoid fever. *J. Hyg. (Camb.)* **51**, 260.

30 Mel D., Gangarosa E. J., Radovanovic M. L., Arsic B. L. and Litvinjenko S. (1971) Studies on vaccination against bacillary dysentery. 6. Protection of children by oral immunization with streptomycin-dependent *Shigella* strains. *Bull. WHO* **45**, 457.

31 McIver J., Grady G. F. and Formal S. B. (1977) Immunization with *Shigella dysenteriae* Type 1: Evaluation of antitoxic immunity in prevention of experimental disease in rhesus monkeys (*Macaca mulatta*). *J. Infect. Dis.* **136**, 416.

32 Mosley W. H. (1969) Vaccines and somatic antigens. The role of immunity in cholera. A review of epidemiological and serological studies. *Tex. Rep. Biol. Med.* **27**, Suppl. 1, 227.

33 Mosley W. H., Aziz K. M. A., Mizanur Rahman A. S. M., Alauddin Chowdhury A. K. M., Ansaruddin Ahmed and Fahimuddin M. (1972) Report of the 1966–67 cholera vaccine trial in rural East Pakistan. *Bull. WHO* **47**, 229.

34 Mosley W. H., Aziz K. M. A., Mizanur Rahman A. S. M., Alauddin Chowdhury A. K. M. and Ansaruddin Ahmed (1973) Field trials of monovalent Ogawa and Inaba cholera vaccines in rural Bangladesh — three years of observation. *Bull. WHO* **49**, 381.

35 Pierce N. F., Cray W. C. Jr and Sircar B. K. (1978) Induction of a mucosal antitoxin response and its role in immunity to experimental canine cholera. *Infect. Immun.* **21**, 185.

36 Polish Typhoid Committee (1965) Evaluation of typhoid vaccines in the laboratory and in a controlled field trial in Poland. *Bull. WHO* **32**, 15.

37 Rowley D. (1977) The problems of oral immunization. *Aust. J. Exp. Biol. Med. Sci.* **55**, 1.

38 Saroso J. S., Bahrawi W., Witjaksono H., Budiarso R. L., Brotowasisto, Bencic Z., Dewitt W. E. and Gomez C. Z. (1978) A controlled field trial of plain and aluminium hydroxide-adsorbed cholera vaccines in Surabaya, Indonesia, during 1973–75. *Bull. WHO* **56**, 619.

39 Sen Gupta P. G., Sircar B. K., Mondal S., De S. P., Gen D., Sikder S. N., Deb B. C. and Pal S. C. (1978) Effect of doxycycline on transmission of *Vibrio cholerae* infection among family contacts of cholera patients in Calcutta. *Bull. WHO* **56**, 323.

40 Sanyal S. C. and Mukerjee S. (1969) Live oral cholera vaccine: report of a trial on human volunteer subjects. *Bull. WHO* **40**, 503.

41 Smith H. W. and Linggood M. A. (1971) Observations on the pathogenic properties of the K88, Hly and Ent plasmids of *Escherichia coli* with particular reference to porcine diarrhoea. *J. Med. Microbiol.* **4**, 467.

42 Tapa S. and Cvjetanovic B. (1975) Controlled field trial on the effectiveness of one and two doses of acetone-inactivated and dried typhoid vaccine. *Bull. WHO* **52**, 75.

43 Typhoid Panel, U.K. Department of Technical Co-operation (1964). A controlled field trial of acetone-dried and inactivated and heat-phenol-inactivated typhoid vaccines in British Guiana. *Bull. WHO* **30**, 631.

44 Wahdan M. H., Sérié C., Cerisier Y., Sallman S. and Germanier R. (1982) A controlled field trial of live *Salmonella typhi* strain Ty 21a oral vaccine against typhoid: Three-year results. *J. Infect. Dis.* **145**, 292.

45 World Health Organization Scientific Working Group (1980) *Escherichia coli* diarrhoea. *Bull. WHO* **58**, 23.

46 Yancey R. J., Willis D. L. and Berry L. J. (1979) Flagella-induced immunity against experimental cholera in adult rabbits. *Infect. Immun.* **25**, 220.

47 Yugoslav Typhoid Commission (1964) A controlled field trial of the effectiveness of acetone-dried and inactivated and heat-phenol-inactivated typhoid vaccines in Yugoslavia. *Bull. WHO* **30**, 623.

13 Public health aspects of gastroenteritis

C. S. Goodwin

Introduction   269
The difference between developed and developing countries   270
Gut bacteria in the water supplies of developing countries   270
Outbreaks of water-borne gastroenteritis in the U.S.A.   271
Human viruses in water and sewage   272
The need in developing countries to link purer water supplies with improved sanitation   274
Bacteriological examination of water   275
Bacteriological examination of milk   276
The control of food-borne disease   277
   Food-handlers and gastroenteritis   279
   Control of enteric diseases   280
Outbreaks of acute gastroenteritis and their investigation   281
   The bacteriological monitoring of sewage   282
Precautions that may be taken by a traveller to prevent gastroenteritis   282
Conclusion   284
References   284

INTRODUCTION

To control disease due to enteric pathogens it is necessary to know the reservoirs and vehicles of infection. Some pathogens, *Salmonella typhi*, *Vibrio cholerae*, and some viruses, exist only in humans, human sewage, and water contaminated by faeces, and therefore sanitary disposal of faeces can greatly reduce the incidence of disease due to these organisms. Other gut pathogens have an animal reservoir such as cattle or dogs. For many of the pathogens mentioned in Chapters 3–11, epidemiological techniques to trace the source of infection, and methods of control have been discussed. The general principles for the control of food-borne disease will be discussed later in this chapter. Because the public health problems of gastroenteritis in developing countries are so large they are discussed in some detail.

THE DIFFERENCE BETWEEN DEVELOPED AND DEVELOPING COUNTRIES

In health matters the gap between developed and developing countries is nowhere near so wide as in the prevention of gastroenteritis. It has been calculated that in 1975 in children under 5 in Asia, Africa, and Latin America, there were probably 500 million episodes of diarrhoea which may have caused 15–20 million deaths (p.188).[29] Such information does not hit the newspaper headlines. On the outskirts of Addis Ababa by the leprosy hospital there was a large encampment with many beggars where in 1968 the mortality rate of children under 1 year old was approximately 90% with many deaths due to gastroenteritis; a typical woman with leprosy would divulge that of her 13 children only one was still surviving. The public health measures required to prevent gastroenteritis involve primarily the provision of sufficient, bacteriologically-clean water, adequate sewage disposal, and control of flies. Near the Addis Ababa leprosy hospital it was not uncommon to see the one stream being used by leprosy patients to wash the bandages provided for their ulcerated feet; and nearby fields were covered with little piles of human faeces each with an attendant swarm of flies.

In developed countries outbreaks of gastroenteritis are dealt with by skilled microbiological and public health personnel and measures to deal with such an outbreak are discussed later in this chapter. However the frequent systematic testing of water supplied to the public is often unappreciated. In developed countries if hands were always washed before food was eaten much diarrhoea would be avoided. The problem is not so simple in developing countries, nor in communities in developed countries without a clean water supply or a good sewage system such as in some Aboriginal communities in Australia, and on some Indian reservations in the USA and Canada. A global programme is being undertaken by the World Health Organization for the control of diarrhoea and the provision of clean water supplies.

GUT BACTERIA IN THE WATER SUPPLIES OF DEVELOPING COUNTRIES

In Jakarta, Indonesia, the isolations of enterobacteria and *Salmonella* sp. from surface waters, rivers and canals were shown in Chapter 9 (Tables 9.10 and 9.11). Of 20 samples of river and canal water 10 samples contained *Salmonella* sp. The bacteriological quality of Nile water in Egypt before and after impoundment in the years 1963–73 has been reviewed.[46] Before 1965 there was a difference in the number of bacteria in Nile water during the flood season compared with the other seasons. During the flood season counts of 10^7 to 10^9 organisms/100 ml were recorded, and at other times 10^5 to 10^7 organisms/100 ml. After impoundment in the Aswan Dam there was no seasonal fluctuation and the count of bacteria was 10^5 to 10^7 organisms/100 ml. However there was a rise in the number of coliforms but not faecal *E. coli*/100 ml, and a slight increase in the incidence of enterococci from 20% to 22% after the establishment of the High Dam.[46] In Malaysia, water supply programmes have been steadily improved. A useful review of the various types of pollution in different communities in Malaysia has been published.[48] The source of water to communities in urban areas in 1970 was a piped supply to 72% of households and in 1980 to 87% of households, while in rural areas it rose from 22% in 1970 to 40% in 1980. The incidence of reported cholera in 1972 was 3 per hundred thousand people and in 1976 was 0.2 per hundred thousand. However the incidence of typhoid and paratyphoid remained at 12 per hundred thousand between 1972 and 1976. This illustrates the difference in epidemiology between cholera, and typhoid and paratyphoid, in that cholera seems to be more frequently spread by contaminated water but typhoid or paratyphoid may also be spread by direct faecal-oral contact; the figures suggest that there are more carriers of typhoid and paratyphoid than carriers of cholera. It was found that in rural areas nearly all rivers were contaminated with *Vibrio cholerae* El Tor.[14] Although the Ministry of Health in Malaysia has taken initiatives to provide technical assistance about water supplies to urban centres, progress was lacking due to the shortage of health workers and to the lack of attention given to this problem at the local authority level. It has been frequently emphasized that there must be acceptance by local authorities at village level of the value of improved sewage disposal and the provision of proper water supplies. As the villagers enjoy improved health they are able to be more productive.

The incidence of human Salmonella carriers in a tropical urban environment has been studied in central Jakarta, Indonesia.[16] *Salmonella* sp. were isolated from rectal swabs from 39 (8.4%) of 464 apparently healthy adults and children in Jakarta. *Salmonella oranienburg* occurred in 22 instances and most of the isolates were resistant to a wide range of antibiotics including ampicillin, neomycin, kanamycin, sulphafurazole and tetracycline, probably because of the widespread and inappropriate administration of antibiotics. The yield of *Salmonella* sp. increased significantly with the use of double enrichment procedures. The high rate of carriage of *Salmonella* sp. in this overcrowded tropical city is probably not atypical, and may be linked with the fact that in Jakarta the surface waters are heavily polluted by faeces. In the mouth and throat of children in Jakarta large numbers of faecal bacteria were detected, which are not present in the oropharynx of children in developed countries.[15] It is of interest that the rate of Salmonella carriage was 9% among 186 Aborigines living in a remote area in the Kimberley region of Western Australia.[16] There is a need for chlorinated water supplies to avoid child mortality and malnutrition in developing countries.[25] Repeated mention of this tragic situation may continue to alert authorities who should be endeavouring to solve the problem.

OUTBREAKS OF WATER-BORNE GASTROENTERITIS IN THE USA

Although water-borne outbreaks of gastroenteritis occur less frequently in developed countries, in 1978 32 outbreaks of water-borne disease involving 11 435 people were reported to the Center for Disease Control in the USA.[43] *Giardia lamblia* affected 5171 people, *Campylobacter* affected 3000 people in one outbreak, and parvovirus-like agents caused disease in 937 people. One outbreak of giardiasis which involved 5000 people was due to sewage contamination of the water supply in a resort in Colorado. Outbreaks of giardiasis have occurred when the water supplies have been shown to contain no coliform bacilli.[51] The presence of coliform organisms is used as an indication of faecal contamination of water supplies and is widely employed in routine surveillance programmes. The outbreak of infection due to *Campylobacter* affecting 3000 people in Vermont was due to the use of two supplementary water sources, neither of which were chlorinated, that were used when the water pressure was low. Routine coliform counts performed during and after the outbreak were negative. Most water-borne outbreaks of gastroenteritis in the USA were due to infrequently used summer camp sites where the water supplies were neither rigidly controlled nor chlorinated.

HUMAN VIRUSES IN WATER AND SEWAGE

More than 100 different enteric viruses have been detected in human faeces, and raw sewage may contain 500 000 infectious particles per litre.[25] All the usual sewage treatment processes reduce viral numbers, but complete elimination is impossible without heavy disinfection. Viruses are protected from the action of chlorine by adsorption onto suspended solids. Water contaminated with enteric viruses may be used for crop irrigation and the crops may become contaminated, and if crops are eaten raw this provides a faecal-oral link. Shellfish may become contaminated, and have led to outbreaks of Hepatitis A. There is much evidence that coliforms or enterobacteria are unreliable indicators of viral contamination; and viruses have been found in water in which faecal coliforms were absent. Treatment methods may destroy faecal bacteria more rapidly than enteric viruses. In Virginia, USA, poliovirus 1 isolates were recovered from finished drinking water which contained free chlorine in excess of 1 mg/l; chlorine was found to be less effective against these isolates than against standard strains of poliovirus.[49] In the laboratory, a strain of poliovirus type I exhibited progressively greater resistance to inactivation by chlorine after repeated exposure of the virus to sublethal doses of chlorine followed by growth of the survivors in cell cultures.[4] However, in water, viruses in contrast to bacteria, do not multiply.

Methods that result in viral removal from water include sedimentation, adsorption, coagulation, and precipitation and filtration.[31] Inactivation of viruses can be produced by a high pH, by chemical oxidation, by disinfectants such as halogens, and photo-oxidation by certain dyes in the presence of light.[31]

In one study enteroviruses were detected in 80% of raw sewage, in 72% of primary effluent, and in 56% of chlorinated effluent samples.[47] Certain enteric viruses can persist for long periods of time in the environment; reported survival times are 2–168 days in tap water, 2–130 days in sea water, 25–125 days in soil, and up to 9 days in oysters.[31]

When water samples are examined for viruses, bacterial and fungal contaminants first have to be removed by centrifugation, or filtering, or treatment with antibiotics before viruses can be assayed in tissue culture. When the virus content of water samples is low as in potable and some surface waters, the viruses must be concentrated by passage of the water through a micropore filter and subsequent dilution into a smaller volume.[41] In Melbourne, Australia, a 5 μm prefilter has been used to remove particulate matter, then the pH is adjusted to 3.5 which is optimal for virus adsorption; sodium thiosulphate is added to neutralize chlorine, and the water is passed through a 0.45 μm epoxy fibreglass pleated cartridge filter.[21] Charges carried by virus particles at acid pH cause attachment to the filter media due to an electrostatic property, not related to the pore size of the filter. The virus is then eluted into an alkaline fluid, which is adjusted to neutral pH and transported to the laboratory for further processing. Filters that carry a positive charge have also been used, which eliminate the need to adjust and maintain an acid pH for virus adsorption.[53]

Outbreaks of gastroenteritis due to water-borne Norwalk virus have been reported in Australia after the consumption of oysters; the virus was found in 32% of stools, and antibody increases demonstrated in seven of ten paired sera.[17] Norwalk virus was identified by immunoelectron microscopy; virus particles were identified as Norwalk virus if they reacted with specific Norwalk antibody, which was present in the convalescent sera but not in the preinfection sera.[17] Heavy rain had preceded the 2 weeks during which the outbreak occurred. Some methods of purification of oysters — depuration — do not eliminate Norwalk virus.[17] It was suggested that oysters should be immersed in depuration tanks for 7 days rather than 48 hours so that viruses would be more effectively removed. Salinity may also have contributed to the failure of depuration in some batches of oysters.

Water used for swimming, including both pool water and sea water, has been associated with the acquisition of virus infections. Sea water does not naturally kill viruses quickly; swimmers in polluted sea water suffer from significantly higher rates of gastrointestinal disease compared to nonswimmers or those who swim in unpolluted sea water. A WHO scientific group considered that the constant exposure of large population groups to even small numbers of enteric viruses in large volumes of water can lead to an endemic state of virus dissemination in the community due to colonization and multiplication in humans;[42] presumably this applies both to drinking water and to water used for recreation. The best method to avoid contamination of sea water is to site sewage outlets away from recreational beaches.

With large cities sited at successive points downstream on a big river, water may be recycled many times. The presence of viruses in drinking water and water for recreation such as swimming pools, will almost certainly become more of an issue in the future. It should not be forgotten that one of the simplest methods of water purification is sand filtration, which was shown to be of value in preventing cholera in Europe in 1892[24] (Chapter 5, p.108). Filtration is also of value in eliminating viruses.

THE NEED IN DEVELOPING COUNTRIES TO LINK PURER WATER
SUPPLIES WITH IMPROVED SANITATION

In 1977 it was recorded that 86% of the rural population in the world lacked an
adequately clean water supply and 92% of the rural population lacked adequate
facilities for excreta disposal, while only 28% of the urban population in the world
had water-borne sewage facilities and 29% had no sanitation facilities of any
kind.[13] With the population explosion — in 1976 the world population increased
by 70 million — the problems of providing a clean water supply in developing
countries will still be the major water problem for many years to come.

It is not possible to separate water-related diseases from those affected by
sanitation.[7] All the 'water-borne' and some of the 'water-based' diseases depend
on faecal access to domestic water sources. The chain of transmission must be
broken by safe disposal of faeces as well as by protection of water supplies.
Sanitation affects some disease vectors too, in that some mosquitoes specifically
favour flooded pit-latrines as breeding sites. Bringing better water supplies into an
area without sanitary disposal of waste water could make the situation worse not
better. Inasmuch as cholera and typhoid have man as their only reservoir, the
elimination of these diseases by the provision of clean water supplies is an
achievable goal.

In addition to bacteria and viruses that are water borne, parasites such as
Giardia lamblia[51] and *Entamoeba histolytica* in the cystic form have been demonstrated to be water borne. The extension of irrigation in Egypt has led to a problem
with *Schistosoma mansoni* which did not exist previously.[7] Because in developing
countries surface waters are still used without treatment directly for water supply
there is a great need to have carefully controlled disposal of waste water
discharge.[36] If treatment facilities are not available for a village water supply then
a 'stream standard' should be imposed to protect the health of public using that
stream, but only as a short-term measure.[36] Stream standards are likely to form
the basis for water quality and management in tropical countries in the foreseeable future. They should be carefully chosen to maintain only the minimum level
of quality for legitimate uses of the water resource. Realistic goals in the planning
and execution of raw water supply programmes in developing countries have
been reviewed.[12] The immediate aims are to improve the quality, quantity,
availability and reliability of water. Benefits that would occur fairly soon would
be the release of labour by improved health of villagers, crop innovation, crop
improvement, and innovation and improvement in animal husbandry. These
would lead to higher cash incomes, increased and more reliable subsistence,
improved health, and increased leisure. It has been found that improving socio-
economic conditions make a community more amenable to population control
measures. Simple measures such as the elimination of a water hole for a village
supply by capping and piping of the water source can greatly reduce the bacterial
numbers in the water. The water will not be chlorinated, and so the major
objection to this piping of poor quality water is that there may be a risk of a
water-borne epidemic. However this risk is probably much less than that to which
the population is normally exposed by unpiped water. Water treatment is always

preferable when the raw water sources are not of excellent quality or are not protected from the risk of pollution. Feachem has provided an algorithm of the decision making process for a water supply in a lower income community.[12] The imortance of community choice and community participation has been emphasized.[56] There needs to be increased understanding of the perception and value frameworks in which communities evaluate alternative schemes. A raw water scheme must be in accord with community dynamics. Self-help programmes for water improvement are emerging in a number of countries, particularly Kenya.[9] The provision of water treatment plants in developing countries is not without problems;[37] in India in 1970 80% of the water treatment plants studied were inoperative because they had not received proper attention. Storage and sedimentation of water can be useful treatments.[37] It is an unfortunate fact that national and international agencies continue to donate items such as a water pump to a village, without any significant coherent effort to improve basic sanitation levels.[30] Simple methods of sanitation, for example water-seal slabs, are unfortunately omitted from village projects. Only after sanitation has been improved would the gift of a water pump to a village probably be a cost-effective way to achieve improved water supply and health.

Ill-health and poverty are inequitably distributed between and within nations.[30] Earlier hopes that benefits obtained by industrial growth in developing countries would spread to rural areas have not been fulfilled. In most tropical regions the present rate of manpower, and budgetary allocation to the improvement of sanitation and water supply is wholly insufficient to meet current demand or even to keep up with population growth. Too much emphasis has been placed on potable water schemes for urban centres, without improvements in urban excreta disposal facilities. The most suitable type of latrine or sanitation system to adopt in many developing countries remains a perplexing question.[30] The pit privy, the bore hole latrine and the septic tank are all efficient methods of excreta disposal. A 'Planning Research Action Institute' latrine has been introduced in India.

BACTERIOLOGICAL EXAMINATION OF WATER

Coliform bacteria have been considered to be the most reliable indicators of faecal pollution of water. Some coliforms may be derived from the intestines of various animals and birds as well as from humans. The presence of sporing anaerobe organisms such as *Clostridium perfringens*, without the presence of coliforms, may indicate that there has been past pollution but it is probably not recent. *Escherichia coli* die in water during the course of several days or weeks after leaving the intestine. The routine tests used for the bacteriological examination of water[39] are firstly a qualitative test for all the coliform bacilli, which is known as the 'presumptive coliform count'. Secondly there is a differential test for faecal or 'type 1' *E. coli* known as the 'differential coliform test'. Thirdly enumeration of viable bacteria by a 'plate count' is done with duplicates at 37° C and 22° C. Because *E. coli* do not multiply except in highly polluted water the number of organisms is probably directly related to the amount of faecal contamination of the water. Specimens are taken in bottles of about 230 ml capacity. If chlorine is present this must be neutralized with sodium thiosulphate. For chlorinated supplies it is recommended that tests should not reveal the presence of coliform bacilli of any kind in 100 ml of water. Sampling techniques for any biological test need to allow a latitude in the reported counts. Throughout the year 95% of samples of unchlorinated water taken from a distribution system for a town should be free from coliform organisms in 100 ml, and no sample should ever contain more than 10 coliform organisms or two *E. coli* in 100 ml.[39] *Clostridium perfringens* may survive chlorination and may give a positive reaction in the 'presumptive coliform test'. Nonchlorinated drinking water is not recommended in developed countries, but if it exists should not contain *E. coli* or enterococci. The demonstration of enterococci is of value in confirming the faecal origin of coliform bacilli in water.[11] The bacteriological quality of swimming water should approximate to that of high purity drinking water.

The details for the bacteriological examination of water supplies are given in two reports.[38,39] Piped water for a population of 100 000 or more should be examined at least once a day, and for a population of less than 20 000 at least once a month.[39] In natural water used for bathing, such as rivers, lakes and the sea, it is impracticable to lay down any bacteriological standards of purity. If sewerages gain access to the water and 'type 1' *E. coli* exceed 1000/ml this will certainly indicate a potential risk to the bathers.[32]

Watercress is a potential source of enteric disease. It should be cultivated in beds supplied with pure water, but this does not always ensure the absence of *E. coli* in samples of watercress. Shellfish become infected by being laid down in polluted water. Large volumes of water enter the shell of oysters and mussels. As indicated above, depuration needs to be carried out for 7 days to eliminate some viruses, although in the past shorter periods have been recommended, combined with ultraviolet light.[59]

BACTERIOLOGICAL EXAMINATION OF MILK

Milk always contains a certain number of bacteria which are derived from the milk ducts of the cow's udder. Mastitis is also quite common. Milk can be contaminated with bacteria from the outside of the udder, from vessels, utensils, and dust in the atmosphere of the milking shed. However of greatest importance is unsterilized milk left in the equipment. Contamination from the hands of human personnel is also important. Bovine tuberculosis can lead to the presence of tubercle bacilli in milk; most developed countries have eliminated this disease. Typhoid, paratyphoid and dysentery bacilli are usually derived from human and animal sources. Some *Salmonella* serotypes occur commonly in cows, and may get into the milk from the faeces of an infected animal or be excreted in the milk should the udder become infected.[58] Raw milk can never be regarded as completely safe for human consumption and the only satisfactory method of eliminating bacteria is by pasteurization or some other form of heat treatment. For

pasteurization milk is retained at between 63° C–66° C for at least
then cooled rapidly to less than 10° C. Flash pasteurization of milk ı
by retaining the milk at a temperature of at least 72° C for at least 15 s
then the milk is cooled to less than 10° C. Pasteurization inactivates
phosphatase which is normally present in raw milk. Laboratory tests
pasteurization are designed to detect the presence of phosphatase.

In ultra-heat-treated milk all bacteria should be nonviable; the milk can be
tested in the laboratory by standard bacteriological methods to detect any
bacteria; the unopened container is stored for 24 hours at between 30° and 37° C,
and 0.02 ml milk is cultured for 48 hours. If less than 10 organisms are present this
conforms to British Standards of satisfactory purity. The presence of antibiotics
in milk is also detected by laboratory tests. Sterilized milk can be assessed by the
fact that the soluble proteins are completely denatured so that when the
caseinogen is precipitated with ammonium sulphate a clear filtrate is obtained
which remains clear after boiling. *Bacillus cereus* may be present in milk; this may
represent dust contamination and suggest that containers and utensils have not
been properly cleaned.

The methylene blue reduction test is a keeping-quality test for raw and
pasteurized milks. The milk is held overnight and incubated at 37°C with
methylene blue. The methylene blue should not be decolourized within 30
minutes. The resazurin test is also a dye-reduction test sometimes used to
determine the hygienic quality of the milk supply.[11] The desire by some members
of the public to drink 'natural' milk exhibits a misplaced trust in the value of this
product, and a minimization of the dangers. In Scotland in 1979 there were 2428
instances of *Salmonella* infection as a result of drinking unpasteurized milk.[50] It is
to be hoped that governments in developed countries will insist that the only milk
consumed is pasteurized.[26] However in the small market that exists for goat's milk
for people allergic to cow's milk, most milk is sold unpasteurized; in New South
Wales, Australia, 13% of 274 samples of goat's milk contained *Yersinia enterocolitica*.[19] Methods for the bacteriological examination of ice cream are similar to
those for milk.[11]

THE CONTROL OF FOOD-BORNE DISEASE

Food-borne gastrointestinal disease has been discussed in Chapters 3–11. Food
may be examined for other organisms, such as *Clostridium botulinum* which is
food-borne but causes non-gastrointestinal symptoms, except in children (see
Chapter 1). The control of food-borne disease depends firstly on public health
measures in the food industries, secondly on meticulous technique in the kitchen,
and thirdly the control of outbreaks of food-borne disease in the community. The
importance of breast-feeding for the safety of infants cannot be overemphasized.[28]
The anti-infective properties of breast milk have been evaluated in India in a
study of 70 high-risk low birth-weight infants delivered in hospital and transferred to a special care nursery.[33] The babies were born to mothers who had
obvious infections, or who had births in unsatisfactory conditions. The babies

ad been breast-fed by their own mothers but required supplementation from donors. Breast milk was manually expressed into autoclaved feeding bottles, transported in ice and fed to the babies within 60 minutes of collection. Other infants given nonhuman milk were compared with this group. The incidence of infection was significantly less in the babies who received breast milk, with two instances of septicaemia among the breast-fed babies, and eight among those receiving nonhuman milk. *Candida albicans* infection did not occur in the breast-fed group, but did occur in five babies in the group not given breast milk.

To ensure the microbiological safety of food many aspects must be considered.[18] Meat is responsible for 80% of all instances of food-borne disease.[8] Thus special attention must be paid to the slaughtering of animals, and to the rapid freezing of uncooked meat. On farms zoonoses should be eliminated from breeding and fattening herds. In abattoirs there must be a clear division between the contaminated section and the clean section. In the home uncooked meat must be stored below 4° C to prevent bacterial multiplication, and before it is cooked it must be thawed fully. Large chickens and turkeys require many hours for complete thawing, otherwise cooking may not destroy bacteria in the centre of the carcass. Cooking must be adequate to kill bacteria even in the interior of the meat. Food that is uneaten must be kept at 4° C or below and reheated quickly when needed again. Rice should be cooked in small quantities to reduce storage time before consumption. After boiling the rice should be kept above 63° C, or if not eaten within 2 hours it should be kept at 4° C or below. *Bacillus cereus* may occur in milk and dairy products. *Salmonella* can be spread from raw to cooked food by hands, surfaces, and equipment; survival of a few organisms after cooking allows multiplication under poor conditions of storage. Especially with bulk-cooked meat and poultry inadequate cooling and cold storage facilities can lead to gastroenteritis due to *Clostridium perfringens*.[18]

Some perishable foods have a limited shelf life due to the incorporation of physical or chemical additives. Such foods are pasteurized meat products with or without brine, fish preserves and sweetened condensed milk.[3]

Meat inspection as practised up to now is similar to that practised approximately a hundred years ago. It has certainly reduced food-borne disease, however, while the methods of farming livestock have changed, the inspection system has not changed in principle, and some of the most important food-borne disease agents today elude the efforts of the meat inspector.[44] The purpose of meat and poultry inspection is to prevent microorganisms present in animals from causing food-borne diseases, to prevent contamination of carcasses by pathogens and to keep other foreign material out of the food. *Salmonella* were found in 16.5% of turkeys condemned by a food inspector but in 12.7% of carcasses passed.[44] Thus food inspection alone was unhelpful with regard to the number of carcasses with *Salmonella* to which the public was exposed. There is no disagreement that inspection is important in the microbiological safety of food; the problem is how to add methods that improve the monitoring process.[44] A most important ideal is to ensure a *Salmonella*-free environment for housing animals, and efficient husbandry practices and waste disposal. *Campylobacter* are frequently present in poultry.[52] However if carcasses are stored at low temperatures, properly thawed before cooking and properly cooked, then pathogens should not remain alive to be eaten.

In England and Wales from 1968 to 1972 there were on average 6000 incidents of gastroenteritis each year, but the reported figure of about 10 000 people affected annually was thought to be a gross underestimate.[18] Meat and poultry were the food vehicles for 80–90% of incidents. In the United Kingdom in 1976, of the reported outbreaks of food-borne gastroenteritis 64% were due to *Salmonella*, 12% to *Clostridium perfringens*, and 3% to *Staphylococcus aureus*.[10] The situation in the USA seems to be that there is even more under-reporting of food-borne gastroenteritis; in 1971 a total of only 320 outbreaks of food-borne illness were reported. The aetiological agents were proved to be bacteria in 63% of outbreaks. *Staphylococcus aureus* accounted for 29% of the outbreaks and 38% of the individuals, whereas *Clostridium perfringens* accounted for 16% of the outbreaks and 29% of the individuals. There was a multi-state outbreak of enteropathogenic *E. coli* gastroenteritis related to imported cheese.[6] In Australia 'food-poisoning' is not a notifiable disease, but the epidemiology appears to be similar to that in Europe and North America.[55] The *Salmonella* serotypes that cause disease in England and Wales have been reviewed by Rowe.[45]

Food-handlers and gastroenteritis

A food-handler may become a carrier of an organism which he or she acquired by handling raw food of animal origin, either meat or poultry. In most outbreaks of food-borne salmonellosis it has been possible to find faults in technique, either inadequate heat treatment of food or cross-contamination from raw to cooked food. The unwashed hands of the food-handler can carry pathogens from raw to cooked food and the pathogen may become resident in the bowel of the food-handler. If such a person is meticulous in their hand washing after defaecation or urination then the pathogen should not be transmitted to another person. Carriers of *Salmonella typhi* for over 30 years have prepared food for their families nearly every day and have never infected any other member of their family.[10]

Microbiological examination of food-handlers on a routine basis has been extensively debated. With regard to *Staphylococcus aureus* many of the strains that are carried by nearly 50% of the human population can produce entero-toxin.[57] Such organisms may be spread to the food without the food-handler being overtly ill. However, obviously a larger number of organisms would be shed by a food-handler with a boil or a staphylococcal lesion. The detection of a *Salmonella* carrier may not be easy. Many enteropathogens are excreted intermittently and not distributed uniformly throughout a stool specimen, so that failure to isolate *Salmonella* from one specimen of faeces is no indication that the patient is not a carrier. Microbiological examination of large numbers of food-handlers is very costly, and no convincing evidence has been put forward to show that routine examination of food-handlers is a cost-effective way of preventing food-borne disease. In fact evidence that is available from countries where this is a routine practice suggests the opposite.[2] Such an attitude does not apply in the epidemiological investigation of an outbreak of food-poisoning when food-handlers must be examined very carefully clinically and microbiologically. In the absence of an outbreak it is probably more important to check that raw food, which enters a food plant, does not become a vehicle for pathogens to be transferred to cooked food by the hands of handlers, without the handlers themselves becoming infected. Money that would be required to pay for the routine examination of food-handlers' faeces may be better spent buying plenty of soap and towels and employing an occupational nurse to teach and check meticulous hand washing, and hygienic practices during food preparation.[10,40] A heavy load of relatively unrewarding work for the laboratory may also be avoided. Microbiological examination of faeces which fails to yield any pathogen may give the food-handlers and the management a false sense of security leading to a failure by the food-handler to appreciate the need for continuous consistent practice of good hygiene.[40] Food-handlers must be meticulous in their handwashing, their handling of cooked food and particularly of cold meats and food eaten raw such as salads and fruit, and their reporting of any incidence of diarrhoea. Any food-handler who develops diarrhoea or a septic skin lesion must be taken off work and not allowed back until the faeces or lesions have been found to be free from intestinal pathogens. The environment of a toilet used by a person suffering from diarrhoea can be a source of infection to others using the toilet.[35] If a food-handler has been on holiday in a country where gastrointestinal diseases are prevalent it is reasonable to question the person on their return to work about any gastrointestinal symptoms, or any contact with other people who had such symptoms. The real value of these procedures may not lie in discovering whether he has had gastrointestinal disease, so much as in continually emphasizing to the food-handler that he can become a carrier of an infection even when he is asymptomatic, and he can infect the food if he does not follow hygienic practices.

Control of enteric diseases

In Chapter 5 a series of measures were outlined for the control of cholera (p.111) and these are of value for the control of all enteric diseases. In general the three basic requirements are: protected and chlorinated public water supplies, sanitary disposal of human excretas, ensuring that they do not contaminate water supplies, and fly control; this is aided by adequate garbage collection and disposal of offal, and screening and spraying which are effective but expensive. Milk and dairy products should be pasteurized or boiled. There should be sanitary transport of commercial milk both to the bottling factory and to consumers, with refrigeration of milk in shops and homes. Shellfish should be supplied only from approved sources after appropriate treatment. The preparation of food in public places, especially uncooked food must be strictly supervised, and attention should be paid to the provision and use of adequate toilet and washing facilities.

In developed countries known excreters of unusual pathogens such as *Salmonella typhi* should be monitored by the public health authorities. When a patient is identified as an excretor of a *Salmonella*, or other enteric pathogen, the family and other contacts of the patient must be examined.

In large institutions, including hospitals, as well as in smaller restaurants, the area where food is prepared must be regularly inspected and occasional microbiological sampling will indicate to workers and public health staff whether good cleaning practices have been followed or not. Trays of sliced cold meat are sometimes stacked on top of each other without any protection from the bottom of the tray above. In the preparation of sausage rolls beaten egg yolk is applied to the edge of the pastry and such a preparation is an ideal culture medium for bacteria which may not be killed by the cooking process; sometimes a paint brush is used to apply the egg yolk and microbiological sampling of such a brush may be revealing. In preparation areas raw meat should be strictly segregated from prepared and cooked foods.

OUTBREAKS OF ACUTE GASTROENTERITIS AND THEIR INVESTIGATION

Outbreaks of gastroenteritis may be either explosive because of a common source of a pathogen, or protracted because of a continuing source, or person-to-person spread. Most reported outbreaks are explosive, people falling ill within hours of each other and usually within 48 hours of eating contaminated food. However where large numbers of people live in common lodging facilities with a limited number of toilets, person-to-person transmission of infection may follow a common source outbreak.[35] Person-to-person spread of *Salmonella* indicates that small numbers of organisms may cause infection, and this is generally thought to be more likely in debilitated persons, the very young and the elderly. Healthy adults are believed to require larger doses such as 10^5–10^8 organisms to produce illness, and such doses usually only result from the proliferation of *Salmonella* in inadequately cooked or unhygienically handled food. However some strains of *Salmonella* may be more virulent and small doses may be sufficient to cause disease.[35]

The initial investigation of an outbreak of gastroenteritis will involve firstly documentation of symptomatically affected people and also everyone in the same group who did not have symptoms of gastroenteritis. Some symptoms may not be due to the pathogen that caused the outbreak, and people with such symptoms may not yield the pathogen in their faeces. Secondly a complete account of all food and liquid consumed by all the people in the group should be compiled; and thirdly bacteriological, toxicological, or viral examination should be made of the food, and specimens such as faeces and vomitus from all members of the group. Especially in a protracted outbreak, the original, contaminated food vehicle may only be recognized when an analysis is made only of people who provided full documentation of symptoms and also a stool sample.[35]

Apart from *Staphylococcus aureus*, which may not be easily detected, the microbiological examination of food for enteric pathogens should only be done after a pathogen has been isolated from affected patients. Examination of a food sample should commence with a careful inspection to determine if there are any abnormalities in appearance or smell; microscopic examination of stained preparations may indicate gross contamination.[11] A total count of viable bacteria per gram of food should be obtained by culture both at 37° C and 22° C, and a selective count should be made for coliform bacilli. Gut pathogens can be detected by standard microbiological techniques.[20] A rapid radiometric method for detection of *Salmonella* in foods has been described.[54] Modified selenite media have been found satisfactory for the isolation of *Yersinia enterocolitica* from meat.[27]

The investigation of an outbreak also requires an examination of faecal specimens from the people who handle the food, and the equipment and kitchen areas used for food preparation. Careful observation of the methods of food preparation should be made, to detect the possibility of cross-contamination from raw to cooked food and bad hygienic practices, as detailed in the earlier section on food-handlers. To diagnose water-borne disease due to the parvovirus Norwalk virus a large volume of stool — 10 g or more — should be collected from each of 6–10 acutely ill patients during the first 48 hours of illness and frozen to −7° C. Acute and convalescent serum specimens should also be collected. Similar specimens should be collected from healthy individuals.[43]

Enterotoxigenic *E. coli* may come from human carriers but are also present in animal faeces, while *Campylobacter*, *Vibrio parahaemolyticus* and *Yersinia* are almost always of animal or environmental origin. *Shigella* organisms are rarely spread by food; usually they are spread by the direct faecal-oral route without the involvement of food. In one outbreak caused by lactose-fermenting *Salmonella newport*, the causal organism was only recognized when primary culture was performed on bismuth sulphite agar.[1] Giardiasis can be food-borne.[34]

The bacteriological monitoring of sewage

The incidence of pathogens in the community can be monitored by the use of the sewer-swab.[32] This technique plays an important role in the epidemiological investigation of enteric disease, to determine the origin of cases of typhoid and other enteric pathogens. The swabs may be inserted in main sewers, branch sewers, house drains, drains from food premises and abattoirs, and individual toilets. The results obtained from the sewer swabs can be used to follow back the organisms to their source in the human or animal carrier, or to animal materials such as processed egg or meat.[58]

PRECAUTIONS THAT MAY BE TAKEN BY A TRAVELLER TO PREVENT GASTROENTERITIS

(Many of the recommendations in this section have been obtained from 'Health Information for International Travel', 1980, published by the US Department of Health and Human Services, Public Health Service, pp. 97–101.)

Chlorinated tap water is considered safe to drink, but chlorine treatment may not kill the protozoa that cause giardiasis and amoebiasis. In areas where chlorinated tap water is not available, water should only be drunk after it has been boiled, or treated with an appropriate tablet that releases chlorine (Steritabs or Halozane) or iodine (Globaline).

Beverages such as tea and coffee made with boiled water, and beer and wine may be drunk. However, canned or bottled carbonated beverages and soft drinks, particularly those manufactured in developing countries are occasionally made with contaminated water and are not always safe to drink. Ice is usually made from raw water and so should be considered to contain pathogens. Such ice should not be placed in beverages, and if ice has been in contact with containers used for drinking, the container should be thoroughly cleaned, preferably with soap and hot water after the ice has been discarded. It is safer to drink directly from a can or bottle than from a container that may be contaminated. Water on the outside of cans or bottles may be contaminated. When there is no method available to make water safe, and water from a hot tap is almost too hot to touch, then such water may be drunk after being left to cool, and such water should be used for brushing the teeth. If cloudy, water of uncertain purity should be strained through a clean cloth before being treated with chemicals or heat. Many foreign workers in developing countries routinely use a filter system for local tap water and then boil it before drinking. In Addis Ababa a simple Berkfeldt filter became rapidly coated with dirt and deposit within 5 or 6 days (Goodwin, personal observation). If water-purifying tablets are not available then liquid chlorine such as laundry bleach with a known percentage of available chlorine can be used to sterilize water. If the bleach has 4–10% of available chlorine then to 1 litre of water 2–4 drops (assumed to be 0.05 ml) of bleach can be added. The water and chlorine should be mixed thoroughly and allowed to stand for 30 minutes. A slight chlorine odour should be detectable in the water. If there is no chlorine odour there may be too many solids in the water which may have absorbed the chlorine, and the dose of bleach can be repeated and the water stood for an additional 15 minutes before being drunk. Tincture of iodine is also useful; 5–10 drops of tincture of iodine should be added to 1 litre of water, and the water mixed and allowed to stand for 30 minutes. The length of time that water should be boiled before it is considered safe varies according to authors consulted. Bringing water to the boil would certainly kill all vegetative organisms, but some authorities recommend that water should be boiled vigorously for at least 10 minutes.

Unpasteurized milk and milk products such as cheese should never be eaten, where hygiene and sanitation are poor. Milk should be brought to the boil. Milk may be sold which may have been diluted with raw water, and this can be detected with a simple instrument to measure specific gravity. Food must be cooked before being eaten, and fruit must be peeled by the traveller himself. If diarrhoea is experienced by a traveller, therapy should not be aimed at suppressing the symptoms, but should focus on correcting or preventing fluid electrolyte imbalances. Oral replacement of fluids can be achieved using two glasses; in one there should be a glass full (225 ml) of orange, or apple, or other fruit juice to supply potassium, plus half a teaspoon of sugar or honey, plus a pinch of table salt. In the other glass, to 225 ml of water should be added a ¼-teaspoon of baking soda which contains sodium bicarbonate. Drinks should be taken alternatively from each glass, and additional carbonated or boiled water can be drunk.

Tetracycline, usually as doxycycline, has been suggested to be of value in preventing traveller's diarrhoea caused by enterotoxigenic *E. coli*. However some strains of *E. coli* are not sensitive to doxycycline, and side-effects of the drug may occur such as photosensitivity to sunlight. Also the drug may eliminate normal flora from the gut which will allow more harmful organisms such as *Salmonella* to cause disease. Drugs that reduce abdominal motility such as diphenoxylate (Lomotil), may cause traveller's diarrhoea to worsen. Iodochlorhydroxyquine (entero-vioform) is of no use in preventing or treating traveller's diarrhoea and prolonged use of it results in severe neurological side-effects in some people. Bismuth subsalicylate has been found to be of value in preventing and treating traveller's diarrhoea in adults. It has to be taken in a dose of 50 ml four times a day. Bicyclomycin or bicozamycin has been reported to reduce the duration of enterotoxigenic diarrhoea to 11–13 hours compared to 50 hours in placebo-treated controls,[23] and it is also active in shigellosis.[22] Bicozamycin shortened the duration of acute diarrhoea due to *Shigella* to 37 hours compared to 90 hours in placebo-treated controls, and to 31 hours in diarrhoea due to *E. coli*, in a study in Mexico.[60] Bicozamycin appears to be specifically active against pathogens without disturbing the normal flora. It may become the drug of choice for traveller's diarrhoea.

CONCLUSION

From the wide range of topics discussed in this chapter it can be seen that gastroenteritis is likely to remain a public health problem in developed countries, and will be of paramount importance in developing countries for many years to come. The fact that chlorination does not destroy some parasites such as *Giardia* and *Entamoeba* is of some concern. In developing countries it is to be hoped that international support will be directed to practical methods of improvement of water supplies and cost-effective sanitation arrangements, which should lead to a considerable reduction in child mortality due to gastroenteritis.

REFERENCES

1 Anand C. M., Finlayson M. C., Garson J. Z. and Larson M. L. (1980) An institutional outbreak of Salmonellosis due to lactose-fermenting *Salmonella newport*. *Am. J. Clin. Pathol.* **74**, 657.
2 Bader R. E. (1972) Are examinations of food handlers for *Salmonellae* and *Shigellae* to be advocated? A suggestion for amendment of section 18 of Federal Communicable Disease Law. *Das Öffentliche Gesundheitswesen* **34**, 283.

3 Bartl V. (1973) Semi-preserved foods: general microbiology in food poisoning. In: *The Microbiological Safety of Food*, p. 89. Eds B. C. Hobbs and J. H. B. Christian, Academic Press, London.

4 Bates R. C., Shaffer P. T. B. and Sutherland S. M. (1977) Development of poliovirus having increased resistance to chlorine inactivation. *Appl. Environ. Microbiol.* **34**, 849.

5 Benenson A. S. (Ed.) (1970) *Control of Communicable Diseases in Man*. 11th edn, p. 54. American Public Health Association, Washington.

6 Brachman P. S., Taylor A., Gangarosa E. J., Merson M. H. and Barker W. H. (1973) Food poisoning in the USA. In: *The Microbiological Safety of Food*, p. 143. Eds B. C. Hobbs and J. H. B. Christian, Academic Press, London.

7 Bradley D. J. (1977) Health aspects of water supplies in tropical countries. In: *Water, Wastes and Health in Hot Climates*, p. 3. Eds R. Feachem, M. McGarry and D. Mara, Wiley, London.

8 Brodhage H. and Anderhub B. (1973) Hygiene in catering. In: *The Microbiological Safety of Food*, p. 47, Eds B. C. Hobbs and J. H. B. Christian, Academic Press, London.

9 Carruthers I. and Brown D. (1973) The economics of community water supply. In: *Water, Wastes and Health in Hot Climates*, p. 130, Eds R. Feachem, M. McGarry and D. Mara, Wiley, London.

10 Charles R. H. G. (1980) Food handlers and food poisoning. In: Health examination of food handling personnel, World Health Organization Report. 1CP/FSP007, p. 11, Copenhagen.

11 Cruickshank R., Duguid J. P., Marmion B. P. and Swain R. H. A. (1975) Bacteriology of water, milk, food, air. In: *Medical Microbiology*, vol. 2, 12th edn, p. 273, Churchill, London.

12 Feachem R. (1977) Water supplies for low-income communities: resource allocation, planning and design for a crisis situation. In: *Water, Wastes and Health in Hot Climates*, p. 75, Eds R. Feachem, M. McGarry and D. Mara, Wiley, London.

13 Feachem R., McGarry M. and Mara D., Eds, (1977) *Water, Wastes and Health in Hot Climates*, p. vii, Wiley, London.

14 Gill G. S. (1976) Cholera in West Malaysia, Ministry of Health, Malaysia.

15 Gracey M., Suharjono, Sutuno and Stone D. E. (1973) Microbial contamination of the gut: another feature of malnutrition. *Am. J. Clin. Nutrition* **26**, 1170.

16 Gracey M. J., Iveson J. B., Sunoto and Suharino (1980) Human Salmonella carriers in a tropical urban environment. *Trans. R. Soc. Trop. Med. Hyg.* **74**, 479.

17 Grohmann G. S., Murphy A. M., Christopher P. J., Auty E. and Greenberg H. B. (1981) Norwalk virus gastroenteritis in volunteers consuming depurated oysters. *Aust. J. Exp. Biol. Med. Sci.* **59**, 219.

18 Hobbs B. C. (1973) Food poisoning in England and Wales. In: *The Microbiological Safety of Food*, p. 129, Eds B. C. Hobbs and J. H. B. Christian, Academic Press, London.

19 Hughes D. and Jensen N. (1981) Yersinia enterocolitica in Raw Goat's Milk. *Appl. Environ. Microbiol.* **41**, 309.

20 International Commission on Microbiological Specification for Foods (1978) *Microorganisms in Foods. 1. Their significance and methods of enumeration*, 2nd edn, University of Toronto Press, Toronto.

21 Irving L. G. (1979) Viruses in water and sewage, and their significance. *Water* **6**, 10.

22 Jarumlinta R., Kradolfer F., Vosbeck K. and Viranuvatti V. (1980) Effect of bicyclomycine in acute diarrhoea of various non-parasitic origins. In: *Curr. Chemoth. Infect. Dis.* Proc. 11th ICC and 19th ICAAC vol 1, p. 435, American Society of Microbiology, Washington.

23 Jarumlinta R., Kradolfer F. and Thanungkul P. (1982) Clinical efficacy of bicozamycin in acute non-parasitic non-dysenteric diarrhea: placebo-controlled study. In: *Current Chemotherapy and Immunotherapy*, Proc. 12th International Congress of Chemotherapy, Florence, 1981, p. 262 American Society of Microbiol., Washington.

24 Koch R. (1894) *The Bacteriological Diagnosis of Cholera*, trans. by Duncan, Edinburgh.

25 Lancet (1978) Viruses in water. *Lancet* **ii**, 1352.

26 Lancet (1981) Hazards of untreated milk. *Lancet* **i**, 705.

27 Lee W. H., Harris M. E., McClain D., Smith R. E. and Johnston R. W. (1980) Two modified selenite media for the recovery of *Yersinia enterocolitica* from meats. *Appl. Environ. Microbiol.* **39**, 205.

28 Lukusa T., Tady M., Makulu M. U. and Muyembe-Tamfum L. (1980) Aspects bactériologiques et cliniques de la salmonellose néonatale à Kinshasa. *Med. Afr. Noire* **27**, 967.

29 Mata L., Kronmal R. A. and Villegas H. (1980) Diarrheal diseases: a leading world health problem. In: *Cholera and Related Diarrhoeas*, p. 1, Eds Ouchterlony and Holmgren, S. Karger, Basel.

30 McGarry M. E. (1977) Institutional development for sanitation and water supply. In: *Water, Wastes and Health in Hot Climates*, p. 195, Eds R. Feachem, M. McGarry and D. Mara, Wiley, London.

31 Melnick J. L., Gerba C. P. and Wallis C. (1978) Viruses in water. *Bull. WHO* **56**, 499.

32 Moore B. (1954) Sewage contamination of coastal bathing water: a review. *Bull. Hyg. (Lond.)* **29**, 689.

33 Narayanan I., Prakash K., Bala S., Verma R. K. and Gujral V. V. (1980) Partial supplementation with expressed breast-milk for prevention of infection in low-birth-weight infants. *Lancet* **ii**, 561.

34 Osterholm M. T., Forfang J. C., Ristinen T. L., Dean A. G., Washburn J. W., Godes J. R., Rude R. A. and McCullough J. G. (1981) An outbreak of foodborne giardiasis. *N. Eng. J. Med.* **304**, 24.

35 Palmer S. R., Jephcott A. E., Rowland A. J. and Sylvester D. G. H. (1981) Person-to-person spread of *Salmonella typhimurium* phage type 10 after a common-source outbreak. *Lancet* **i**, 881.

36 Pescod M. B. (1973) Surface water quality criteria for tropical developing countries. In: *Water, Wastes and Health in Hot Climates*, p. 52, Eds R. Feachem, M. McGarry and D. Mara, Wiley, London.

37 Pickford J. (1977) Water treatment in developing countries. In: *Water, Wastes and Health in Hot Climates*, p. 162, Eds R. Feachem, M. McGarry and D. Mara, Wiley, London.

38 Report (1962) *Recommended Procedures for the Bacteriological Examination of Sea Water and Shellfish*, 3rd edn, American Public Health Association, New York.

39 Report (1969) The bacteriological examination of water supplies, Reports on Public Health and Medical Subjects No. 71, HMSO, London.

40 Report (1971) Food hygiene report on a Seminar. World Health Organization Regional Office for Europe, Copenhagen, Euro 0389, p. 20.

41 Report (1975) Micropore filter technic for enteric virus concentration and detection in finished waters. In: *Standard Methods for the Examination of Water and Waste Water*, 14th edn, p. 971, American Public Health Association and American Water Association.

42 Report (1979) Human viruses in water, waste water and soil. World Health Organization tech. rep. series No. 639, WHO, Geneva.

43 Report (1980) Water-related disease outbreaks, US Department of Health and Human Services. HHS Publication No. (CDC) 80-8385, p. 1.

44 Riemann H. (1973) Means and Methods. In: *The Microbiological Safety of Food*, p. 121, Eds B. C. Hobbs and J. H. B. Christian, Academic Press, London.

45 Rowe B. (1973) Salmonellosis in England and Wales. In: *The Microbiological Safety of Food*, p. 165, Eds B. C. Hobbs and J. H. B. Christian, Academic Press, London.

46 Saleh F. A. (1980) Bacteriological quality of Nile water before and after impoundment (1963–1973): a review. *Zentralb. Bakteriol. II Abt*, **135**, 123.

47 Sattar S. A. and Westwood J. C. N. (1978) Viral pollution of surface waters due to chlorinated primary effluents. *Appl. Env. Microbiol.* **36**, 427.

48 Sekarajasekaran Ira (1979) Physical changes of the environment and health effects with special reference to water pollution and sanitation in Malaysia. *Southest Asia J. Trop. Med. Public Health* **10**, 634.

49 Shaffer P. T. B., Metcalf T. G. and Sproul O. J. (1980) Chlorine resistance of poliovirus isolants recovered from drinking water. *Appl. Env. Microbiol.* **40**, 1115.

50 Sharp J. C. M., Paterson G. M. and Forbes G. I. (1980) Milk-borne salmonellosis in Scotland. *J. Infect.* **2**, 333.

51 Shaw P. K., Brodskyre, Lyman, D. O., Wood B. T., Hibler C. P., Healy G. R., MacLeod K. I. E., Stahl W. and Schultz M. G. (1977) A community wide outbreak of giardiasis with evidence of transmission by a municipal water supply. *Ann Int. Med.* **87**, 426.

52 Simmons N. A. and Gibbs F. J. (1979) Campylobacter spp. in oven-ready poultry. *J. Infect.* **1**, 159.

53 Sobsey M. D. and Glass J. S. (1980) Poliovirus concentration from tap water with electropositive adsorbent filters. *Appl. Env. Microbiol.* **40**, 201.

54 Stewart B. J., Eyles M. J. and Murrell W. G. (1980) Rapid radiometric method for detection of Salmonella in foods. *Appl. Env. Microbiol.* **40**, 223.

55 Sutton R. G. A. (1973) Food poisoning and Salmonella infections in Australia. In: *The Microbiological Safety of Food*, p. 153, Eds B. C. Hobbs and J. H. B. Christian, Academic Press, London.

56 White A. and Burton I. (1973) Water supply and community choice. In: *Water, Wastes and Health in Hot Climates*, p. 113, Eds R. Feachem, M. McGarry and D. Mara, Wiley, London.

57 Wieneke A. A. (1974) Enterotoxin production by strains of *Staphylococcus aureus* isolated from food and human beings. *J. Hyg. (Camb.)* **73**, 255.

58 Wilson G. S. and Miles A. A. (1975) The bacteriology of water, shellfish and sewage. In: *Topley and Wilson's Principles of Bacteriology Virology and Immunity*, 6th edn, p. 2641, Edward Arnold, London.

59 Wood P. C. (1961) The principles of water sterilisation by ultraviolet light, and their application in the purification of oysters. Fishery Invest, Ser. II, 23, No. 6, Minist. Agric., Fish, Food. HMSO, London.

60 Ericsson C. D., DuPont H. L., Sullivan P., Galindo E., Evans D. G. and Evans D. J. (1983) Bicozamycin, a poorly absorbable antibiotic, effectively treats travelers' diarrhea. *Ann. Int. Med.* **98**, 20.

14 The functions and the regulation of normal gut bacteria, and bacterial overgrowth syndromes

P. J. McDonald

Introduction	289
Selection factors for 'normal' gastrointestinal bacteria	291
Environmental	291
Oxygen tension	291
pH	291
Flow	291
Bacteria found in different regions of the gut	292
Stomach	292
Upper small bowel	292
Lower ileum	292
Colon	292
Mucosal flora	293
Functions of the normal gut flora	294
Overgrowth of gut bacteria	296
Aetiological factors	296
Clinical presentations	298
Diagnosis	299
Indirect tests for bacterial overgrowth	299
Breath tests	299
Assays for products of bacterial metabolism	300
Direct tests for bacterial overgrowth	300
Collection of samples	301
Laboratory processing	301
Interpretation of results	301
Identification of species and detection of enterotoxigenicity	301
Treatment	302
Appendix	303
Laboratory processing of luminal contents	303
References	303

INTRODUCTION

A very full description of the distribution and metabolic activities of gut bacteria, and the aetiology and consequences of bacterial overgrowth are found in a book by Drasar and Hill.[8] This chapter attempts to summarize some of the clinically relevant data. Cancer of the colon and gut bacteria are discussed in Chapter 17.

The human colon contains approximately 1.5 kg (wet weight) of bacteria. Obligate anaerobes predominate in the large intestine; in one study 113 distinct species of organisms were detected.[26] If stepwise proximal sampling is undertaken from the rectum, the density of intraluminal bacteria diminishes proximally from the colon where there are 10^{10} to 10^{12} bacteria/ml. The ileocaecal valve is a major partition between the large and small intestine. There is a reduction of approximately 10^2 to 10^5 anaerobes/ml between the colon and distal ileum.[12] The bacterial species in the ileum are similar to those observed in the colon but occur in smaller numbers. The jejunum and duodenum however contain relatively small numbers of bacteria — up to 10^3 to 10^4/ml;[16] the types of bacteria represent swallowed oral bacteria and organisms ingested with food.

It has generally been assumed that intestinal bacteria perform useful functions,[37] and protect against oral infection.[3] Germ-free animals, however, tend to live longer,[20] and seem healthier than normally-bred animals who have residual flora. Germ-free animals on the other hand are susceptible to infection with bacteria that are harmless to conventional animals,[13] and after an oral dose of 10^2 *Salmonella panama* the count in the caecum was 10^9/g, whereas in conventional mice the count was only 10^5/g.[27] Man cannot live separately from microorganisms, and from the time of birth, a complex relationship evolves between man and a variety of microorganisms which come to populate epithelial and mucosal surfaces. Should this relationship become disturbed then disease may result. This is seen after the use of wide-spectrum antibiotics, which may selectively kill certain enteric bacteria.[30,36] This allows overgrowth of organisms which disturb the metabolic function of man, as well as other organisms which populate the gut. Paradoxically, there is evidence to suggest that gut bacteria predispose to some infections. For example, guinea pigs cannot be infected with *Entamoeba histolytica* unless their gut is colonized with *Escherichia coli*. Because these intestinal parasites feed on Enterobacteriaceae such as *E. coli* they are unable to establish an infection unless these organisms are present in the colon of animals. The gut bacteria engage in a variety of metabolic activities which contribute to normal human homeostasis.[8] If the numbers of bacteria increase in the upper gut, their metabolism alters the availability of nutrients or destroys aids to digestion such as bile salts, and disease may result.[23] These disease syndromes are essentially an expression of excessive bacterial metabolism.[5,7] Obligate anaerobic bacteria seem to be the main contributors to the metabolic processes which produce the physiological abnormalities of bacterial overgrowth syndromes.[19] Enterotoxigenic enterobacteria may cause tropical sprue.[18,21]

Bacterial overgrowth syndromes are expressed clinically as malabsorption particularly with steatorrhoea, and vitamin B_{12} deficiency.[8,19] The terms 'stagnant loop' and 'intestinal stasis' refer to overgrowth within the intact but usually diseased small intestine. The 'blind-loop' syndrome is a specific entity which describes bacterial overgrowth in a loop of intestine disconnected from the main flow of gut contents; blind loops are usually the result of surgery or inflammatory bowel diseases such as Crohn's ileitis.

SELECTION FACTORS FOR 'NORMAL' GASTROINTESTINAL BACTERIA

Environmental

Bacteria are ingested with food. The type of bacterium ingested tends to differ with the environment, eating habits, methods of food preparation and the nature of food ingested.

Oxygen tension

The mouth and oesophagus are generally aerobic or oxygenated. The stomach and small bowel are generally anaerobic or unoxygenated, as also are the colon and rectum. Anaerobiosis favours the establishment of anaerobic bacteria in the colon and faeces.

pH

At the levels of acidity found in the stomach most bacteria are destroyed.[9] Some bacteria survive passage through the stomach either because the transit time is rapid, the pH is not lowered to the antibacterial levels required, or the organisms are specially adapted to survive in an acid environment. Mycobacteria and spores can survive passage through the stomach. After the pylorus, the pH changes abruptly and bacteria suited to an acid survival are adversely affected by exposure to the relatively alkaline environment. This factor, together with rapid transit in the upper small bowel[17] tends to prevent the establishment of flora in this segment of the gut.

Flow

There is rapid transmission of luminal contents from the pylorus to the caecum. Experimental evidence with flow systems in which bacteria are growing indicates that organisms tend to accumulate in the down stream portion of flow. In the human gut when motility is normal and transit time rapid, bacteria are unable to establish themselves in the upper small intestine. If motility is disturbed, then bacteria migrate from the lower gut and multiply throughout the stagnant portion of the small intestine.[28] In the colon, transit is relatively slow and this factor, in association with anaerobiosis and plentiful nutrients allows certain types of bacteria to flourish.

BACTERIA FOUND IN DIFFERENT REGIONS OF THE GUT

Stomach

Fewer than 10^3 organisms/ml of viridans streptococci, lactobacilli and *Candida* species are found in the normal fasting stomach. Two hours after a meal, the number of these bacteria increases up to 10^5 organisms/ml.[9] When the gastric pH is greater than 4, or in association with gastric carcinoma, numbers are also increased. The types of bacteria found in the stomach are similar to those present in the mouth and probably represent bacteria ingested with food.

Upper small bowel

Gram-positive aerobic bacteria are found in very small numbers. The anaerobic species commonly found in the lower small intestine and colon have been reported to be absent in the duodenum or jejunum.[6] However a study in India of 10 apparently normal individuals found some variation between the bacteria cultured from fluid aspirated from the lumen of the first part of the jejunum and bacteria grown by culture of mucosal tissue obtained by biopsy from the same site.[2] The most common organisms in jejunal juice and the biopsy were enterobacteria, streptococci, veillonellae, fusobacteria, and *Bacteroides*. In some subjects fusobacteria were found only in the biopsy but in other individuals only in the juice. However spiral bacteria, which are difficult to grow, were not reported. The significance of mucosal flora is discussed in a later section of this chapter.

Lower ileum

Approximately equal numbers of aerobic and anaerobic bacteria are present. The aerobic bacteria are members of the Enterobacteriaceae, and the anaerobic bacteria are members of the bacteroides and bifidobacterium genera, plus lactobacilli.[12]

Colon

The normal colonic flora is usually inferred by analysis of normal faeces. Suitable techniques for sampling various levels of the human colon have yet to be developed. Data from animal studies support the assumption that the flora does not alter during defaecation, indicating that the faecal flora adequately represent that of the rectosigmoid colon. It is known that the flora of the rectosigmoid area differs from that of the ileo-caecal junction and this suggests that a change takes place in the upper part of the colon. The number of different species of bacteria in the various parts of the colon is shown in Table 14.1.

Table 14.1 The bacterial flora of the lower intestine in man

Species	Mean $\log_{10}$ viable count/gram Intestinal material		
	Terminal ileum	Caecum	Faeces
Enterobacteria	3	6	7
Enterococci	2	4	5
Lactobacilli	2	6	6
Clostridia	2	3	5
Bacteroides	6	8	10
Gram-positive non-sporing anaerobes (Eubacteria and Bifidobacteria)	5	8	10

Non-sporing anaerobic rod-shaped organisms predominate in the human faeces, accounting for more than 99% of the total organisms. Differences have been found between Japanese-Hawaiians[26] and white North American men.[22] The major species present are *Bacteroides fragilis, Eubacterium aerofaciens, Peptostreptococcus productus, Fusobacterium prausnitzii,* and *Bifidobacterium adolescentis,* and 113 different species have been found in all.[26] It must be stressed that, although facultative anaerobes such as *E. coli* and *Klebsiella* species are apparently minor components of the average normal flora, they may be of major importance in a person at risk of gut-originated sepsis.

MUCOSAL FLORA

Studies in rodents have shown that a range of bacteria are adherent to the gastro-intestinal mucosa, which are different from the bacteria in the lumen.[10] They play an important role in maintaining the gut ecosystem. Four main groups of bacteria can be found adherent to the mucosa in rodents; firstly, species related to *Campylobacter* sp., secondly bacteria resembling *Selemonas* sp., thirdly *Borrelia* sp., and fourthly spiral bacteria which have not been satisfactorily speciated. In addition, filamentous organisms have been described. In humans, the mucosally-attached gut flora have not been well characterized, but one study has demonstrated that bacteria obtained from a biopsy of the jejunum could differ from bacteria obtained in a luminal aspirate;[2] however, none of the species described above for rodents was mentioned in this study. Many bacteria are known to possess specific adhesive factors such as the K88 antigen of *Escherichia coli.*

'Human mucosally-associated bacteria' seem to be embedded in tags of mucus attached to the mucosa, especially at the tips or folds of the villi. As this is the site for shedding of epithelial cells, the relationship of these bacteria to the mucosa may be due to one of four possibilities. Bacteria may participate directly in the process of shedding cells; or the extruded cells may be a suitable habitat for bacteria; or pumping actions of villi may bring about an accumulation of bacteria and mucus at the apex of the villus; or the appearances may be artefacts. The second possibility is the most probable in humans because bacteria are seen to attach to 'dying' cells, and these bacteria are the same as those detected in the gut lumen. Longitudinal studies of human gut microflora have not been undertaken, but there appears to be significant variation between individuals.[2,22] Stabilization of the gut flora occurs over the period of weaning, but by about 4 weeks postpartum an adult-type population is established. The development of the infant gut flora is fully discussed in Chapter 1. Some anomalies are observed. For instance up to 60% of children are colonized by *Clostridium difficile* during the first year of life, whereas possibly 2% of healthy adults appear to harbour this organism (see Chapter 16). The inability to detect this organism in adults may reflect inadequate culture techniques, but when disease occurs from *Clostridium difficile* toxin production, small epidemics are observed, suggesting cross-infection rather than overgrowth of endogenous bacteria.

The role of mucosal organisms in human health and disease remains speculative. Nevertheless, mucosal organisms may play a role in preventing attachment of pathogenic organisms and also in provoking intestinal immunity. In terms of producing physiological abnormalities due to overgrowth it is difficult to envisage the upward migration of mucosally-attached organisms in the same way as intraluminal bacteria. Humans may differ from rodents and the observed human mucosal bacteria may merely be luminal organisms that become firmly trapped in mucin and effete epithelial cells.

FUNCTIONS OF THE NORMAL GUT FLORA

Bacteria possess a variety of enzymes and it would be surprising if they did not play a significant role in the overall function of the human body. Colonic bacteria constitute the bulk of the gut flora. Their metabolic activities include the following.

CONVERSION OF BILIRUBIN TO UROBILINOGEN[8]

VITAMIN SYNTHESIS

Vitamin K is synthesized by bacteria but colonic absorption occurs only slowly.[37] The organisms principally involved in vitamin K synthesis are *Bacteroides* sp. and *E. coli*. Since *Bacteroides* sp. outnumber *E. coli* by 100 to 1, anaerobic organisms are the principal mechanism of vitamin K synthesis in the gut.

DECONJUGATION OF BILE SALTS[8]

Only free bile acids are found in faeces. Cholic acid is converted to deoxycholic acid in the colon and both of these bile acids are absorbed from this site.

Gram-positive anaerobes probably contribute more to the deconjugation of bile acids than do the Gram-negative anaerobes.[7]

AMMONIA METABOLISM

Intestinal bacteria produce ammonia partly by deamination of amino acids, but principally by urea hydrolysis. Urea undergoes an enterohepatic circulation, being absorbed in the liver, then entering the colon by passive diffusion where it is hydrolysed to ammonia and carbon dioxide. The ammonia re-enters the portal blood by diffusion and returns to the liver to be converted back to urea or incorporated into protein. It appears that the mucosal flora of the colon is important in urea metabolism. Very little urea is detectable in faeces, presumably because all urea entering the gut is hydrolysed to ammonia. In normal persons, the ammonia generated in the gut is restricted to the portal blood system but in liver disease there is diminished capacity to detoxify the ammonia, which enters the general circulation and causes many of the effects that are attributed to liver failure. Although 'harmful' in liver failure, intestinal bacteria are useful in renal failure because they hydrolyse urea to ammonia and thereby reduce the circulating blood urea level which is responsible for toxicity in renal failure.

PROTECTION AGAINST SOME ENTERIC PATHOGENS

The pre-treatment of mice with antibiotics kills some of the bacterial flora and increases their susceptibility to oral challenge with salmonellae,[3] shigellae or *Vibrio cholerae*.[15] In patients given neomycin, there is prolonged carriage of salmonellae.[1]

METABOLISM OF DRUGS

Bacteria possess certain enzymes that are responsible for a variety of effects on drugs. For example, senna and cascara are degraded to active ingredients by colonic bacteria. Chloramphenicol, aspirin, steroids (of all types), sulphonamides, salicylate derivatives, and caffein are all able to be degraded by intestinal bacteria.[8]

CARCINOGENESIS

Colon cancer and gut bacteria are discussed in great detail in Chapter 17. In brief, the incidence of colon cancer seems to be correlated with both total faecal bile acid concentration and concentration of dihydroxycholanic acid. It has been postulated that colon cancer is produced by production of a carcinogen *in situ* from a benign substrate such as bile acid, which becomes polyunsaturated by bacterial degradation. Only certain clostridia are able to complete this alteration of bile acids, and a causative role has been attributed to these organisms because they occur in high frequency in populations with a high incidence of colon cancer (see Chapter 17).

BORBORYGMI AND HALITOSIS

These are due to gut bacteria, at least in part. Borborygmi may be due to excess production of intraluminal gas by bacteria, and halitosis represents the incomplete degradation of substrates. As stated earlier, the components of the gut flora tend to be fixed early in life and some individuals are colonized by flora which are better able than others to degrade organic matter. Methane production by colonic bacteria is well recognized both as a hazard in the operating room when occasional unfortunate explosions occur with diathermy applications, and also as a college cult where the ability to expel inflammable gas per rectum entitles one to membership of the 'order of the royal blue flame'.

OVERGROWTH OF GUT BACTERIA

Aetiological factors

Any factor that inhibits peristalsis, diminishes secretions, or disturbs the anatomical integrity of the gut may lead to the overgrowth syndrome.[4]

ABNORMAL PERISTALSIS

The intact myoenteric plexus is responsible for coordinated peristalsis, thus any neurological disorder which disturbs gut innervation may induce overgrowth of the flora. As the vagus nerve has a major effect on gut function, overgrowth of bacteria occurs as a problem after nonselective vagotomy. Less frequently, diabetic neuropathy may involve the autonomic nervous system including the myoenteric plexus, and bacterial overgrowth in the small gut may result.

Obstructions to flow by tumours or even foreign bodies will prevent normal peristalsis; malignant tumours of the small intestine are relatively rare, and are mainly due to lymphatic tumours.

LACK OF SECRETIONS

IgA deficiency is associated with overgrowth. This may be due to the uninhibited growth of ingested organisms such as *Salmonella* or *Escherichia coli* which would normally not attach to the mucosa because secretory IgA coats the bacterial attachment sites. Pancreatic insufficiency can produce a malabsorption

Table 14.2 Conditions associated with bacterial overgrowth

Stasis	Afferent loop
	Strictures
	Blind loop
	Diverticulae
	Hypomotility — diabetes, scleroderma
Reflux of colonic material	Fistulae connecting with colon
	Incompetent ileo-caecal valve
Impaired decontamination of luminal contents	Achlorhydria
	IgA deficiency
	Rapid stomach transit
Enterotoxigenic enterobacteria in upper intestine	Tropical sprue
Related sepsis	Cholangitis

syndrome; and excess metabolic substrates are available to bacteria, which overgrow.

ANATOMICAL ABNORMALITIES

Surgical procedures that produce a 'blind loop' — a noncontiguous section of gut — account for a significant proportion of cases of bacterial overgrowth. Peptic ulcer surgery has been the main contributor to this problem by producing a blind loop after gastro-jejunostomy procedures; the duodenum and proximal jejunum form the blind loop.

The problems associated with bacterial overgrowth have been a major factor in choosing alternative forms of surgical attack on peptic ulcers. Vagotomy and drainage is a popular operation for peptic ulceration, but unless the vagotomy spares the vagal fibres supplying the small intestine, peristalsis will be impaired. Various bypass procedures are undertaken for gut obstruction, biliary drainage and even diversion of urine flow. Each of these procedures carries the risk of bacterial colonization in the segment of gut which is not contiguous with the normal stream. Other conditions that allow bacterial overgrowth in 'blind' or stagnant sections of gut, fall into two categories; diverticula that may occur in the duodenum and small bowel, and fistulae from inflammatory bowel disease, or less commonly malignant tumours. Malabsorption due to bacterial overgrowth may be a presenting symptom of Crohn's ileitis. A list of the diseases and conditions leading to bacterial overgrowth is given in Table 14.2.

TROPICAL SPRUE

Enterotoxigenic enterobacteria, and occasionally anaerobes, have been found in large numbers in the upper intestine of adults with mild and severe diarrhoea and malabsorption who have been resident in developing countries.[2,18,21,24,33,34] In mild sprue enterobacteria including *Klebsiella* sp. and *Citrobacter* sp. were found in the luminal fluid or mucosal samples in numbers ranging from 10^3 to 10^8 per ml or g.[8,35] In severe tropical sprue colonization of the mucosa was a particular feature;[34] in 26 such patients in India 14 of 16 strains of *Klebsiella, Enterobacter* or *E. coli* obtained from the upper intestine produced enterotoxins.[21]

Clinical presentations

Malabsorption is the major feature of bacterial overgrowth. The symptoms are the result of excessive bacterial metabolism.

STEATORRHOEA

Anaerobic organisms are especially active in deconjugating bile salts to produce free bile acids[7,19] which may be absorbed in the proximal small intestine by nonionic diffusion. The absence of bile salts results in impaired micelle formation and fat malabsorption. Experimental studies also indicate that triglyceride absorption is impaired in blind loops.

ANAEMIA

Intraluminal bacteria degrade vitamin B_{12} and thus this vitamin may not be available in sufficient quantities for absorption in the lower ileum. Vitamin B_{12} malabsorption appears to be related to the total number of bacteria in the small bowel rather than to overgrowth of one specific type of microorganism.[19] Macrocytic anaemia with a megaloblastic bone marrow can occur. This deficiency of vitamin B_{12} is not corrected by intrinsic factors in the Schilling test.

DIARRHOEA

This may result not only from steatorrhoea but also from impaired peristalsis which is produced by diseases such as scleroderma.[28] Scleroderma or diabetes[38] are very likely to produce extragastrointestinal symptoms and the pathophysiology of overgrowth in these diseases relates to the degeneration of neural transmission, or thickening of the intestinal wall.

WEIGHT LOSS

The outcome of malabsorption will be weight loss which is primarily due to inadequate digestion of foodstuffs.

GLOSSITIS, PERIPHERAL NEUROPATHY, AMENORRHOEA, BLEEDING, OEDEMA AND BONE PAIN

All these may occur in the end stage of malabsorption.

Diagnosis

The clinical diagnosis of malabsorption is suggested by the symptoms described above, but there are numerous causes of malabsorption. The first aspect of diagnosis is to establish that malabsorption or steatorrhoea is present. Quantitative determination of faecal fat excretion is the single most important test to confirm steatorrhoea. A normal individual should excrete less than 6 g/24 h or achieve greater than 95% absorption of ingested fat.

Laboratory tests to distinguish bacterial overgrowth syndromes from other causes of malabsorption either utilize indirect methods for demonstrating bacterial overgrowth or involve direct sampling techniques.

INDIRECT TESTS FOR BACTERIAL OVERGROWTH

A series of techniques that depend upon the properties of gut bacteria to metabolize specific substances such as radioactive labelled bile salts, indican, volatile phenols and fatty acids have been devised. A quantitative estimation of the metabolites is then used to distinguish the normal from abnormal. Unfortunately, the sensitivity of these tests is variable, and the results must be cautiously interpreted.

Breath tests

The advantage of breath tests is that they are noninvasive techniques which can be used to distinguish many causes of malabsorption. The most reliable breath tests for bacterial overgrowth are those which utilize radiolabelled substrates.

BILE-ACID BREATH TEST[11,23,25,29]

C^{14} labelled glycine cholate (cholylglycine-1-C^{14}) is administered orally. In normal subjects the bile acid is absorbed at the terminal ileum and enters the enterohepatic circulation. If the glycine cholate encounters bacteria, then $C^{14}O_2$ is liberated and detected in exhaled air. Initially this test was thought to be valuable in determining bacterial overgrowth of the small intestine as well as indicating disease of the terminal ileum. The value of this test in determining ileal disease is dubious unless the breath analysis is accompanied by faecal bile acid excretion. Nevertheless, for detecting bacterial overgrowth the $C^{14}O_2$ estimation is a satisfactory initial investigation. False negatives will occur if the bacteria in the

test patient fail to deconjugate glycine cholate, which is unusual, and false positive
results may occur not only with terminal ileal disease but also in cholangitis and
after cholecystectomy when the turnover of bile salts is high.

In normal subjects, ingested glucose is fully absorbed but if there are large
numbers of bacteria in the upper small bowel, hydrogen may be produced by
bacterial fermentation prior to absorption. This hydrogen production can be
detected in exhaled gases and the usual glucose test dose is 50 g.

Detection of products of bacterial metabolism

Gut bacteria may produce detectable quantities of volatile fatty acids which can
be detected by chromatography of jejunal aspirates.[5] Obligate anaerobes are
predominantly responsible for production of these substances.

   Jejunal samples are obtained by direct aspiration and assayed for acetic,
propionic and butyric acids which are specific metabolites of anaerobes. Results
of these analyses can be rapidly available, and most laboratories that undertake
identification of anaerobes by chromatography should be able to apply the same
techniques to analysis of jejunal aspirates.

URINARY INDICAN

This is the most widely used and perhaps simplest method of detecting overgrowth.[14] This test depends upon the ability of bacteria to metabolize ingested
tryptophan to indole which is hydroxylated and sulphated by the host and
excreted in the urine as indoxylsulphate (indican). However the concentration of
urinary indican is influenced by many factors including the amount of
endogenous or exogenous tryptophan in the gut, gut pH, the carbohydrate content
of the gut, and bacterial species in the gut flora.

   The correlation between bacterial overgrowth and excess urinary indican is
quite poor and a positive test should merely result in a request for direct bacterial
sampling. The indirect tests are relatively insensitive, and they do not indicate the
site of disease.

DIRECT TESTS FOR BACTERIAL OVERGROWTH

There is a surprising difference between different patients suffering from overgrowth of gut bacteria, as far as the species of colonizing bacteria is concerned.
One patient may have predominant *Klebsiella* sp. colonizing the upper intestine
because of drainage from a biliary focus whereas another may demonstrate a

predominance of *Bacteroides* sp. Culture techniques are valuable for isolating the specific bacteria and this allows antibiotic therapy to be specific.

Collection of samples

Luminal aspirates should be collected from several sections of the intestine and the specimens processed immediately.[2,33,34] Very little work has been undertaken on transport systems and it is advisable to obviate any delays between collection and processing, to avoid loss of fastidious organisms on the one hand and prevent overgrowth of enterobacteria on the other hand. Anaerobic transport conditions can be achieved by aspirating into a syringe and then expelling all air and sealing the shank with an air-tight cap. Some workers have aspirated samples directly into a cooled CO_2-containing tube. Biopsy samples should be transported in bottles containing carbon dioxide, or in oxygen-free tubes.

Laboratory processing

Aspirates or biopsy specimens should be cultured in ways that will enable a total aerobic and anaerobic bacterial count to be achieved[31] (see Appendix). Processing of samples in an anaerobic cabinet is ideal, but strict anaerobes in fresh clinical specimens have been shown to tolerate exposure to air for up to 8 hours such as might occur during bench techniques in clinical laboratories.[32] The media chosen should grow lactobacilli, *Bacteroides* sp., *Veillonella* sp., and clostridia as well as facultative enterobacteria.

Interpretation of results

The problems of 'double-counting' can be avoided by using selective media in conjunction with nonselective media and ensuring that the additive counts on the selective media approximate to the total count on nonselective media. Interpretation is usually not difficult because the jejunum should contain less than 10^3/ml of bacteria; and greater than 10^5 can usually be distinguished with ease, providing that appropriate anaerobic techniques are used. A useful check on results is to undertake a wet mount and Gram stain of material cultured. Counts in excess of 10^5/ml should be detected microscopically, and the morphology of the bacteria will assist in indicating appropriate culture techniques.

Identification of species and detection of enterotoxigenicity

There is little value in speciating the various components of mixed bacteria which are usually observed in overgrowth syndromes. If one bacterial type predominates then speciation and sensitivity testing is warranted. Detection of enterotoxin production may be valuable.[21]

TREATMENT

When possible, diseased segments, stagnant loops or fistulae should be surgically corrected. Siting of the pathological segment may require segmental aspiration and or biopsy, however most blind loops can be visualized by contrast radiology or endoscopy.

With inflammatory bowel disease, scleroderma, diabetes and multiple diverticulae of the small bowel, surgical removal is impractical and antibiotic therapy is indicated, although its use is fraught with problems. There is a paucity of clinical trials to evaluate the most effective agents. Different individuals yield differing proportions of bacterial types. Prolonged antibiotic administration will not eradicate the gut flora but merely predispose to superinfection.

If analysis of the aspirate indicates the presence of a single strain then an antibiotic should be prescribed based upon sensitivity testing. This circumstance most frequently occurs with biliary sepsis leaking into the upper intestine. When antibiotics are selected to treat biliary sepsis it is important that agents are used that are concentrated or secreted in bile, e.g. ampicillin, tetracycline, cefamandole, or trimethoprim. When a single strain is in the lumen of the bowel an antibiotic which is not absorbed may be useful, such as colistin sulphate.

Most bacterial overgrowth syndromes are associated with mixed anaerobic flora, and in these circumstances intermittent courses of antibiotics should be given to reduce bacterial numbers rather than continuous antibiotic treatment which will only result in colonization by resistant bacteria. Tetracycline compounds are the substances most frequently used and they are a logical choice because tetracyclines inactivate most of the anaerobic as well as the aerobic flora. The dosage of tetracycline base is 500 mg–1 g/day in adults. Tetracycline has also been used, usually successfully, in tropical sprue.[34] However, there are no data to indicate that tetracyclines are more or less successful than the antimicrobials used to prevent gut-derived sepsis in surgery, such as metronidazole, plus a cephalosporin or an oral aminoglycoside.

Therapy should be maintained until symptoms improve or laboratory parameters such as vitamin B_{12} concentration return to normal. The length of therapy should not exceed 3–4 weeks, and cyclical courses of treatment are advised.

Prevention is preferable to cure, and surgical procedures should be modified or selected to avoid the creation of blind loops. Advances in the medical and surgical management of peptic ulcer have reduced the numbers of patients with this problem. Much more information is required about optimal antimicrobial treatment regimens, and adequate comparative studies need to be undertaken. However, the principles detailed in the approach to management of postoperative sepsis (see Chapter 15) are very likely to apply to the bacterial overgrowth syndrome.

APPENDIX

Laboratory processing of luminal contents

Either a gram or a millilitre of the specimen, depending on its consistency, is homogenized in freshly-reduced thioglycollate medium without added dextrose. Serial 1 in 10 dilutions to 10^{-8} are made in the thioglycollate medium. 0.1 ml volumes of each of the eight dilutions are plated on the range of media tabulated below. Incubation under appropriate conditions is allowed to proceed for 1–3 days under aerobic conditions, and 3–7 days under anaerobic conditions. After adequate incubations, plates with discrete colonies are examined with a lens and representatives of every type of colonial morphology streaked on nonselective blood agar for aerobic and anaerobic incubation, and then identification.

Medium	Purpose
Sheep blood agar*	To determine *total* aerobic and anaerobic counts
Kanamycin laked horse blood agar	To suppress facultative Gram-negative rods
Kanamycin-vancomycin laked horse blood agar	To suppress bacteria other than *Bacteroides* sp. and *Fusobacterium* sp.
Egg-yolk neomycin agar	To detect lecithinase-producing *Clostridium* sp., e.g. *Cl. perfringens*
Bile-aesculin-azide agar	To enumerate Group D streptococci (enterococci); other bacteria are suppressed
LBS (Rogosa) agar	To enumerate *Lactobacillus* sp.; other bacteria are suppressed

*Enriched with haemin, vitamin K and yeast extract. Sheep blood allows easy detection of the double zone of haemolysis characteristic of *Cl. perfringens*.

REFERENCES

1   Association for the study of infectious disease (1970) *Lancet* **ii**, 1159.
2   Bhat P., Albert M. J., Rajan D., Ponniah J., Mathan V. I. and Baker S. J. (1980) Bacterial flora of the jejunum: A comparison of luminal aspirate and mucosal biopsy. *J. Med. Microbiol.* **13**, 247.
3   Bohnhoff M., Miller C. P. and Martin W. R. (1964) Resistance of the mouse's intestinal tract to experimental Salmonella infection. I. Factors which interfere with the initiation of infection by oral inoculation. *J. Exp. Med.* **120**, 805.
4   Borriello P., Hudson M. and Hill M. (1978) Investigation of the gastro-intestinal bacterial flora. *Clin. Gastroenterol.* **7**, 329.
5   Campbell C. B., Cowan A. E. and Harper J. (1973) Duodenal bacterial flora and bile salt patterns in patients with gastrointestinal disease. *Aust. N.Z. J. Med.* **3**, 339.
6   Dellipiani A. W. and Girdwood R. H. (1964) Bacterial changes in the small intestine in malabsorptive states and in pernicious anaemia. *Clin. Sci.* **26**, 359.
7   Drasar B. S., Hill M. J. and Shiner M. (1966) The deconjugation of bile salts by human intestinal bacteria. *Lancet* **i**, 1237.
8   Drasar B. S. and Hill M. J. (1974) *Human Intestinal Flora*, Academic Press, London.

9   Drasar B. S., Shiner M. and McLeod G. M. (1969) Studies on the intestinal flora. I. The bacterial flora of the gastrointestinal tract in healthy and achlorhydric persons. *Gastroenterology* **56**, 71.

10 Dubos R., Schaedler R. W., Costello R. and Hoet P. (1965) Indigenous, normal, and autochthonous flora of the gastrointestinal tract. *J. Exp. Med.* **122**, 67.

11 Faviar S., Fromm H., Schindler D. and Schmidt F. W. (1979) Sensitivity of bile acid breath test in the diagnosis of bacterial overgrowth in the small intestine with and without stagnant (blind) loop. *Dig. Dis. Sci.* **24**, 33.

12 Finegold S. M., Sutter V. L., Boyle J. D. and Shimada K. (1970) The normal flora of ileostomy and tranverse colostomy effluents. *J. Infect. Dis.* **122**, 376.

13 Formal S. B., Dammin G., Sprinz H., Schneider H., Horowitz R. E. and Forbes M. (1961) Experimental shigella infections V, studies in germ-free guinea pigs. *J. Bact.* **82**, 284.

14 Frankel S., Reitman S. and Sonnenwirth A. C. (1970) *Gradwohl's Clinical Laboratory Methods and Diagnosis*, 7th edn, p. 1861, C. V. Mosby, St Louis.

15 Freter R. (1956) Experimental enteric shigella and vibrio infections in mice and guinea pigs. *J. Exp. Med.* **104**, 411.

16 Goldstein F., Wirts C. W. and Josephs L. (1962) The bacterial flora of the small intestine. *Gastroenterology* **42**, 755.

17 Gorbach S. L. (1967) Population control in the small bowel. *Gut* **8**, 530.

18 Gorbach S. L., Banwell J. G., Jacobs B., Chatterjee B. D., Mitra R., Brigham K. L. and Neogy K. N. (1970) Intestinal microflora in Asiatic cholera. II. The small bowel. *J. Infect. Dis.* **121**, 38.

19 Gorbach S. L. and Tabaqchali S. (1969) Bacteria, bile and the small bowel. *Gut* **10**, 963.

20 Gordon H. A., Bruckner-Kardross E. and Wostmann B. S. (1966) Aging in germ-free mice: life tables and lesions observed at natural death. *J. Gerontol.* **21**, 380.

21 Gracey M. (1979) The contaminated small bowel syndrome: pathogenesis, diagnosis and treatment. *Am. J. Clin. Nutr.* **32**, 234.

22 Holdeman L. V., Good I. J. and Moore W. E. C. (1976) Human fecal flora: Variation in bacterial composition within individuals and a possible effect of emotional stress. *Appl. Environ. Microbiol.* **31**, 359.

23 James O. F. W., Agnew J. E. and Bouchier I. A. D. (1973) Assessment of the ^{14}C-Glycocholic acid breath test. *Br. Med. J.* **3**, 191.

24 Klipstein F. A., Engert R. F. and Short H. B. (1978) Enterotoxigenicity of colonising coliform bacteria in tropical sprue and blind-loop syndrome. *Lancet* **ii**, 342.

25 Metz G., Gassull M. A., Drasar B. S., Jenkins D. J. A. and Blendis L. M. (1976) Breath-hydrogen test for small-intestinal bacterial colonisation. *Lancet* **i**, 668.

26 Moore W. E. C. and Holdeman L. V. (1974) Human fecal flora: The normal flora of 20 Japanese-Hawaiians. *Appl. Microbiol.* **27**, 961.

27 Ruitenberg E. J., Guinee P. A. and Kruyt B. C. (1971) Salmonella pathogenesis in germ-free mice. A bacteriological and histological study. *Br. J. Exp. Pathol.* **52**, 192.

28 Salen G., Goldstein F. and Wirts C. W. (1966) Malabsorption in intestinal scleroderma. Relation to bacterial flora and treatment with antibiotics. *Ann. Int. Med.* **64**, 834.

29 Sherr H. P., Sasaki Y., Newman A., Banwell J. G., Wagner H. N. and Hendrix T. R. (1971) Detection of bacterial deconjugation of bile salts by a convenient breath-analysis technic. *N. Eng. J. Med.* **285**, 656.

30 Sutter V. L. and Finegold S. M. (1974) The effect of antimicrobial agents on human faecal flora: Studies with cephalexin, cyclacillin and clindamycin. Soc. Appl. Bacteriol. Symp. Ser. 3(0), 229.

31 Sutter V. L., Vargo V. L. and Finegold S. M. (1975) *Wadsworth Anaerobic Bacteriology Manual*, 2nd edn, p. 68, University of California, Los Angeles.

32 Tally F. P., Stewart P. R., Sutter V. L. and Rosenblatt J. E. (1975) Oxygen tolerance of fresh clinical anaerobic bacteria. *J. Clin. Microbiol.* **1**, 161.

33 Tomkins A. M., Drasar B. S. and James W. P. T. (1975) Bacterial colonisation of jejunal mucosa in acute tropical sprue. *Lancet* **i**, 59.

34   Tomkins A. M., James W. P. T., Cole A. C. E. and Walters J. H. (1974) Malabsorption in overland travellers to India. *Br. Med. J.* **3**, 380.
35   Tomkins A. M., Wright S. G. and Drasar B. S. (1980) Bacterial colonization of the upper intestine in mild tropical malabsorption. *Trans. R. Soc. Trop. Med. Hyg.* **74**, 752.
36   Valtonen M. V., Suomalainen R. J., Ylikahri R. H. and Valtonen V. V. (1977) Selection for multiresistant coliforms by long-term treatment of hypercholesterolaemia with neomycin. *Br. Med. J.* **1**, 683.
37   Wiseman G. (1964) *Absorption from the Intestine*, Academic Press, London.
38   Gorbach S. L. (1971) Intestinal microflora. *Gastroenterology* **60**, 1110.

15 The antimicrobial management of gut-derived sepsis complicating surgery and cancer chemotherapy

P. J. McDonald, J. McK. Watts and
J. J. Finlay-Jones

Pathogenesis	308
Gastrointestinal surgery	308
Risk of sepsis according to operation	309
Pathology	309
Bacterial virulence factors	310
Nonspecific factors in intra-abdominal sepsis	311
Host factors	311
Summary	311
Leukaemia, neutropaenia and sepsis	312
The pathogens	312
The role of antimicrobials	313
Therapeutic or preventive antimicrobial regimens?	314
Prevention of surgical sepsis	314
Selection of antimicrobial	315
Which operations warrant preventive antimicrobials?	316
Timing of antimicrobial administration	317
Colo-rectal surgery	318
Reduction of colonic flora	319
Systemic prophylaxis	319
Appendicectomy	320
Gastroduodenal surgery	322
Biliary surgery	322
Leukemia and granulocytopenia	323
Prophylactic antimicrobial regimens	325
References	326

After operations on the lower gut approximately half of all patients will develop septic complications unless antimicrobials are prescribed appropriately. In leukaemia, infection is a common cause of death and a frequent complication of antineoplastic chemotherapy. In both these circumstances, gut micro-organisms are the major source of the bacteria that cause wound infection, bacteraemia or metastatic sepsis.

When appropriate measures are taken to modify the gut flora during the 'risk' period of surgery or during the induction of cancer chemotherapy, the incidence of septic complications can be reduced substantially. However, the indiscriminate and especially the prolonged use of antimicrobials in these conditions may increase the septic complications of surgery and leukaemia by predisposing to superinfection with resistant strains of micro-organisms.

PATHOGENESIS

Gastrointestinal surgery

Postoperative wound infections are either a result of tissue contamination during surgery or of micro-organisms entering the wound in the postoperative period. The only bacteria that penetrate an intact surgical wound are the invasive pathogens. The main sources of operative contamination of the wound are gut bacteria and skin bacteria.

WHICH BACTERIA ARE THE PATHOGENS?

In a study of 601 patients undergoing elective surgery at Flinders Medical Centre, quantitative samples were collected from the edges of the incision just prior to closure. The samples were immediately cultured for aerobic and anaerobic bacteria. The bacteria detected in the wound at the conclusion of surgery are listed in Table 15.1. These represent the contaminating inoculum.

Table 15.1   Bacteria detected in the incision at the conclusion of 601 enterotomy operations

Bacterial type	No. of patients with isolate*	%
Staphylococci		
Coagulase negative	342	57
Coagulase positive	21	3
Diphtheroids	88	15
Enterococci	59	10
Enterobacteriaceae	107	18
Bacteroides fragilis group	86†	14
Bacteroides melaninogenicus group	5	1

*More than one species was isolated from some patients. †*B. fragilis* 30, *B. vulgatus* 17, *B. distasonis* 7, *B. thetaiotaomicron* 5, *B. ovatus* 4, unspeciated 34.

Table 15.2   Bacteriology of septic wounds

Bacteria in pus	No.	No. with same organism in incision wound
Staphylococcus aureus	6	1 (17%)
Facultative Gram-negative aerobes (one or more species)	11	8 (73%)
Obligate anaerobes (one or more species)	21	16 (76%)
No growth	7	—
Not done*	23	

*Approximately one-third of all wound infections occurred after patients had left hospital.

Septic postoperative wounds occurred in 68 (11%) of these patients. The bacterial types isolated from these infected wounds are listed in Table 15.2, together with a correlation between the contaminating inoculum and bacteria present at sepsis.

Clearly, not all the contaminants in Table 15.1 persisted to cause sepsis, and there was a higher risk of sepsis with some bacteria than others. The bacteria that demonstrated a close correlation between contamination at operation and presence in the septic wound can be considered as the primary gut pathogens. Further analysis of the data indicated that firstly when *Bacteroides* sp. or the Enterobacteriaceae were present in postoperative pus, the same organisms were present in the wound at the time of surgery. Secondly, in the majority of wounds there was more than one species of bacteria. Thirdly, the chance of developing postoperative sepsis was proportional to the numbers of contaminating bacteria, and was related to the types of contaminating bacteria. When Enterobacteriaceae were present in numbers $> 10^4$/ml at the conclusion of operation, then 50% of wounds became septic. If *Bacteroides fragilis* were present in numbers $> 10^4$/ml, 60% of wounds became septic. Fourthly, of the six patients with *Staphylococcus aureus* in postoperative pus, only one patient had this organism detected as a 'contaminant' during surgery, suggesting that *Staphylococcus aureus* enters the wound in the postoperative period. This corroborates epidemiologic information which indicates that *Staphylococcus aureus* is a cross-infecting nosocomial organism in surgical sepsis which often colonizes the skin and mucous membranes of patients, and staff.

Risk of sepsis according to operation

The determinants of postoperative sepsis are the nature and extent of bacterial contamination together with host response. Some operations are more prone to intraoperative contamination, and this is reflected in the wound infection rates observed in gut operations when no antibiotic cover is provided (Table 15.3). These statistics have been taken from the 'placebo' groups in drug trials reported in 1978 and 1979.

Table 15.3 Infection rate according to type of operation — no antibiotic prophylaxis

Operation	Rate of wound sepsis
Appendicectomy	23%
Gastroduodenal operation	20%
Biliary	11%
Large bowel	40%
Other enterotomy	16%

Pathology

Obligate anaerobic pathogens, such as *Bacteroides fragilis* alone or in combination with facultative enteric bacteria, usually produce abscesses when inoculated into sterile tissue such as a surgical wound or the peritoneal cavity.

When facultative enteric bacteria such as *E. coli* contaminate such tissue in sufficient numbers then bacteraemia without localization is the usual outcome. This has been shown in animal models by Bartlett *et al.*[1] Rats challenged with an intraperitoneal inoculum of caecal material mixed with an adjuvant such as barium sulphate responded in one of four ways. Firstly, immediate death from endotoxic shock; *E. coli* was cultured from the blood in these animals. Secondly, 1–5 days after challenge a diffuse peritonitis occurred in conjunction with bacteraemia due to *E. coli*. Septicaemic death usually followed. Thirdly, 7–14 days after challenge localized intra-abdominal abscesses occurred. Obligate anaerobes such as *B. fragilis* were present in the abscesses. Fourthly, there was complete recovery.

Human response to intraperitoneal faecal challenge is somewhat similar. Colon rupture with gross faecal soiling is sometimes rapidly fatal due to endotoxic shock. In patients with a less overwhelming challenge such as a leaking anastomosis, general peritonitis with or without bacteraemia is likely. Despite the fact that the faecal challenge is predominantly 'anaerobic', bacteria cultured from the bloodstream usually belong to the Enterobacteriaceae. It has been suggested that anaerobic bacteria may impair local immune responses and allow the enterobacteria to become invasive.

Abscess formation is the hallmark of infection due to obligately anaerobic bacteria and this process is observed typically in diverticular and appendiceal abscesses. Cultures of these lesions will usually yield anaerobic pathogens such as *B. fragilis* either alone or in combination with facultative enteric bacteria.

The sites of intraperitoneal sepsis are determined by gravitational and physiological factors. The diaphragmatic action and recumbent posture will favour a cephalic spread of material, hence the frequency of 'subphrenic' abscess. Other favoured sites of collection are the para-colic spaces, the pelvis, including the pouch of Douglas in females, the retro-peritoneum, and the lesser sac.

Bacterial virulence factors

Although anaerobes and aerobes can be major pathogens in postenterotomy surgical sepsis it has been found that bacteraemia is associated with enterobacteria such as *E. coli*, but abscess formation is due to either anaerobes alone or a mixture of facultative and obligately anaerobic bacteria. The virulence factors of the gut pathogens are endotoxin or capsules. Facultative Gram-negative bacteria contain endotoxin which when released has myriad adverse effects on mammalian physiology. Cell wall extracts or heat-inactivated Gram-negative anaerobes such as *Bacteroides* sp., however, do not demonstrate the same biological effect as facultative Gram-negatives. Patients with bacteroides bacteraemia rarely demonstrate intravascular coagulation. However the factor associated with *Bacteroides* which most closely correlates with virulence is the capsule. Nonencapsulated strains of *B. fragilis* do not alone induce abscess formation in animal models, but heat-killed suspensions of encapsulated *Bacteroides fragilis* do so. In the course of infection with *Bacteroides fragilis*, capsule antibody titres rise, as the capsule is mildly immunogenic. The bacteroides capsule is composed of polysaccharide, and it may be demonstrated occasionally by negative staining such as with India-ink, or more reliably by electron microscopy.

BACTERIAL SYNERGY

A hallmark of endogenous surgical infections is that more than one species of bacteria is found. There is some evidence that facultative bacteria act synergistically with obligate anaerobes to produce pathology. Postulated mechanisms include the reduction of tissue redox potentials by facultative bacteria, thereby allowing anaerobes to proliferate, or the provision of growth factors or interference with immune mechanisms.

Nonspecific factors in intra-abdominal sepsis

In animal models some form of adjuvant is required to produce intra-abdominal sepsis. Barium sulphate has been widely used in such experiments. In disease states, a likely 'adjuvant' is faecal fibre. Autoclaved faeces have been shown to act as an adjuvant in animal experiments.[1] Gastric acid and bile may also act similarly in human disease and predispose to mixed anaerobic/aerobic sepsis because peritonitis is a frequent accompaniment of ruptured peptic ulcer and perforated gallbladder.

Host factors

Surgery itself produces at least a minor local interference with nonspecific immune defences by breaching mucous membranes, by interfering with peristaltic movement, by inserting sutures or other foreign material, and by creating haematomata. The extent of perturbation produced by the operation itself is related to the nature of the operation, the technique of the operating team, and the general health of the patient (Table 15.4).

Table 15.4 Host factors which influence susceptibility to infection

Age
Thickness of abdominal fat
Length of incision
Foreign body insertion
Innate or acquired immunodeficiency
Local ischaemia
Immunosuppressive drugs (steroids)
Alcoholism
Diabetes
Malignancy

Summary

Sepsis following gut surgery is usually due to endogenous bacteria being transferred to normally sterile sites such as the peritoneum or operative wound. Certain endogenous bacteria such as *Bacteroides fragilis* and *E. coli* are able to overcome host defences, perhaps with the aid of adjuvants such as faecal fibre and gastric mucin. The nature of postoperative sepsis depends on the extent and type of bacterial challenge and host defence factors. However, both of these fundamental factors are modified significantly by surgical technique and the nature of the operation being undertaken.

LEUKAEMIA, NEUTROPAENIA AND SEPSIS

The underlying cause of sepsis in leukaemia is undoubtedly immunosuppression produced either by the disease process itself due to infiltration of the bone marrow, or by therapy. This chapter is devoted mainly to a consideration of the role of antimicrobials in preventing the septic complications of surgery and leukaemia. The approach to the prevention of sepsis in leukaemia differs according to whether or not one is dealing with the intercurrent infections to which the leukaemic patient is susceptible or whether one is considering the problem of preventing infection while antineoplastic therapy is being administered, especially during the induction of remission with combination chemotherapy which will produce profound neutropaenia.

This section considers the nature of sepsis, and methods for the prevention of sepsis that occurs when antineoplastic drugs produce granulocytopaenia.

The pathogens

Susceptibility to infection is closely related to the degree of immunosuppression. After the peripheral blood granulocyte count falls below 1000/cmm, then infectious episodes are common. Numerous studies have been undertaken with a view to demonstrating the opportunistic pathogens in granulocytopaenic patients. Predictably, the results of such studies varied widely depending on the extent and frequency of microbiological sampling and the manner in which the patient was nursed. Cross-infection is a special hazard for immunosuppressed patients, and it has now become common for such patients to be treated in 'reverse isolation' under circumstances that will prevent nosocomial microorganisms being acquired by the patient.

The incidence of infection during granulocytopaenia is high. Approximately 90% of patients with peripheral blood granulocyte counts below 1000/cmm will develop fever. A definite cause for this fever can be found in approximately 50% of such patients. The European Organization for Research on Treatment of Cancer (EORTC[5]) has undertaken large-scale prospective trials with a view to defining the aetiology and optimal antimicrobial therapy for febrile granulocytopaenic patients. In 625 patients reviewed by EORTC the frequency of pathogens was comparable to other published series.[5] Table 15.5 outlines the pathogens that occurred in these patients.

Table 15.5 Pathogenic microorganisms isolated from febrile granulocytopaenic patients (data from EORTC study[5])

Organism	Frequency in patients (%)
Escherichia coli	23
Staphylococcus aureus	16
Klebsiella species	16
Pseudomonas aeruginosa	11
Candida species	5
Enterococci	4.8
Proteus species	4.8
Staphylococcus epidermidis	2.2
Enterobacter species	2.2
Serratia marcescens	2.0
Streptococcus pneumoniae	1.7
Other bacteria	6
Hepatitis B virus antigen	1.1
Yeasts/fungi	0.5
Other viruses	0.5
Pneumocystis carinii	0.5

Clearly the Enterobacteriaceae and other bacteria found in the gut were major causes of sepsis but it is by no means certain that the Enterobacteriaceae that produced bacteraemia took direct origin from the gut.

The EORTC study suggested that the oral cavity, skin and soft-tissues, lung and urinary tract were the most frequent clinical sources of infection. As a consequence of hospitalization and illness the normal flora of the skin and oral cavity tend to become colonized with Enterobacteriaceae. The role of bowel organisms as primary sources of bacteraemia in these patients is unresolved. In summary, while almost any organisms may produce infection during granulocytopaenia, facultative Gram-negative bacteria are responsible for the majority of such infections, with *Staphylococcus aureus* as the next most frequent cause.

THE ROLE OF ANTIMICROBIALS

In surgery and leukaemia, a clear distinction must be drawn between preventive and therapeutic antimicrobial therapy. The choice of antimicrobial and dosage schedule in both these situations should take account of the following principles:

(a) Antimicrobials must penetrate to the site of presumed contamination or infection in concentrations which exert an antimicrobial effect.

(b) The antimicrobials must retain their activity at the site of infection. Aminoglycosides are inactivated by acid pH; clindamycin is tightly bound to α_1 acid glycoprotein at sites of acute inflammation.

(c) The target bacteria must be able to assimilate the antibiotic; resting or L-phase bacteria may not provide the active transport mechanisms required.

(d) No single antibiotic or combination of antibiotics is able to eradicate completely all micro-organisms which constitute 'normal' flora.

(e) The predisposition to superinfection with resistant strains is related to the spectrum of activity of the chosen antimicrobial and the length of time for which it is given.

(f) Whether therapeutic or preventive, the choice of antimicrobial must be determined by the known or predicted susceptibility profile of the bacteria producing infection or challenging the host.

The untoward consequences of antimicrobial therapy usually result from prolonged administration of broad spectrum agents which provoke major changes in the patient's normal flora and select out resistant strains of bacteria; the latter constitute a risk to the individual and can contaminate the hospital environment.

Therapeutic or preventive antimicrobial regimens?

This chapter discusses the use of preventive antimicrobials in surgery and leukaemia, but it is important to realize that in some circumstances it is difficult to judge whether infection is already established in common conditions such as appendicitis and cholecystitis. Similarly, in the febrile, leukaemic patient with infiltration of tissues it is not possible to decide immediately whether the fever is due to infection or neoplastic infiltrate.

If infection is already established, then the choice of antimicrobial and duration of therapy needs to be modified according to the invading pathogen and nature of pathology. A ruptured gangrenous appendix will already have established at least a local peritonitis, and antimicrobials administered more than a few hours after appendix rupture cannot be expected to prevent the formation of localized collections of pus.

Prevention of surgical sepsis

Approximately 60% of antibiotics used in hospitals are prescribed by surgeons, and a significant proportion of these are for the prevention of infection. The use of antibiotics in surgery, however, constitutes only a secondary aspect of infection prevention; the primary role of surgical technique, adequate nutrition and control of cross-infection needs to be recognized.

Antimicrobials have a role in the prevention of surgical sepsis, and the circumstances in which they have been shown to be effective are when postoperative infection is due to intraoperative contamination, when the antimicrobials used are active against the contaminating pathogens, and when a high concentration of active antibiotic is present in the operative site at the time of tissue contamination.

The efficacy of prophylactic antimicrobials, particularly in gut surgery, was not established until recent times. This was due in part to the lack of adequate, controlled studies, and in part to the untoward effects observed with certain pre-scribing practices which resulted in increased morbidity. At one time it was popular to prescribe penicillin and streptomycin for 2–3 days preoperatively and then for a further 5 days postoperatively. The result of this prescribing pattern was to diminish the patient's susceptible normal flora in the preoperative period and allow colonization, often with strains of resistant bacteria. In the postoperative period this selection pressure was maintained by the continuation of antibiotics which allowed the super-infecting bacteria to flourish in the operative wound, urinary catheter, endotracheal tube or other perturbations of normal defences such as intravenous cannulae.

It is interesting to analyse the rationale behind the use of penicillin and streptomycin. The choice of antibiotic was undoubtedly determined by the pathogens found in postoperative sepsis. Neither penicillin nor streptomycin is active against *Bacteroides fragilis* which has been realized to be a common pathogen. The timing of doses was probably aimed at 'eradication' of the putative pathogens. However, it is now clear that total eradication of such bacteria from the gut is almost impossible, and the intraoperative concentrations of antibiotic achieved with 'pre' and 'post' administration are very likely to be inadequate. Resistant bacterial overgrowth was probably overlooked or accepted as a penalty to be incurred occasionally in order to prevent serious sepsis.

To prevent sepsis after gut surgery several approaches are logical. The con-taminating inoculum of pathogenic bacteria should be reduced. The normal physiological processes responsible for local and systemic homeostasis and immunity should be maintained or restored. The natural mechanisms of anti-bacterial resistance should be supplemented with antibiotics. Exposure of the patient's normal flora to antibiotics should be minimized.

Selection of antimicrobial

The antimicrobials administered must be active against the potentially pathogenic micro-organisms which contaminate the operative field. At the time of surgery it is impractical to determine the exact extent and nature of contamina-tion. In biliary surgery, some centres have adopted a practice of doing a Gram stain on the bile, and if organisms are seen, appropriate antibiotics are administered. Generally, the choice of antimicrobials must be based on empirical knowledge of the likely contaminating flora.

Earlier in this chapter it was demonstrated that the major pathogenic endogenous bacteria in gut surgery are facultative enteric bacteria (Entero-bacteriaceae, enterococci) and obligately anaerobic bacteria (*Bacteroides fragilis, Bacteroides melaninogenicus*). Also, the risk of postoperative sepsis is propor-tional to the degree of contamination with these pathogens. The type of operation is therefore a major determinant of operative contamination (Table 15.3).

The antibiotic susceptibility profile of the major pathogens associated with gut surgery is predictable, and a variety of effective agents can be listed. The choice of agents should be based on cumulative susceptibility data for a given hospital or

Table 15.6 Antimicrobial susceptibility of antibiotics used in gut surgery

Antimicrobial	Activity against Enterobacteriaceae	Enterococci	*Bacteroides fragilis*	*Bacteroides* species other than *B. fragilis*
Aminoglycosides	+ +	±	−	−
Ampicillin	+	±	−	+ +
Cephalosporins*	+ +	−	−*	+ +
Clindamycin/lincomycin	−	−	+ +	+ +
Imidazoles (metronidazole, tinidazole)	−	−	+ +	+ +
Tetracycline	+	±	+	+ +
Chloramphenicol	+ +	+	+ +	+ +
Cefoxitin	+ +	−	+ +	+ +
Trimethoprim/sulpha-methoxazole	+ +	+	±	±

+ + Fully effective; + effective in most circumstances; ± variable; − ineffective;
* moxalactam is effective against *B. fragilis*.

geographic area because the susceptibility profile, particularly of the Entero-bacteriaceae may vary according to local patterns of antibiotic usage. A list of antimicrobials and their activity against the pathogens in gut surgery is given in Table 15.6. There are important factors to consider in selecting antibiotics. Firstly, aminoglycosides administered orally reduce intraluminal Entero-bacteriaceae but they have no impact on intraluminal anaerobes. In some hospitals aminoglycoside-resistant Gram-negative bacteria are quite prevalent and there is a danger that oral aminoglycosides may induce colonization with resistant strains. Secondly, patterns of antimicrobial use may modify the prevailing sensitivity patterns of any of the bacteria. Thirdly, the nitro-imidazoles — metronidazole and tinidazole — do not have any activity against facultative enteric bacteria such as *E. coli*. Fourthly, resistance of *Bacteroides fragilis* to beta-lactam antibiotics is due to beta-lactamase production. Of recent antimicrobials only cefoxitin, moxalactam and thienamycin have adequate resistance to the beta-lactamase of *B. fragilis*.

A review of the antibiotics used in enterotomy operations indicates that the best effect is achieved when antimicrobials active against all contaminating pathogens are administered. Nevertheless, there is some good effect gained from the use of an agent which is active against only some of the pathogens contaminating the wound. It is evident that postoperative sepsis is related to the degree of operative contamination, and is most likely to be prevented by antimicrobials that are directed specifically against the contaminating pathogens.

Which operations warrant preventive antimicrobials?

Any operation where endogenous bacterial contamination is 'significant' deserves a prophylactic antimicrobial in addition to meticulous surgical technique. In abdominal surgery any procedure which opens a contaminated viscus usually has a postoperative septic complication rate which can be reduced by appropriate antimicrobial prophylaxis. A useful classification of operations for the purposes of determining when to use antibiotics is that of Cruse and Foord,[4] who analysed 23 649 operations; Table 15.7 shows the wound infection rate with each type of procedure in the absence of antibiotic cover.

Table 15.7 Incidence of postoperative wound sepsis according to degree of contamination (after Cruse and Foord 1973[4])

Operation type	Criteria	No.	% Infected
Clean	No infected viscus opened. No acute inflammation	18 090	1.8
Clean-contaminated	No apparent contamination. Viscus containing normal flora	4106	8.9
Contaminated	Spillage from heavily contaminated or infected viscus. Acute inflammation	770	21.5
Dirty	Pus Perforated viscus	683	38.5

Placebo-controlled double-blind studies in clean-contaminated, contaminated and 'dirty' surgery have now been undertaken with a variety of antibiotics and there is clear evidence that appropriate antimicrobial combinations can diminish the postoperative septic complication rate in each of the categories listed.

Before discussing specific types of operation and prophylaxis, the timing of antibiotic administration needs to be analysed.

Timing of antimicrobial administration

By definition, prophylactic antimicrobials are given to inhibit the development of sepsis rather than treat established bacterial lesions. It takes only about 4 hours for contaminating bacteria to become localized and antibiotics administered after this period cannot prevent the development of a septic process. The classic experiments of Miles[8] and Burke[3] illustrate clearly that timing is crucial. When a penicillin-sensitive staphylococcus was injected into animals in whom the plasma concentration of penicillin was above the minimal inhibitory concentration, then a lesion did not develop. If penicillin was injected after the tissues were challenged with staphylococci, then the size of the subsequent lesion was proportional to the time interval between inoculation and antibiotic administration.

The best effect from an antibiotic is achieved if an adequate concentration is present in the tissues prior to bacterial challenge. No effect can be anticipated after the infection is localized, which is as early as 4 hours after inoculation. Thus postoperative antibiotics cannot be expected to prevent sepsis. The reasons why antibiotics are inactive in localized collections (abscesses) are listed in Table 15.8.

Table 15.8   Reasons for the ineffectiveness of antimicrobials in an abscess

---

1   Inadequate drug penetration
2   Breakdown of drug within the abscess. Beta-lactamase enzymes of bacteria can destroy many beta-lactam antibiotics
3   pH prevents antibiotic activity; for example in an acid pH aminoglycosides are less effective
4   The drug becomes bound to proteins; for example clindamycin is bound to α_1-acid glycoprotein
5   Oxygen tension; aminoglycosides require oxygen-dependent bacterial transport; metronidazole works only under anaerobic conditions
6   Organisms persist within phagocytes
7   L-phase or non-metabolizing bacteria fail to take up drug
8   High bacterial inoculum

Prolonged preoperative administration of antibiotics should be avoided to prevent superinfection with resistant strains.

In summary, optimal regimens of prophylactic antibiotics should achieve adequate concentrations of circulating antibiotic during the period of operative contamination and for the short postoperative period during which further contamination may occur. The latter may be either locally, for example before a gut anastomosis seals over, or via the systemic route, for example bacteraemia induced by instrumentation such as sigmoidoscopy, or an operative cholangiogram. Thus selected antimicrobials should be administered preoperatively. This can be achieved with parenteral, oral or even topical administration.

Specific approaches to prophylactic antimicrobials in particular types of surgery will now be considered.

COLO-RECTAL SURGERY

In the absence of antimicrobial prophylaxis the incidence of postoperative sepsis in elective colon surgery is as high as 50%.[2] Postoperative infections are due either to intraoperative contamination which is usually high (primary infection), or anastomotic dehiscence (secondary infection). The secondary infections are due to inadequate surgical technique or poor wound healing. Antimicrobials cannot prevent anastomotic dehiscence but they can almost abolish the primary sepsis due to intraoperative contamination.

To prevent primary sepsis after colectomy three approaches are possible. First, preoperatively the number of colonic bacterial pathogens may be reduced. Second, therapeutic blood concentrations of effective antibacterial agents may be achieved intraoperatively. Third, topical agents may be put in the peritoneal cavity and the wound at operation.

Reduction of colonic flora

It has been traditional to minimize operative faecal soiling by preparing the patient with enemas or other mechanical forms of bowel washout such as anterograde lavage or a mannitol purge. Controlled studies have failed to vindicate these mechanical preparations as significant factors in reducing post-operative sepsis. Nevertheless there is some advantage from the operator's point of view in having a 'clean' colon. Mechanical preparations may reduce bacterial numbers by 50–99%. However, when this reduction is viewed in logarithmic terms, there is merely a diminution of bacteria from 10^{10} bacteria/ml to perhaps 10^8/ml. The latter is still a highly significant concentration of bacteria.

The aesthetic and technical advantages of mechanical preparations have to be weighed against the inconvenience to the patient and consequences of additional preoperative hospitalization. One important aspect of preoperative hospitalization is the opportunity this provides for colonization with resistant hospital bacteria. This colonization is aided by preoperative antimicrobial therapy.

A number of regimens have been studied which reduce intraluminal bacterial concentrations preoperatively. In the USA and Canada the most widely reported bowel preparation is oral neomycin plus erythromycin. The US Veterans Co-operative Study[2] assessed oral neomycin plus erythromycin versus placebo in elective colon surgery and noted a significant reduction not only in wound infection rates from 35% (placebo) to 9%, but there was also a significant reduction in the incidence of intra-abdominal sepsis, anastomotic leak and septicaemia. This regimen consisted of oral erythromycin base 1 g plus oral neomycin 1 g at 1.00 p.m., 2.00 p.m. and 11.00 p.m. on the day prior to surgery. This combined oral regimen achieved a reduction of faecal aerobes and anaerobes by a factor of about 10^5, from approximately 10^7–10^9 bacteria/ml down to $<10^4$ bacteria/ml. Earlier in this chapter it was pointed out that 'significant' infection rates are seen only with bacterial contamination in excess of 10^4/ml.

SYSTEMIC PROPHYLAXIS

Antimicrobials like tetracycline, metronidazole and clindamycin when administered orally also have an impact on bowel flora but they achieve quite high serum concentrations. In the assessment of many trials it is difficult to distinguish between the relative contributions of reduction of bowel flora and the effect of antibiotics which achieve adequate peroperative serum concentrations. Adequate serum concentrations may be achieved by parenteral or oral administration.

Regimens which provide a systemic concentration of antibiotic without reducing the bowel flora appear to be at least as effective as 'oral' regimens. The crucial aspect of successful 'systemic' regimens is that a high concentration of antibiotic, active against both anaerobes and aerobes, is maintained throughout the operative period. A list of adequate and effective drug regimens is given in Table 15.9.

Table 15.9   Preventive antimicrobial regimens in elective colo-rectal surgery

Agents	Duration	% Sepsis in treated group
Oral regimens		
Neomycin + erythromycin	1 day perop.	9%
Kanamycin + meronidazole	3 days preop.	8%
Neomycin + metronidazole	3 days preop.	10–15%
Thalazole + metronidazole	4 days preop.	10–15%
Tetracycline + neomycin	2 days preop.	5%
Systemic regimens		
*Lincomycin i.m.	24 h perop.	16%
*Metronidazole i.v.	24 h perop.	14%
Clindamycin + cephalothin i.v. (or gentamicin)	48 h perop.	8%
Cefoxitin	8 h perop.	5%

*Regimens active against anaerobes alone are not as effective as regimens active against aerobes and anaerobes.

A substantial reduction in primary sepsis after colo-rectal surgery can be achieved with either oral or systemic regimens. The advantages of intravenous administration are reliability of dosing and a minimal antibiotic effect on patient or hospital flora. Advantages of oral regimens which reduce intraluminal bacteria are mainly drug-cost factors. Oral regimens which reduce bacterial flora should not be administered for more than 24 hours preoperatively because there is a possibility of resistant bacterial overgrowth. Antimicrobials such as metronidazole, tinidazole and doxycycline have long half-lives, longer than 6–8 hours, and after high-dose preoperative oral or rectal administration adequate concentrations can be sustained throughout the operative period. The chosen drug or combination should be active against the pathogenic aerobes and also anaerobes, and the dosage regimen must achieve satisfactory peroperative concentrations. When reduction of bowel flora is attempted with oral regimens, the course of therapy should be brief, with a maximum of 24–36 hours, and should be immediately prior to operation.

APPENDICECTOMY

The micro-organisms causing sepsis after appendicectomy are the same as those associated with colo-rectal surgery. However there is a major difference between the results which can be anticipated with preventive antimicrobials in appendicectomy and elective colo-rectal surgery.

The septic complication rate after appendicectomy is related to the nature of the underlying pathology. After removal of a normal appendix, the overall septic complication rate is 5–10%. If simple acute appendicitis is present, then the infection rate rises to 15%; gangrenous appendicitis is accompanied by a septic complication rate up to 30%, and if appendiceal perforation occurs, then up to 50% of all patients will develop sepsis.

As previously indicated, the efficacy of antimicrobials in already established sepsis is limited. Thus, by the time a patient with a ruptured or gangrenous appendix reaches hospital, localized purulent collections may already have formed, and the most that can be expected of antimicrobials is to limit the spread of the established sepsis. Antimicrobials should be used in three situations but they are not prophylactic. The type of antimicrobial selected, however, should be active against both aerobic and anaerobic pathogens. Unlike elective colon surgery, there is no opportunity to reduce the bacterial flora in the appendix preoperatively. If operation is delayed in the presence of appendiceal inflammation, then an abscess will develop and antimicrobials will not affect the organisms in the abscess. The thrust of antimicrobial prophylaxis with appendicitis must therefore be to achieve effective systemic concentrations at the time of operation. A list of effective regimens is given in Table 15.10.

Table 15.10 Suggested preventive antimicrobial regimens for appendicectomy

Agent	Route	Duration
Metronidazole +	i.v.	
Gentamicin	i.v.	Immediately preop. and for 24 hours postop. at
or		8-hourly intervals
Cephalosporin		
or		
Trimethoprim		
Metronidazole	Rectal	As above
or	(or oral)	
Tinidazole +		
Cephalosporin	i.v./i.m.	
or	or oral	
Ampicillin		
or		
Trimethoprim		
Clindamycin +	i.v.	Perop. and for 24 hours postop.
Gentamicin	i.v.	
Cefoxitin	i.v.	Perop. and 12–24 hours postop.
Tetracycline	i.v.	Perop. and for 12 hours postop.

Effective peroperative concentrations of antimicrobial may be achieved with either systemic or parenteral administration. In appendicitis, intravenous administration is preferable because the patient may experience nausea and vomiting. Rectal administration of agents such as metronidazole is an alternative, but the bioavailability of such preparations must be ensured. There is no place for oral, nonabsorbable aminoglycosides in appendicitis.

The value of preventive antimicrobials during the removal of an uninflamed appendix is dubious, and preventive regimens for appendicectomy are only advised for patients with clinical preoperative evidence of peritonitis or complications such as perforation, gangrene and rupture.

GASTRODUODENAL SURGERY

The normal fasting stomach contains very few micro-organisms, and the healthy duodenum is unlikely to harbour the numbers of pathogenic organisms likely to cause postoperative sepsis. According to the underlying disease state, however, the density of micro-organisms in the stomach and duodenum will vary. High numbers of pathogenic anaerobes and aerobes can be expected with a carcinoma. Achlorhydria is also accompanied by high numbers of bacteria in the stomach, though these organisms tend to reflect mouth flora rather than faecal flora.

The risk of developing sepsis in gastric surgery is therefore dependent on the underlying pathology, and preventive antimicrobials should be administered to all patients with cancer and those with achlorhydria. Gut ulcer surgery is accompanied by septic complications in about 10% of cases, and preventive antimicrobials in these operations are warranted on the basis that the underlying pathology and technical problems encountered at operation cannot be fully anticipated. An exception to this is simple vagotomy and drainage in circumstances where the underlying pathology has been clearly delineated by laparoscopy. The antimicrobials and dosage regimens recommended are the systemic peroperative regimens outlined for colo-rectal or appendix surgery.

BILIARY SURGERY

The septic complications of biliary surgery are dependent on the underlying pathology. It is therefore unwise to make a general recommendation that preventive antibiotics be administered to all patients undergoing cholecystectomy. In a survey of 275 consecutive patients undergoing biliary surgery at Flinders Medical Centre, South Australia, the overall wound infection rate was 5.5%. For cholecystectomy alone it was 3.6%, and for operations involving the common bile duct, with or without cholecystectomy, it was 10.7%. There was a significant association between wound infection and the presence of bacteria in bile whether infection was in the gall bladder or in the common bile duct. Bile was more likely to contain bacteria if there was acute cholecystitis, or if stones were in the common bile duct, with or without obstruction, or if the patient was aged 60 years or more. An analysis of other series reveals that factors which predispose to infection in biliary surgery include the presence of stones, obstruction, a carcinoma, acute cholecystitis, advancing age, an emergency operation, reoperation on the biliary tract, or recurrent cholangitis.

The bacteria isolated from bile and associated with biliary sepsis during acute cholecystitis and in the postoperative period seem to be very different from the mixtures of anaerobes and aerobes commonly complicating gut surgery. Obligate anaerobes such as *Bacteroides fragilis* and clostridia seem to play a relatively minor role in biliary sepsis. The circumstances under which obligate anaerobes become important biliary pathogens are in circumstances where abnormal communication exists with the gut, such as cholecystojejunostomy, when reoperation is undertaken, or when carcinoma is present. The important biliary pathogens are the Enterobacteriaceae and enterococci, with the obligate anaerobes posing a problem only in complicated biliary surgery, carcinoma, and the 'necrotic' gallbladder. A reasonable approach to the use of preventive antibiotics in biliary surgery is that for simple elective cholecystectomy antibiotics are unnecessary. Antibiotics active against enterobacteria can be used in gallbladder operations involving calculi, obstruction, and in the elderly patient; such antibiotics would be ampicillin plus gentamicin, or cefamandole, or tetracycline. For reoperation, carcinoma and necrotic gallbladders, a regimen in Table 15.10 is recommended.

If pus is found at operation, then some should be sent to the laboratory. A gram stain and appropriate culture will indicate the appropriate choice of antimicrobials. Selection of antimicrobials also needs to take account of their ability to achieve adequate concentrations in bile. The antibiotics that are concentrated in bile are shown in Table 15.11. However, in the presence of obstruction none of these agents achieve adequate concentrations.

Table 15.11   Antimicrobials and bile concentrations

High concentrations	Adequate	Minimal
Tetracyclines	Ampicillin/amoxycillin	Sulphonamides
Lincomycin/clindamycin	Carbenicillin	Gentamicin
Rifamide	Most cephalosporins	Amikacin
Cefamandole	Chloramphenicol	Streptomycin
Cefoxitin*	Cefoxitin*	
Trimethoprim*	Trimethoprim*	

*The concentrations achieved by these drugs are moderately high but they are not concentrated in bile to the same extent as the other antibiotics in the left-hand column.

In summary, simple cholecystectomy does not involve entry into a contaminated viscus therefore routine antimicrobial prophylaxis is unwarranted. In the presence of stones, obstruction, or other gallbladder pathology, significant operative contamination is likely to occur, and appropriate preoperative antimicrobials should be administered. Obligate anaerobes such as *Bacteroides* are uncommon biliary pathogens, and specific agents directed at these bacteria are required only for reoperations, cancer, and situations where abnormal communication exists between the biliary tract and gut.

LEUKAEMIA AND GRANULOCYTOPAENIA

The principles of antimicrobial therapy in surgery apply equally to the use of antimicrobials in granulocytopaenia. The choice of antimicrobial must be determined by the susceptibility profile of the anticipated or demonstrated pathogens. Prolonged use of antimicrobials will alter normal host flora and predispose to superinfection. A distinction must be drawn between therapeutic and preventive use of antimicrobials in so far as dosage regimens are concerned. Host defences are required to supplement antimicrobial action.

Unfortunately it is difficult to undertake controlled studies of antimicrobial regimens in immunosuppressed patients because disease processes and responses to antineoplastic therapy vary widely, and the invading pathogens tend to differ between institutions because nosocomial infection in leukaemia is a significant problem. It has already been indicated that granulocytopaenic patients frequently suffer infection and in any patient wih a peripheral blood granulocyte count below 1000/cmm a constant surveillance must be maintained for infection. Unfortunately the clinical signs may be relatively nonspecific and therapy should be commenced immediately fever occurs whilst at the same time undertaking the necessary investigations to detect pathogens. The approach to management of presumptive sepsis in the granulocytopaenic patient should be as follows. If possible all drugs including immunosuppressive drugs should be ceased. Specimens of blood, urine, throat, sputum, faeces, and CSF if applicable, should be taken for bacteriological investigations. Fungal and viral analyses on appropriate specimens are also recommended. Therapy should be started with antibiotic combinations which will be active against the likely pathogens as outlined in Table 15.5. Appropriate combinations for initial therapy are gentamicin plus carbenicillin, or a cephalosporin plus aminoglycoside or any drug combination which is active against the organisms most frequently causing problems in a particular unit. For example, if gentamicin-resistant *Klebsiella* sp. were causing infections in a unit then the first choice of agents would need to include a recent cephalosporin such as moxalactam or cefotaxime, or an aminoglycoside such as amikacin. The importance of careful microbiological monitoring and the modification of therapeutic antibiotic regimens according to prevailing sensitivity patterns is crucial.

Therapy should be modified in accordance with information available after microscopic examination of initial specimens. Additional immediate investigations which are useful in these circumstances include rapid antigen detection, by latex agglutination or countercurrent immunoelectrophoresis, for bacterial polysaccharide antigens in blood, urine and CSF. If no clinical response has occurred after 48 hours, and there is no clue to the microbiological cause from initial investigations, the spectrum of antibacterial therapy should be widened to include most of the bacteria listed in Table 15.5. This may necessitate adding a third agent such as a penicillinase-resistant penicillin, or the substitution of a recent cephalosporin or aminoglycoside instead of the initial agent of choice. Concurrently, investigations should be initiated to demonstrate invasive viral, fungal or parasitic infection. Depending on clinical and radiological manifestations, bronchoscopy, lung biopsy, liver biopsy and lymph-node biopsy deserve consideration. It is important to pursue actively an aetiological diagnosis at an early stage because success of treatment is much higher when a pathogen can be specifically demonstrated.

The role of leukocyte transfusion remains debatable because clinical trials have not convincingly demonstrated its efficacy. Nevertheless, it is a logical approach in the face of opportunistic infection to reinforce host defences, and leukocyte transfusion appears most effective with Gram-positive infections. Cessation of immunosuppressive agents however is more important.

In recent times a more aggressive approach has been taken with antineoplastic therapy, and an inevitable outcome of these treatments is severe granulocytopaenia and immunosuppression. The advent of bone marrow transplantation and cyclical antineoplastic drug regimens warrant an approach to prevent infection in leukaemia similar to that outlined for contaminated elective surgery. This approach includes a minimization of cross-infection, administration of antimicrobials active against the commonly observed pathogens, and avoidance of excessive periods of antimicrobial therapy, particularly with broad spectrum agents.

Prophylactic antimicrobial regimens

Two approaches have been tried. Firstly, eradication of normal flora and complete isolation within a germ-free environment, and secondly selective antimicrobial regimens with agents active against the common pathogens found during induction of remissions in leukaemia; the latter are mainly the Enterobacteriaceae.

The eradication approach is difficult to manage outside special units with appropriately trained staff and sophisticated facilities to produce laminar airflow, sterile food and complete reverse-isolation nursing within the protected environment. Even in units with such facilities the costs and adverse effects of attempted microbiological sterilization tend to outweigh any benefits of these regimens over the antimicrobial regimens that are specifically directed at Gramnegative bacteria which are the common pathogens.

In order to achieve gut 'sterilization' a variety of regimens have been used, but basically these regimens include nonabsorbable oral antimicrobials to eliminate all bacteria and fungi from the gut, such as polymyxin-B sulphate, vancomycin, and mycostatin; antimicrobials which achieve high circulating concentrations, such as cephalosporins plus aminoglycosides plus 5-fluorocytosine plus clindamycin, and rectal, nasal, vaginal and skin antiseptics. The reader is referred to Rodriguez *et al.*[9] for a complete description of such regimens, but the success of these multiple antimicrobial applications to achieve total sterilization is incomplete, and such regimens should only be considered in special units where cross-infection can be totally prevented. A preferred approach for hospitals without special facilities for total isolation is the selective regimens which are directed at suppression of the common pathogens in granulocytopaenic patients.

Trimethoprim-sulphamethoxazole (TMP-SMZ) administered as two tablets twice daily (320 mg trimethoprim and 1600 mg sulphamethoxazole daily in adults) has been widely assessed. The results of TMP-SMZ are as good as those of the 'sterilization' regimens described above. TMP-SMZ, or TMP alone, has the ability to suppress gut Enterobacteriaceae almost completely during the period of administration and for many days thereafter. Therapy should be maintained only whilst remission is being induced with anticancer drugs and while the granulocyte count is below 1000/cmm. Concurrently, the patient must be protected from cross-infection, and surveillance maintained for super-infection. An additional advantage of TMP is its activity against *Pneumocystis carinii*, but the doses required are much higher than those used in suppressing gut Entero-bacteriaceae.

Other selective antimicrobial regimens are currently being assessed in various centres. Nalidixic acid, chloramphenicol and cephalosporin regimens are under scrutiny, but to the present time, results do not exceed the reported efficacy of TMP-SMZ.[6,7]

In summary, preventive antimicrobials should be used selectively, in adequate doses and for limited periods of time. Such an approach to prevention, or prophylaxis, will minimize drug resistance and reduce morbidity due to infection.

REFERENCES

1   Bartlett J. G. (1981) The pathophysiology of intra-abdominal sepsis. In: *Infection in Surgery*, p. 47, Eds J. McK. Watts, P. J. McDonald, P. E. O'Brien, V. R. Marshall and J. J. Finlay-Jones, Churchill-Livingstone, Edinburgh.
2   Bartlett J. G., Condon R. E., Gorbach S. L., Clark J. S., Nichols R. L. and Ochi S. (1978) Veterans administration study on bowel preparation for elective colo-rectal operations: impact of oral antibiotics regimen on colonic flora, wound irrigation cultures and bacteriology of septic complications. *Ann. Surgery* **188**, 249.
3   Burke J. F. (1961) The effective period of preventive antibiotic action in experimental incisions and dermal lesions. *Surgery* **50**, 161, 184.
4   Cruse P. J. E. and Foord R. (1973) A five year prospective study of 23 649 wounds. *Arch. Surgery* **197**, 206.
5   EORTC (1978) The EORTC International Antimicrobial Therapy Project Group 'Three antibiotic regimens in the treatment of infection in febrile granulocytopaenic patients with cancer'. *J. Infect. Dis.* **137**, 14.
6   Gruse W. E. and Bodey G. (1980) Intravenous trimethoprim-sulphamethoxazole alone or combined with tobramycin for infections in cancer patients. *Am. J. Med Sci.* **279**, 4.
7   Gurwith M. J., Brunton J. L., Lank B. A., Harding G. K. and Ronald A. R. (1978) A prospective controlled investigation of prophylactic trimethoprim/sulphamethoxazole in hospitalized granulocytopaenic patients. *Am. J. Med.* **66**, 248.
8   Miles A. A., Miles E. M. and Burke J. F. (1957) The value and duration of defence reactions of the skin to the primary lodgement of bacteria. *Br. J. Exp. Pathol.* **38**, 79.
9   Rodriguez V., Bodey G. P., Freidreich E. J., McCredie K. B., Gutterman J. U., Keating M. J., Smith T. L. and Gehan E. A. (1978) Randomized trial of protected environ-ment-prophylactic antibiotics in 145 adults with acute leukaemia. *Medicine* **57**, 253.

16 *Clostridium difficile* and gut disease

S. P. Borriello

Introduction   327
Pathogenesis   328
Seasonal variation and age and sex associations   329
Diagnosis   330
Interpretation of laboratory findings   331
Treatment   331
  Antimicrobials   332
  Ion-binding resins   334
  Manipulation of bowel flora   335
  Other methods   337
Prevention   337
The second toxin   338
Appendix
  Detection and identification of *C. difficile*   339
  Detection of *C. difficile* cytotoxin   341
References   342

INTRODUCTION

The first isolation of the organism now known as *Clostridium difficile* was reported in 1935 by Hall and O'Toole.[45] During their study of the faecal flora of breast-fed infants these workers analysed 63 faecal specimens obtained from 10 infants during the first 10 days of life. They isolated a Gram-positive spore-forming anaerobic bacillus from 13 samples obtained from four of the infants. Because of the general characteristics of this organism and the difficulty experienced in its isolation and study the organism was called *Bacillus difficilis*. In addition, it was shown that these strains of *B. difficilis* (*C. difficile*) were highly pathogenic for rabbits as demonstrated by subcutaneous inoculation of 48 hour broth cultures. Inoculation of broth culture filtrates of four of these isolates also caused disease in guinea pigs. These observations prompted Hall and O'Toole to suggest that the organism produced a soluble exotoxin and to 'suspect that convulsions in babies may sometimes be due to the absorption of the toxin of *B. difficilis* from the intestinal tract where there may have been, for one reason or another, a failure in the development of the normal milk stool flora and an abnormal persistence of the organism. This, of course, presents an interesting problem for the future'. It is interesting that their idea that a clostridial toxin produced in the gut may be absorbed and cause disease, was to be subsequently proven for infant botulism and *Clostridium botulinum* (see Chapter 1). However, indirect evidence of *C. difficile* (*B. difficilis*) involvement in gastrointestinal disease did not occur until 1977 when Larson *et al.*[59] described the presence of a cytotoxin detected in 1975 in the faeces of a girl who developed pseudo-membranous colitis (PMC) after oral penicillin. It was shown in hamsters by Bartlett *et al.*[9] that *C. difficile* was the probable source of the toxin in PMC, and a number of workers in rapid succession implicated *C. difficile* and its associated cytotoxin as the aetiological agent of PMC.[6,34,60] Subsequently, *C. difficile* has been shown to be associated with a spectrum of gastrointestinal disorders ranging from mild diarrhoea to the life-threatening pseudomembranous colitis.[18,43]

PATHOGENESIS

Many antibiotics have been associated with the induction of *C. difficile*-mediated disease,[5,18] in particular clindamycin, ampicillin and the cephalosporins. There is as yet no discernible correlation between the incidence of pseudomembranous colitis, and dose or duration of antibiotic treatment. In addition to antibiotics, 'nonantimicrobial chemotherapeutic agents' such as antineoplastic agents have been shown to be associated with this disease.[32]

Both *C. difficile* and its associated cytotoxin are invariably present in the faeces of patients with pseudomembranous colitis. The current thinking is that certain factors, such as administration of antibiotics, disrupt the normal defence mechanisms that operate to exclude *C. difficile* from the gut thereby making any such patient susceptible to infection by this organism. However, not all adult subjects who have been shown to have *C. difficile* present in their faeces have disease,[39,70] and in some people the organism disappears after only mild diarrhoea during the transient *C. difficile* carriage.[18] In addition it has been known for many years that this organism can be isolated frequently from the stools of healthy infants,[45] and it has recently been shown that *C. difficile* cytotoxin may also be present in both term and pre-term infants.[15,60,84] It is evident that in these individuals the full pathogenic potential of the organism is not expressed. A number of these strains have been examined in our laboratory and have induced a fatal enterocaecitis when administered to hamsters. Although this is not an ideal guide to the pathogenic potential in man, it implies that the 'resistance' to disease in asymptomatic carriers is not due to an inability on the part of the organism to cause disease but to other factors such as host susceptibility to the effects of toxin(s). Other explanations include the possibilities that other unknown components of the gut flora must be present for the full expression of pathogenicity or, more probably, these asymptomatic carriers still possess sufficient components of their normal gastrointestinal flora to suppress the full expression of pathogenicity. An interesting possibility is that *C. difficile* must associate with the gut wall to cause disease. This may help to explain the localized plaques seen in the early stages of pseudomembranous colitis. It is known that

C. difficile can become intimately associated with the gut mucosa in man,[15] and we have also recently shown this to be the case in the hamster model of *C. difficile*-induced ileocaecitis (Fig. 16.1). Transient and asymptomatic carriage may be explained by exclusion of *C. difficile* from the gut wall by normal components of the mucosal flora. It is interesting to note that the K88 antigen of *E. coli* appears to be associated with the ability to adhere to gut mucosa and the subsequent induction of neonatal diarrhoea in pigs;[50] piglets suckled by dams that had been vaccinated with K88 antigen were significantly more resistant to deaths caused by neonatal diarrhoea after challenge with a large dose of a K88-positive enteropathogenic strain of *E. coli* than piglets suckled by nonvaccinated dams.[78]

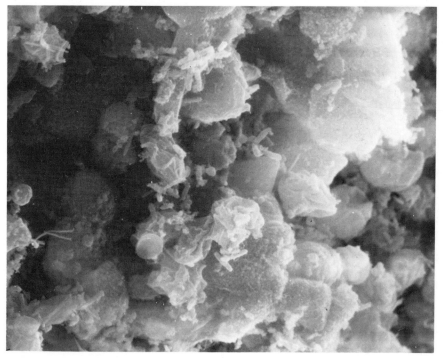

Fig. 16.1 Association of *C. difficile* with mucosal surface of hamster caecum (magnification × 3750).

SEASONAL VARIATION AND AGE AND SEX ASSOCIATIONS

Analysis of faecal specimens during a 2-year period for the presence of *C. difficile* and its associated cytotoxin showed no seasonal variation with respect to this infection (Fig. 16.2).

Associations of age and sex with *C. difficile* carriage, faecal cytotoxin and pseudomembranous colitis have been investigated by Borriello and Larson,[18] who found that there were more female than male patients 'positive' for *C. difficile* and/or its associated cytotoxin, and for histologically confirmed

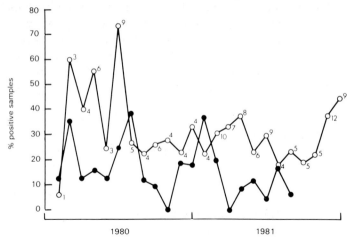

Fig. 16.2 Isolation rates of *C. difficile* on a monthly basis from faeces over a two-year period. ● samples from patients at Northwick Park Hospital, ○ samples from centres throughout the United Kingdom. Accompanying numbers represent the number of centres from which the positive samples were obtained

pseudomembranous colitis. In addition, most of the 'positive' samples came from patients in the older age groups, with patients who were older than 50, accounting for 73% of the positive samples and 71% of the histologically proven PMC cases.

DIAGNOSIS

The vast majority of patients have diarrhoea[89] and have recently received antibiotics. The diarrhoea may be bloody, and this seems to occur most frequently after penicillin or ampicillin. Other typical symptoms are nausea, vomiting, fever and abdominal pain, and in some patients a polymorphonuclear leukocytosis is found.

Definitive diagnosis is based on a combination of pathological features in the colon and the demonstration of *C. difficile* and its associated cytotoxin in a stool specimen. Sigmoidoscopic examination usually reveals elevated plaques distributed over the colonic mucous membrane. Histological examination of biopsies obtained from suspicious lesions reveals distinctive features on which, in most cases, a reliable diagnosis can be made.[75] There have been cases of pseudo-membranous colitis in which there was rectal sparing[52] and some cases of right-sided colitis associated with ampicillin.[80] These findings highlight the potential use of colonoscopy and this method has been advocated by Seppälä and coworkers.[81] In their prospective study the characteristic endoscopic changes of pseudomembranous colitis with pseudomembranes present were observed in only five of 16 patients by sigmoidoscopy but in 11 of 13 of these patients in whom colonoscopy was also performed. George[36] has suggested that as a negative result on sigmoidoscopic examination does not exclude the diagnosis of pseudo-membranous colitis, a barium enema examination[91] or colonoscopy should be performed unless contraindicated. The situation is now complicated by the recognition of the spectrum of gastrointestinal disease associated with *C. difficile* infection[18,62] and that pseudomembranous colitis is probably the most severe form. It is at present unknown what proportion of patients with *C. difficile* diarrhoea would go on to develop pseudomembranous colitis if left untreated. The detection and identification of *C. difficile* and its toxins in faeces are fully discussed in the appendix to this chapter.

INTERPRETATION OF LABORATORY FINDINGS

The presence of faecal cytotoxin and *C. difficile* does not always indicate gastro-intestinal disease. Both the organism and the toxin have been demonstrated in the faeces of healthy infants[15,60,84] (see also Chapter 1) and the organism has been isolated from 2% of normal adult faeces.[70] It is also true that not all patients with antibiotic associated pseudomembranous colitis have *C. difficile* or cytotoxin present at the time of examination.[18] In some patients this may be due to inadequate technique or the fact that the patient has been given specific chemo-therapy directed against the organism.[18] There have been cases strongly suggestive of antibiotic associated pseudomembranous colitis in which neither organism nor toxin have been detected although adequate techniques were employed.[71,85,92] In all of these cases the patient responded to vancomycin.

Interpretation of the laboratory findings can only be made against a back-ground of the clinical findings and patient details such as age and prior chemo-therapy. Although cytotoxin titres of 6400 or more tend to be associated with the presence of pseudomembranes[21] severity of disease is best judged by clinical criteria. However toxin titres can be used to monitor response to therapy.[52,60]

TREATMENT

Prior to the recognition of *C. difficile* as the aetiological agent of pseudo-membranous colitis (PMC) the mortality rate of severe disease was relatively high. Treatment consisted of rehydration, electrolyte replacement, steroids, surgery, and for a brief period during the 1950s vancomycin therapy. Vancomycin had been used with good effect during this period for the treatment of *Staphylococcus aureus* enterocolitis[51] which was frequently associated with tetracycline therapy. The major breakthrough in developing a rational and specific approach to the treatment of PMC came with the discovery of *C. difficile* as the aetiological agent of the disease.

Antimicrobials

VANCOMYCIN

The most widely used antibiotic for the treatment of PMC is vancomycin. This antibiotic was first used in the treatment of antibiotic-associated colitis in the 1950s (see above) and was shown to be effective in protecting hamsters from clindamycin-associated ileocaecitis.[7,8] Vancomycin is poorly absorbed from the gastrointestinal tract[90] and high concentrations can be readily achieved in the faeces after oral administration.[20,90] In addition, all strains of *C. difficile* tested to date (over 200) have been shown to be uniformly sensitive *in vitro* to vancomycin at a minimal inhibitory concentration (MIC) of 16 µg/ml or less.[20,30,33,37,82] Of the 236 strains in these studies only three had MICs of greater than 4 µg/ml.

In 1978 Tedesco *et al.*[90] treated nine patients with PMC with oral vancomycin in a dose of 500 mg every 6 hours for at least 7 days. All patients in this study showed a good clinical response with resolution of diarrhoea during 7 days and a decrease in concentrations of cytotoxin in the stool. In seven patients follow-up sigmoidoscopy showed major improvements or complete clearing of lesions after 7–10 days' treatment. In their study an oral dose of 2 g of vancomycin daily resulted in a mean faecal concentration of 3100 µg/g. Resolution of diarrhoea and overall clinical improvement after the use of vancomycin for the treatment of PMC was also reported in 1978 by Larson *et al.*;[58] there was concomitant disappearance of both cytotoxin and *C. difficile* from the stool of a patient with PMC, with clinical improvement.

A report of the findings of a prospective randomized controlled trial was published in the same year by Keighley.[54] Forty-four patients with postoperative diarrhoea were allocated 5 days' treatment with either 125 mg vancomycin by mouth 6 hourly or a placebo. Only the patients with faecal cytotoxin showed any response to vancomycin. Of the 16 patients with faecal cytotoxin nine received vancomycin and five received placebo. There was a significant response in the treatment group when compared to the control group with respect to disappearance of stool cytotoxin and *C. difficile*, normalization of bowel habits and disappearance of histological evidence of PMC. Although vancomycin is generally accepted as the treatment of first choice, relapses following its use have been reported.[11,42,63]

In the majority of cases patients respond to a second course of vancomycin, although occasionally three courses of vancomycin treatment have been required.[11] In some cases from the study by Bartlett *et al.*[11] vancomycin treated patients continued to excrete *C. difficile* and its associated cytotoxin even when asymptomatic. One patient relapsed then recovered spontaneously, which raises a very important point; treatment of this patient with a second course of vancomycin could have induced a relapse as it is known that administration of vancomycin to hamsters makes them susceptible to *C. difficile* colonization,[60] presumably by disruption of those components of the caecal flora that confer colonization-resistance. A similar mechanism probably exists in man; where immediately after vancomycin treatment the patient is still susceptible to colonization by *C. difficile* either from an exogenous or endogenous source, and patients who respond to treatment are those who are either not exposed to *C. difficile* during this period or those in whom relevant components of the normal gut flora re-establish themselves sufficiently quickly to confer protection against colonization by *C. difficile*. In fact induced normalization of the gut flora has been used in the successful treatment of pseudomembranous colitis (see below). If relapse is due to exposure to *C. difficile* in the immediate environment strict cross-infection measures may help to prevent relapse. However, *C. difficile* has been recovered from faecal specimens during and after vancomycin therapy[11],[18] and relapses may be due to out-growth of spores of *C. difficile* that have survived in the gut. More recently, the small bowel has been indicated as a possible source for large bowel recolonization.[88] There have been other reports of spontaneous disappearance of *C. difficile* and toxin from patients' stools.[18] These observations imply that careful monitoring of faecal numbers of *C. difficile* and the patient's condition may in some cases obviate the need for specific chemo-therapy directed against *C. difficile* as this organism may be spontaneously eradicated. The decision to treat or not must in the end lie with the clinician in charge of the case.

BACITRACIN

Bacitracin is an antibiotic that exhibits a similar spectrum of activity to vancomycin, being mainly directed towards Gram-positive organisms. Like vancomycin, it is poorly absorbed from the intestine ensuring high faecal levels after oral administration and avoiding the possibility of systemic toxicity. Bacitracin has a number of advantages over vancomycin in that it is much more readily available worldwide and is cheaper. This antibiotic has been used to successfully protect hamsters from clindamycin-associated colitis[8] and to be active against *C. difficile in vitro*.[37] In 1980 bacitracin was used for the treatment of antibiotic-associated colitis and diarrhoea.[24] Diarrhoea resolved in all four treated cases within 2 days, with disappearance of *Clostridium difficile* cytotoxin in the stools of three of the patients sampled; treatment was 25 000 units of oral bacitracin four times daily for 7–10 days. Two of the patients treated were post-vancomycin relapse cases. One of the patients treated with bacitracin also relapsed and was then successfully treated with vancomycin.

METRONIDAZOLE

Metronidazole is as active as vancomycin against *C. difficile in vitro*.[30,33,37,82] Although no controlled trials have been performed, effective use of metronidazole in the treatment of *C. difficile*-mediated disease has been well documented, with symptomatic and clinical improvement being accompanied by the elimination of both *C. difficile* and its associated cytotoxin.[12,13,64,68,93]

Metronidazole has also been used for the successful treatment of a post-vancomycin relapse case.[67] A dosage regimen of 200–400 mg orally every 8 hours for 5–7 days has been suggested as adequate in most cases for successful treatment.[13] Theoretical objections to the use of metronidazole have been raised due to its characteristic rapid absorption high in the gastrointestinal tract possibly resulting in sub-inhibitory colonic levels. However, metronidazole has proved to be effective, and in cases of diarrhoea therapeutic levels can be detected in the stool with levels as high as 55 µg/g reported.[13] There have been rare cases of the development of PMC following metronidazole use, however in the majority of cases metronidazole had been administered in combination with other antibiotics.[5,18,52,53] There has however been one documented case of metronidazole-associated PMC.[92] In this patient neither *C. difficile* nor its associated cytotoxin could be detected although the patient responded to vancomycin. A metronidazole-associated case has also been mentioned by Bartlett.[5] The major advantage of metronidazole over vancomycin is that it is cheap and well tolerated.

OTHER ANTIBIOTICS

A number of other antibiotics have been suggested as possibly useful agents for the treatment of PMC. These include the imidazole antifungal agent, miconazole,[20] thiostrepton[38] and tetracycline.[29] Of these antimicrobials only tetracycline has been clinically assessed. In these studies[29,69] 12 patients with antibiotic-associated diarrhoea responded to 250 mg of oral tetracycline 3–4 times a day for 5 days. However, in 11 of the 12 patients there was no evidence of colitis, although investigators could not rule out microscopic evidence of antibiotic associated colitis. In addition, *C. difficile* and its associated cytotoxin were not looked for as this work predated recognition of this aetiological agent. The authors conclude 'It is possible that tetracycline may be helpful in obvious cases of antibiotic-associated colitis. Our experiences, however, do not warrant such a conclusion and this should be evaluated in the future'. Although strains of *C. difficile* have been found to be inhibited by concentrations of tetracycline that can be achieved in faeces,[30,33,37,82] there is evidence for transferable tetracycline resistance between strains of *C. difficile*.[49,83]

Ion-binding resins

C. difficile cytotoxin is bound *in vitro* by the anion-exchange resins cholestyramine and colestipol.[26,35,86] This activity probably explains the apparent effective use of cholestyramine in the treatment of PMC.[56] However, these agents also bind vancomycin *in vitro*,[35,86] and when administered to hamsters they decrease the amount of active vancomycin expected in the stool indicating that binding also occurs *in vivo*.[86] It would probably be advisable to avoid the use of these anion-exchange resins during vancomycin therapy. Despite these disadvantages it has been suggested that cholestyramine may be considered as a possible therapeutic agent for mild cases.[11]

Manipulation of bowel flora

It is generally accepted that events, such as the administration of antibiotics, that result in alteration of the normal flora and physicochemical milieu of the bowel, predispose subjects to *C. difficile*-mediated disease. This indicates the important role played by components of the normal gut flora in protecting the host from *C. difficile* infection or overgrowth. On this basis it could be postulated that normalization of the gut flora may be an effective method of preventing or treating *C. difficile*-associated gastrointestinal disease. Indications of the importance of the normal flora in regulating *C. difficile* colonization come from a number of studies in animals and humans. Hamsters that have not had antibiotics administered to disrupt their gut flora do not succumb to disease when challenged with *C. difficile*.[60] Again in animals, *C. difficile*-mediated disease of newly-born hares does not involve adult animals.[28] It is probable that the newly-born hare is susceptible to *C. difficile* colonization as a result of an incompletely developed intestinal flora. In normal healthy adults *C. difficile* is extremely rare,[18,41] however this organism can be frequently recovered from the stools of infants when the normal gastrointestinal flora is not fully developed.[15,45,60,84] An observation from our laboratory that adds weight to the importance of the normal gut flora is that growth of *C. difficile* is inhibited when the organism is incubated in a 1 in 20 dilution of stool from a healthy donor. No such growth inhibition occurs in filtrates or heat sterilized aliquots of these faecal suspensions. Interestingly, there was person-to-person variation in the inhibitory capability of the faecal suspensions used although there is as yet no data on week-to-week variation in a given subject. In the one situation studied in detail there was a large decrease in vegetative forms and a concomitant increase in the number of spores during the first 24 hours and then a steady decrease during 9 days with the proportion of spores to vegetative forms remaining roughly the same. Detectable levels of cytotoxin had also disappeared by day 9 (Borriello and Barclay, unpublished data). If a similar *C. difficile* inhibition effect occurs *in vivo* then it is probable that the organism would be eradicated by the normal mechanical clearing mechanisms.

Recent work by Wilson and coworkers[98] demonstrated that daily administration of caecal contents (*per os* or by enema) from healthy animals was effective in preventing *C. difficile* induced ileocaecitis in hamsters. More importantly, 16 patients with pseudomembranous colitis were treated by administration of faecal enemas by Bowden and coworkers.[19] In this study during an 18-year period 13 of 16 patients with pseudomembranous enterocolitis were successfully treated by administration of faecal enemas. Of the three patients who died, two did not have pseudomembranes at death and one had involvement of the small bowel. This report is both encouraging and exciting, and indicates that a search for the minimum components of the normal faecal flora required to cause the same effect is warranted. Some work in this respect has been done.

In vitro inhibition of *C. difficile* by faecal isolates belonging to the genera *Bifidobacterium*, *Lactobacillus* and group D enterococci[76] and inhibition of 50 strains of *C. difficile* by a faecal strain of *Clostridium beijerinkii*[3] have been noted. A recent interesting observation in this laboratory is that prior colonization of antibiotic treated hamsters with noncytotoxigenic strains of *C. difficile*, prior to subsequent challenge with cytotoxigenic strains, significantly prolongs survival (Fig. 16.3). The mechanism operative is probably one of exclusion of the cytotoxigenic strain by occupation of the ecological niches required for its establishment (e.g. muosal receptors). In addition, it has recently been demonstrated that a commercial preparation of lyophilized *L. acidophilus* and *L. bulgaricus* (Lactinex) was effective in preventing ampicillin-associated diarrhoea in man[44] and the development of *C. difficile* induced ileocaecitis in hamsters treated with antibiotics.[100]

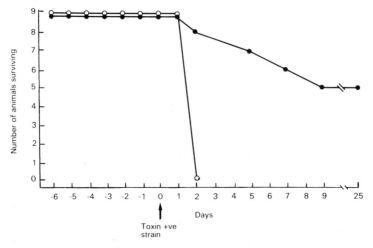

Fig. 16.3   Protection of hamsters from ileocaecitis by prior colonization with non-cytotoxigenic *C. difficile*. All animals received a single dose of 5 mg of Clindamycin phosphate i.p. They were housed singly in sterile conditions. After 5 days nine animals received 10^7 noncytotoxigenic *C. difficile* p.o. (●) and nine animals received sterile broth (○). On day 7 following this procedure all animals were challenged with 10^7 cytotoxigenic *C. difficile*

It may prove possible to find a faecal marker that is indicative of colonization resistance. This has proved to be the case in mice where there is a direct correlation between the presence of faecal β-aspartylglycine and susceptibility to colonization by *E. coli*.[96] Preliminary investigations in this laboratory indicate that a significant decrease in faecal β-glucosidase is associated with many cases of antibiotic-associated diarrhoea and also with pseudomembranous colitis. It has also been shown that the relative concentrations of the volatile phenolics, phenol and *p*-cresol, are altered in the stools of patients with pseudomembranous colitis, with concentrations of phenol being greater than those of *p*-cresol in PMC patients and the converse situation being found in healthy individuals. It may prove possible in the near future to be able to recognize patients at increased risk for the development of *C. difficile* associated disease by analysis for specific faecal markers indicative of the state of colonization resistance. It is probable that restoration of specific components of the normal bowel flora will be used in the future for both the prevention and treatment of *C. difficile*-associated gastro-intestinal disease and that the success of this treatment will be monitored by measurement of faecal markers of colonization resistance. This sort of approach may also be useful in the prevention of other gastrointestinal disorders of suspected microbial, but as yet unknown, aetiology.

Other methods

Antiperistaltic agents such as diphenoxylate-atropine (Lomotil), loperamide and codeine have been used for the symptomatic treatment of antibiotic-associated diarrhoea.[94] There is a suggestion that these agents may prolong or exacerbate symptoms[66] and predispose to toxic megacolon.[72] However, there is a lack of controlled studies so that the possible beneficial or detrimental effects of these agents is difficult to assess.

Systemic or local corticosteroids have been used in the treatment of PMC,[94] however results have been variable and data available are limited. With the well documented agents available for treatment (see above) and the potential hazards of systemic steroid therapy, corticosteroids probably have no place in the treatment of this condition.

There are a number of *in vitro* and animal model observations that may prove to be applicable to the treatment of this disease. For example, it has been demonstrated that the administration of *C. sordellii* antitoxin before clindamycin challenge is effective in protecting hamsters from the development of ileocaecitis.[1] These workers conclude 'Our data suggest that immunization via the systemic route alone may be adequate for protection against this disease in humans'. The observation that several heavy metal compounds inactivate *C. difficile* toxin *in vitro*[77] also merits further research.

Finally, it must be remembered that in many cases discontinuation of the offending chemotherapeutic agent(s), when possible, is sufficient to induce symptoms to resolve within 1–2 weeks.[89]

PREVENTION

The evidence generated to date indicates that the most likely course of events is that chemotherapy renders a patient susceptible to colonization by exogenously acquired *C. difficile*. If this is the case then attempts can be made to prevent *C. difficile* infection, in a number of ways. The most obvious is to prevent exposure of the patient to the organism. It has been suggested that patients shown to be excreting *C. difficile* should be isolated.[55,65] It may also prove possible to recolonize patients with specific components of a normal faecal flora to remove their susceptibility to *C. difficile* infections (see Treatment). An additional

Table 16.1   Comparison of the two toxins of *C. difficile* (compiled from Banno *et al.*,[2] Bartlett *et al.*,[10] Burdon *et al.*,[22] Taylor *et al.*,[87] Libby *et al.*,[102] Lyerly *et al.*[103])

	Enterotoxin	Cytotoxin
Acid stability	+	−
Heat lability	+	+
Inactivation by		
trypsin	∓	+
pronase	+	+
Fluid accumulation in the rabbit ligated ileal loop	+	−
Fluid response in infant mice	+	+
Mouse lethality	+	∓
Lethal to hamsters on intracaecal injection	+	+
Inflammatory response to intracaecal injection	+	+
Increased vascular permeabiity	+	+
Cytotoxicity	∓	+
Neutralization by *C. sordellii* antitoxin	+	+
Molecular weight	600 000	480 000

∓ represent conflicting results.

approach to the prevention of disease would be the development of a vaccine. In fact a vaccine has recently been developed which prevents pig-bel (enteritis necroticans), a disease caused by *C. perfringens* type C.[61]

THE SECOND TOXIN

A number of workers have described the existence of a second toxin produced by *C. difficile in vitro*.[2,10,87,105] Although this toxin is less cytopathic to cells in tissue culture compared to the cytotoxin, it does increase vascular permeability, causes fluid accumulation in the rabbit ligated loop test, and is lethal for mice and hamsters (Table 16.1). To what extent this toxin is involved in human disease is as yet unknown. However, these recent observations may help to explain the apparent lack of association between faecal cytotoxin titres and severity of disease. It is also possible that the presence of a second toxin may help to explain a group of 22 patients with antibiotic-associated diarrhoea studied in our laboratory who had no faecal pathogens present on routine examination, no demonstrable faecal cytotoxin and carried noncytotoxigenic strains of *C. difficile*. The recent development of an ELISA technique for the detection of the enterotoxin should facilitate this type of analysis.[104] These types of investigations offer useful areas for future research.

APPENDIX

Detection and identification of *C. difficile*

An obvious aid in diagnosis is the demonstration of *C. difficile* in the faeces. This procedure has been greatly facilitated by the development of a selective medium.[40,97] George *et al.*[40] used 500 µg/ml of cycloserine, and 16 µg/ml of cefoxitin as selective agents whereas Willey and Bartlett[97] used 250 µg/ml and 10 µg/ml respectively, of these two antibiotics. There is now a commercially available selective medium based on these findings (Oxoid Ltd, Basingstoke, England). The basic procedure employed is to seed the selective agar with a low dilution of the faecal material under investigation and to incubate the plate at 37° C under an anaerobic atmosphere for 24–48 hours. An alternative to the use of a selective medium is the alcohol treatment method.[17] In this method an aliquot of the faecal dilution is mixed with an equal volume of absolute ethanol and left on the open bench at room temperature for 1 hour. The sample can then be used to seed an ordinary blood plate which is incubated as indicated for the selective medium. Whichever method is employed the plates must be screened carefully for presumptive *C. difficile* colonies. This procedure is simplified by the use of long wave ultraviolet light (360 nm). Colonies of *C. difficile* exhibit a characteristic low green/chartreuse fluorescence when exposed to ultraviolet light of this wavelength.[17,40] A number of workers have used the fact that *C. difficile* can produce *p*-cresol from L-tyrosine[31] as a selective and presumptive identification procedure. As *p*-cresol is toxic to most organisms Hafiz and Oakley[46] assumed that an organism that produced *p*-cresol must be resistant to that compound; they recommend 0.2% of phenol or *p*-cresol in reinforced clostridial medium (RCM) for the isolation of this organism. However, *C. difficile* is not the only clostridium than can produce *p*-cresol from tyrosine[14,31] and the so-called characteristic 'cornfield' growth in RCM containing *p*-cresol and 0.05% agar is not restricted to this organism (unpublished observations). In addition, it has been found that many strains of *C. difficile* are sensitive to 0.2% *p*-cresol[40] and the use of this medium as a screen prior to subculture onto a selective medium for the isolation of *C. difficile* from faeces has proved to be disappointing.[97] A modification of the selective medium developed by George *et al.*[40] has been developed by Phillips and Rogers.[70] The latter medium has half the concentration of selective antibiotic agents recommended by George *et al.*[40] and the addition of *p*-hydroxyphenyl acetic acid (0.1% wt/vol) as indicated, which is metabolized by *C. difficile* to yield *p*-cresol. The *p*-cresol produced can be detected by gas liquid chromatography (GLC) after extraction from agar plugs removed from an area of confluent growth or from beneath five discrete colonies. The distinct odour of *p*-cresol apparently is often discernible on examination of culture plates, which can make GLC essentially confirmatory. This technique appears to offer little advantage over the media and methods described by Willey and Bartlett[97] and Borriello and Honour[17] because the amount of tyrosine normally present in a blood base medium is sufficient for the production of *p*-cresol, and unless very few colonies of *C. difficile* are present the characteristic odour of *p*-cresol ('horsey' smell) is easily discernible.

Recognition of *C. difficile* obviously becomes easier with experience and it is recommended that people unfamiliar with the organism obtain a known culture of *C. difficile* to familiarize themselves with its cultural and biochemical characteristics. As already stated its ability to grow on agars incorporating cycloserine and cefoxitin and its characteristic smell and fluorescence properties can all be useful aids in its presumptive identification. In addition, *C. difficile* has a characteristic cellular morphology at 48 hours as seen by Gram film, with subterminal spores at both ends of the Gram-positive rod to give a 'dumb-bell' appearance.[17] This will not be noted on Gram films prepared from colonies grown on the cycloserine-cefoxitin selective agars as spore formation is inhibited. Presumptive *C. difficile* colonies should be isolated, and identification confirmed. Tests that can be used to confirm identification include biochemical reaction patterns, and gas liquid chromatography profiles of the volatile fatty acid products of carbohydrate metabolism,[47] and the detection of cytotoxin (see below). However, despite the claim of others,[46] our experience has been that there is a great deal of strain to strain variability in the biochemical reaction patterns generated by *C. difficile* when performed by conventional methods using anaerobic media. This has also been noted by others,[73] and also extends to commercially available identification kits such as the API 20A System (Borriello and Cohen, unpublished observations). Although we have always found the volatile fatty acid profile to be characteristic there is a report that asaccharolytic strains fail to produce valeric acid.[73] Many strains of *C. difficile* produce a cytotoxin that is specifically neutralized by the cross-reacting *C. sordellii* antitoxin (see below) and this test can be an aid in the identification of this organism. It must be remembered however that not all strains of *C. difficile* are cytotoxigenic.[18]

The detection of the associated cytotoxin has also formed the basis of a counter-immunoelectrophoresis test for the identification of toxigenic *C. difficile*.[95] This system failed to differentiate *C. bifermentans* and *C. sordellii* from *C. difficile*, and it has been suggested that the system used is detecting a common cell surface antigen.[74]

There have been a number of attempts to develop methods which would allow the direct visualization of *C. difficile* in clinical specimens by use of immuno-fluorescence (IFA) techniques. Wilson and coworkers[99] studied a direct IFA technique to determine its usefulness in the rapid detection of *C. difficile* in stools. The fluorescein-conjugated sera reacted with three other species of clostridia and *S. aureus*. Although it gave positive results for 83% of patients with *C. difficile* colitis it also gave positive results for 62% of stools from which *C. difficile* was not cultured. An immunofluorescent technique has also been described by Hubert *et al.*[48] Problems encountered in IFA applied directly to faecal specimens include a high proportion of positive results probably due to the presence of Fc receptors on cellular debris in faeces. If the bacteria are antibody-coated this would add another problem in the use of IFA for the detection of *C. difficile* in faeces.

Detection of *C. difficile* cytotoxin

The presence of a cytotoxin in the stools of a patient with pseudomembranous colitis was first described by Larson *et al.*[59] It was rapidly shown that this toxin was neutralized by *C. sordellii* antitoxin[23] and that the source of this toxin was *C. difficile.*[9] Almost all patients with histologically proven pseudomembranous colitis have this toxin in their stools[4,18] and there is a very good correlation between the presence of this toxin and isolation of *C. difficile* from the specimen.[18] Thus tissue culture assay for the detection of faecal cytotoxin that is neutralized by *C. sordellii* antitoxin has become a favoured diagnostic test in patients in which a *C. difficile*-mediated gastrointestinal disease is suspected. The following method has proven to be of use in our laboratory. The stool specimen is diluted in glycerol transport broth[27] to yield a 1:10 dilution. This is centrifuged at 14 000 g for 30 minutes and the supernatant removed. An aliquot of this supernatant (100 μl) is added to a tissue culture tube containing a confluent monolayer of 2–3 day old human embryonic lung fibroblasts (MRC V) cells. The inoculated tubes are incubated at 37° C on a tissue culture roller drum for a maximum of 48 hours. All the cell lines used for this work contain penicillin G (100 units/ml) and streptomycin (100 μg/ml). The cells are examined under an inverted tissue culture microscope for the presence of a cytopathic effect at 24 and 48 hours. All positive samples are repeated in duplicate and one of the duplicates tested for neutralization by *C. sordellii* antitoxin (Wellcome Research Laboratories). An equal volume of *C. sordellii* antitoxin is added to 100 μl of faecal supernatant and left to equilibrate for 1 hour at room temperature, before being added to the cell monolayer.

Although we use MRC V cells all cell types appear to be susceptible to this toxin.[25] When large numbers of stool specimens and culture filtrates are to be screened a micromethod is used.[16] Not all laboratories have tissue culture facilities and this has stimulated interest in the development of alternative methods for the detection of this toxin. Two groups of workers have investigated the possible use of counterimmunoelectrophoresis (CIE). The method described by Welch *et al.*[95] was designed to detect toxin in culture filtrates only. The use of CIE for the detection of toxin in faeces was described by Ryan *et al.*[79] In their hands the technique proved to be reliable with positive results in 15 patients from whom *C. difficile* was isolated, and in one patient with antibiotic-associated diarrhoea but negative for both *C. difficile* and its toxin as detected by tissue culture. Five of the 15 CIE-positive samples were negative for toxin by the tissue culture assay, although strains of *C. difficile* from these samples produced a cytopathic toxin *in vitro.* Thus this system appears useful but it needs to be evaluated by other workers.

A recent method described for the detection of this toxin is an enzyme-immunoassay (EIA) system.[101] A comparison was made of EIA and the tissue culture cytotoxicity assay for the detection of *C. difficile* antigen in specimens of human stool; EIA was shown to be a rapid sensitive technique. Of 277 specimens analysed 84 samples were positive and 190 negative by both techniques. Three specimens were positive only by EIA. Of these three specimens, *C. difficile* was isolated from two, and the third specimen of this group was from a patient with pseudomembranous colitis who was treated with vancomycin and who had cytotoxin present in stool specimens obtained before treatment.

REFERENCES

1 Allo M., Silva J. Jr, Fekety R., Rifkin G. D. and Waskin H. (1979) Prevention of clindamycin-induced colitis in hamsters by *Clostridium sordellii antitoxin. Gastroenterology* **76**, 351.
2 Banno Y., Kobayashi T., Watanabe K., Ueno K. and Nozawa Y. (1981) Two toxins (D-1 and D-2) of *Clostridium difficile* causing antibiotic-associated colitis: purification and some characterization. *Biochem. Int.* **2**, 629.
3 Barclay F. E. and Borriello S. P. (1982) *In vitro* inhibition of *C. difficile. Europ. J. Chemother. Antibiot.* Supplement, **2**, 155.
4 Bartlett J. G. (1979) Antibiotic-associated colitis. *Clin. Gastroenterology* **8**, 783.
5 Bartlett J. G. (1981) Antimicrobial agents implicated in *Clostridium difficile* toxin-associated diarrhea or colitis. *Johns Hop. Med. J.* **149**, 6.
6 Bartlett J. G., Chang T. W., Gurwith M., Gorbach S. L. and Onderonk A. B. (1978) Antibiotic-associated pseudomembranous colitis due to toxin producing clostridia. *N. Engl. J. Med.* **298**, 531.
7 Bartlett J. G., Chang T. W. and Onderdonk A. B. (1978) Comparison of five regimens of treatment of experimental clindamycin-associated colitis. *J. Infect. Dis.* **138**, 81.
8 Bartlett J. G., Onderdonk A. B. and Cisneros R. L. (1977) Clindamycin-associated colitis in hamsters. Protection with Vancomycin. *Gastroenterology* **73**, 772.
9 Bartlett J. G., Onderdonk A. B., Cisneros R. L. and Kasper D. L. (1977) Clindamycin-associated colitis due to a toxin-producing species of *Clostridium* in hamsters. *J. Infect. Dis.* **136**, 701.
10 Bartlett J. G., Taylor N. S., Chang T. W. and Dzink J. (1980) Clinical and laboratory observations in *Clostridium difficile* colitis. *Am. J. Clin. Nutr.* **33**, 2521.
11 Bartlett J. G., Tedesco F. J., Shull S., Lowe B. and Chang T. W. (1980) Symptomatic relapse after oral treatment of antibiotic associated colitis. *Gastroenterology* **78**, 431.
12 Bolton R. P. (1979) *Clostridium dificile* associated colitis after neomycin — treated with metronidazole. *Br. Med. J.* **2**, 1479.
13 Bolton R. P. (1982) Pseudomembranous colitis — diseases, aetiology and treatment. *Europ. J. Chemother. Antibiot.* Supplement **2**, 115.
14 Bone E., Tamm A. and Hill M. (1976) The production of urinary phenols by gut bacteria and their possible role in the causation of large bowel cancer. *Am. J. Clin. Nutr.* **29**, 1448.
15 Borriello S. P. (1979) *Clostridium difficile* and its toxin in the gastrointestinal tract in health and disease. *Res. Clin. Forums.* **1**, 33.
16 Borriello S. P. (1979) An evaluated micromethod for the detection of *Clostridium difficile* enterotoxin. *Microbios Let.* **7**, 25.
17 Borriello S. P. and Honour P. (1981) Simplified procedure for the routine isolation of *Clostridium difficile* from faeces. *J. Clin. Pathol.* **34**, 1124.
18 Borriello S. P. and Larson H. E. (1981) Antibiotics and Pseudomembranous Colitis. *J. Antimicrob. Chemother.* **7**, Suppl. A, 53.
19 Bowden T. A., Mansberger A. R. and Lykins L. E. (1981) Pseudomembranous enterocolitis: Mechanisms of restoring floral homeostasis. *Am. Surg.* **47**, 178.
20 Burdon D. W., Brown J. D., Youngs D. J., Arabi Y., Shinagawa N., Alexander-Williams J. and Keighley M. R. B. (1979) Antibiotic susceptibility of *Clostridium difficile. J. Antimicrob. Chemother.* **5**, 307.

21 Burdon D. W., George R. H., Mogg G. A. G., Arabi Y., Thompson H., Johnson M., Alexander-Williams J. and Keighley M. R. B. (1981) Faecal toxin and severity of antibiotic-associated pseudomembranous colitis. *J. Clin. Path.* **34**, 548.

22 Burdon D. W., Thompson H., Candy D. C. A., Kearns M., Lees D. and Stephen J. (1981) Enterotoxin(s) of *Clostridium difficile. Lancet* **ii**, 258.

23 Chang T. W., Gorbach S. L. and Bartlett J. G. (1978) Neutralisation of *Clostridium difficile* toxin by *Clostridium sordelli* antitoxin. *Infect. Immun.* **22**, 418.

24 Chang T. W., Gorbach S. L., Bartlett J. G. and Saginur R. (1980) Bacitracin treatment of antibiotic-associated colitis and diarrhoea caused by *Clostridium difficile* toxin. *Gastroenterology* **78**, 1584.

25 Chang T. W., Lauermann M. and Bartlett J. G. (1979) Cytotoxicity assay in antibiotic-associated colitis. *J. Infect. Dis.* **140**, 765.

26 Chang T. W., Onderdonk A. B. and Bartlett J. G. (1978) Anion-exchange resins in antibiotic-associated colitis. *Lancet* **ii**, 258.

27 Crowther J. S. (1971) Transport and storage of faeces for bacteriological examination. *J. Appl. Bacteriol.* **34**, 477.

28 Dabard J., Dubos F., Martinet L. and Ducluzeau R. (1979) Experimental reproduction of neonatal diarrhea in young gnotobiotic hares simultaneously associated with *Clostridium difficile* and other *Clostridium* strains. *Infect. Immun.* **24**, 7.

29 DeJesus R. and Peternel W. W. (1978) Antibiotic associated diarrhoea treated with oral tetracyclin. *Gastroenterology* **74**, 818.

30 Dzink J. and Bartlett J. G. (1980) In vitro susceptibility of *Clostridium difficile* isolated from patients with antibiotic-associated diarrhoea or colitis. *Antimicrob. Agents Chemother.* **17**, 695.

31 Elsden S. R., Hilton M. G. and Waller J. M. (1976) The end products of the metabolism of aromatic amino acids by clostridia. *Arch. Microbiol.* **107**, 283.

32 Fainstein V., Bodey G. P. and Fekety R. (1981) Relapsing pseudomembranous colitis associated with cancer chemotherapy. *J. Infect. Dis.* **143**, 865.

33 Fekety R. (1979) Prevention and treatment of antibiotic associated colitis. In: Schlessinger D. (Ed.): *Microbiology — 1979*, p. 276, American Society for Microbiology, Washington D.C.

34 George R. H., Symonds J. M., Dimock F. *et al.* (1978*a*) Identfication of *Clostridium difficile* as a cause of pseudomembranous colitis. *Br. Med. J.* **1**, 695.

35 George R. H., Youngs D. J., Johnson E. M. and Burdon D. W. (1978) Anion-exchange resins in pseudomembranous colitis. *Lancet* **ii**, 624.

36 George W. L. (1980) Antimicrobiol agent-associated colitis and diarrhea (Medical Progress) *West. J. Med.* **133**, 115

37 George W. L., Kirby B. D., Sutter V. L. and Finegold S. M. (1979) Antimicrobial susceptibility of *Clostridium difficile*. In: Schlessinger D. (Ed.): *Microbiology — 1979*, p. 267. American Society for Microbiology, Washington D.C.

38 George W. L., Rolfe R. D. and Finegold S. M. (1980) Treatment and prevention of antimicrobial agent-induced colitis and diarrhea. *Gastroenterology* **79**, 366.

39 George L., Rolfe R. and Mulligan M. (1979*b*) Presence of *Clostridium difficile* and its toxin in feces of asymptomatic subjects receiving cefoxitin (Abstract). *Clin. Res.* **27**, 344A.

40 George W. L., Sutter V. L., Citron D. and Finegold S. M. (1979) Selective and differential medium for isolation of *Clostridium difficile*. *J. Clin. Microbiol.* **9**, 214.

41 George W. L., Sutter V. L. and Finegold S. M. (1977) Antimicrobial agent-induced diarrhoea — a bacterial disease. *J. Infect. Dis.* **136**, 822.

42 George W. L., Volpicelli N. A., Stiner D. B., Richman D. D., Liechty E. J., Mok H. Y. I., Rolfe R. D. and Finegold S. M. (1979) Relapse of pseudomembranous colitis after vancomycin therapy. *N. Engl. J. Med.* **301**, 414.

43 Gilligan P. H., McCarthy L. R. and Genta V. M. (1981) Relative frequency of *Clostridium difficile* in patients with diarrheal disease. *J. Clin. Microbiol.* **14**, 26.

44 Gotz V., Romankiewicz J. A., Moss J. and Murray H. W. (1979) Prophylaxis against ampicillin-associated diarrhoea with a lactobacillus preparation. *Am. J. Hosp. Pharm.* **36**, 754.

45 Hall I. C. and O'Toole E. (1935) Intestinal flora in new-born infants. *Am. J. Dis. Child.* **49**, 390.

46 Hafiz S. and Oakley C. L. (1976) *Clostridium difficile*: Isolation and characteristics. *J. Med. Microbiol.* **9**, 129.

47 Holdeman L. V., Cato E. P. and Moore W. E. C. (Eds) (1977) *Anaerobe Laboratory Manual*, 4th edn, Virginia Polytechnic Institute and State University, Blacksburg.

48 Hubert J., Ionesco H. and Sebald M. (1981) Détection de *Clostridium difficile* par isolement sur milieu minimal sélectif et par immunofluorescence. *Ann. Microbiol.* (Paris), **132A**, 149.

49 Ionesco H. (1980) Transfert de la résistance à la tétracycline chez *Clostridium difficile. Ann. Microbiol (Paris)* **131A** (2), 171.

50 Jones G. W. and Rutter J. M. (1972) Role of the K88 Antigen in the pathogenesis of neonatal diarrhea caused by *Escherichia coli* in piglets. *Infect. Immun.* **6**, 918.

51 Kahn M. Y. and Hall W. H. (1966) Staphylococcal enteritis treated with oral vancomycin. *Ann. Int. Med* **65**, 1.

52 Kappas A., Shinagawa N., Arabi Y., Thompson H., Burdon D. W., Dimock F., George R. H., Alexander-Williams J. and Keighley M. R. B. (1978) Diagnosis of pseudomembranous colitis. *Br. Med. J.* **1**, 675.

53 Keighley M. R. B. and Burdon D. W. (1979) Metronidazole in the aetiology of pseudomembranous colitis. *Lancet* **ii**, 607.

54 Keighley M. R. B., Burdon D. W., Arabi Y., *et al.* (1978) Randomised controlled trial of vancomycin for pseudomembranous colitis and postoperative diarrhoea. *Br. Med. J.* **2**, 1667.

55 Kim K. H., Fekety R., Batts D H., Brown D., Cudmore M., Silva J. Jr and Waters D. (1981) Isolation of *Clostridium difficile* from the environment and contacts of patients with antibiotic-associated colitis. *J. Inf. Dis.* **143**, 42.

56 Kreutzer E. W. and Milligan F. D. (1978) Treatment of antibiotic-associated pseudomembranous colitis with cholestyramine resin. *John Hopkins Med. J.* **143**, 67.

58 Larson H. E., Levi A. J. and Boriello S. P. (1978) Vancomycin for pseudomembranous colitis. *Lancet* **ii**, 48.

59 Larson H. E., Parry J. V., Price A. B., Davies D. R., Dolby J. and Tyrrell D. A. J. (1977) Undescribed toxin in pseudomembranous colitis. *B. Med. J.* **1**, 1246.

60 Larson H. E., Price A. B., Honour P. and Borriello S. P. (1978) *Clostridium difficile* and the aetiology of pseudomembranous colitis. *Lancet* **i**, 1063.

61 Lawrence G., Shann F., Freestone D. S. and Walker P. D. (1979) Prevention of necrotising enteritis in Papua New Guinea by active immunisation. *Lancet* **i**, 227.

62 Lishman A. H., Al-Jumaili I. J. and Record C. O. (1981) Spectrum of antibiotic-associated diarrhoea. *Gut* **22**, 34.

63 Marrie T. J., Faulkner R. S., Badley B. W. D., Hartlen M. R., Comeau S. A. and Miller H. R. (1978) Pseudomembranous colitis: isolation of two species of cytotoxic clostridia and successful treatment with vancomycin. *J. Can. Med. Assoc.* **119**, 1058.

64 Matuchansky C., Aries J. and Maire P. (1978) Metronidazole for antibiotic-associated pseudomembranous colitis. *Lancet* **ii**, 580.

65 Mulligan M. E., George W. L., Rolf R. D. and Finegold S. M. (1980) Epidemiological aspects of *Clostridium difficile*-induced diarrhea and colitis. *Am. J. Clin. Nutr.* **33**, 2533.

66 Novak E., Lee J. G., Seckman C. E., Phillips J. P. and Disanto A. R. (1976) Unfavourable effect of atropine — diphenoxylate (Lomotil) treatment in lincomycin caused diarrhoea. *J. Am. Med. Assoc.* **235**, 1451.

67 Oldenburger D. and Miller J. A. (1980) Treatment of pseudomembranous colitis with oral metronidazole after relapse following vancomycin. *Am. J. Gastroenterology* **74**, 359.

68 Pashby N. L., Bolton R. P. and Sherriff R. I. (1979) Oral metronidazole in *Clostridium difficile* colitis. *Br. Med. J.* **2**, 1605.

69 Peternel W. W. (1975) Ampicillin associated diarrhea. *Am. J. Dig. Dis.* **20**, 191.

70 Phillips K. D. and Rogers P. A. (1981) Rapid detection and presumptive identification of *Clostridium difficile* by *p*-cresol production on a selective medium. *J. Clin. Pathol.* **34**, 642.

71 Phillips R. K. S., Glazer G. and Borriello S. P. (1981) Non-clostridium difficile pseudo-membranous colitis responding to both vancomycin and metronidazole. *Br. Med. J.* **283**, 823.

72 Pitman F. E. (1974) Adverse effects of lomotil. *Gastroenterology* **67**, 408.

73 Poxton I. R. (1982) Detection and isolation of *Clostridium difficile. Europ. J. Chemother. Antibiot.* Suppl. **2**, 123.

74 Poxton I. R. and Byrne M. D. (1981) Detection of *Clostridium difficile* toxin by counter-immunoelectrophoresis: a note of caution. *J. Clin. Microbiol.* **14**, 349.

75 Price A. B. and Davies D. R. (1977) Pseudomembranous colitis. *J. Clin. Pathol.* **30**, 1.

76 Rolfe R. D., Helebian S. and Finegold S. M. (1981) Bacterial interference between *Clostridium difficile* and normal faecal flora. *J. Infect. Dis.* **143**, 470.

77 Rolfe R. D. and Finegold S. M. (1979) Purification and charaterization of *Clostridium difficile* toxin. *Infect. Immun.* **25**, 191.

78 Rutter J. M., Jones G. W., Brown G. T. H., Burrows M. R. and Luther P. D. (1976) Antibacterial activity in colostrum and milk associated with protection of piglets against enteric disease caused by K88-positive *Escherichia coli. Infect. Immun.* **13**, 667.

79 Ryan R. W., Kwasnik I. and Tilton R. C. (1980) Rapid detection of *Clostridium difficile* toxin in human faeces. *J. Clin. Microbiol.* **12**, 776.

80 Sakurai Y., Tsuchiya H., Ikegami F., Funatomi T., Takasu S. and Uchikoshi T. (1979) Acute right-sided hemorrhagic colitis associated with oral administration of ampicillin. *Dig. Dis. Sci.* **24**, 910.

81 Seppälä K., Hjelt L. and Sipponen P. (1981) Colonoscopy in the diagnosis of antibiotic-associated colitis. A prospective study. *Scand. J. Gastroenterol.* **16**, 466.

82 Shuttleworth R., Taylor M. and Jones D. M. (1980) Antimicrobial susceptibilities of *Clostridium difficile. J. Clin. Pathol.* **33**, 1002.

83 Smith C. J., Markowitz S. M. and Macrina F. L. (1981) Transferable tetracycline resistance in *Clostridium difficile. Antimicrob. Agents Chemother.* **19**, 997.

84 Smith M. F., Borriello S. P., Claydon G. S. and Casewell M. W. (1980) Clinical and bacteriological findings in necrotising enterocolitis: A controlled study. *J. Infect.* **2**, 23.

85 Schwartz J. N., Hamilton J. P., Fekety R., Green E. G., Stamper L., Batts D. H. and Silva J. (1980) Ampicillin induced enterocolitis: implications of toxigenic *Clostridium perfringens,* type C. *J. Pediatr.* **97**, 661.

86 Taylor N. and Bartlett J. G. (1980) Binding of *Clostridium difficile* cytotoxin and vancomycin by anion-exchange resins. *J. Infect. Dis.* **141**, 92.

87 Taylor N. S., Thorne G. M. and Bartlett J. G. (1981) Comparison of two toxins produced by *Clostridium difficile. Infect. Immun.* **34**, 1036.

88 Taylor R. H., Borriello S. P. and Taylor A. J. (1981) Isolation of *Clostridium difficile* from the small bowel. *Br. Med. J.* **283**, 412.

89 Tedesco F. (1976) Clindamycin-associated colitis: Review of the clinical spectrum of 47 cases. *Am. J. Digest Dis.* **21**, 26.

90 Tedesco F., Markham R., Gurwith M., Christie D. and Bartlett J. G. (1978) Oral vancomycin for antibiotic associated pseudomembranous colitis. *Lancet* **ii**, 226.

91 Tedesco F. J., Stanley R. J. and Alpers D. H. (1974) Diagnostic features of clindamycin-associated pseudomembranous colitis. *N. Eng. J. Med.* **290**, 841.

92 Thomson G., Clark A. H., Hare K. and Spilg W. G. S. (1981) Pseudomembranous colitis after treatment with metronidazole. *Br. Med. J.* **282**, 864.

93 Trinh Dinh H., Kernbaum S. and Frottier J. (1978) Treatment of antibiotic-induced colitis by metronidazole. *Lancet* **i**, 338.

94 Viteri A. L., Howard P. H. and Dyck W. P. (1974) The spectrum of lincomycin-clindamycin colitis. *Gastroenterology* **66**, 1137.

95 Welch D. F., Menge S. K. and Matsen J. M. (1980) Identification of toxigenic *Clostridium difficile* by counterimmunoelectrophoresis. *J. Clin. Microbiol.* **11**, 470.

96 Welling G. W., Groen G., Tuinte J. H. M., Koopman J. P. and Kennis H. M. (1980) Biochemical effects on germ-free mice of association with several strains of anaerobic bacteria. *J. Gen. Microbiol.* **117**, 57.

 97 Willey S. H. and Bartlett J. G. (1979) Cultures for *Clostridium difficile* in stools containing a cytotoxin neutralised by *Clostridium sordelli* antitoxin. *J. Clin. Microbiol.* **10**, 880.

 98 Wilson K. H., Fekety R. and Silva J. (1980) Prevention of antibiotic-associated colitis by recolonization with normal colonic flora. *Clin. Res.* **28**, 382A.

 99 Wilson K. H., Silva J. and Fekety R. (1980) Fluorescent antibody to *Clostridium difficile* as an aid to diagnosis of antibiotic-associated colitis (AAC). 20th Interscience Conf. Antimicrob. Agents Chemoth., Abstract 206.

100 Winans L. Jr, Thornton G. B. and Carski T. R. (1980) The effect of Lactinex granules on *Clostridium difficile* induced pseudomembranous colitis. Abstracts of Annual Meeting Am. Soc. Microbiol. Abstract A4.

101 Yolken R. H., Whitcomb L. S., Marien G., Bartlett J. G., Libby J., Ehrich M. and Wilkins T. (1981) Enzyme immunoassay for the detection of *Clostridium difficile* antigen. *J. Infect. Dis.* **144**, 378.

102 Libby J. M., Jortner B. S. and Wilkins T. D. (1982) Effects of the two toxins of *Clostridium difficile* in antibiotic-associated cecitis in animals. *Infect. Immun.* **36**, 822.

103 Lyerly D. M., Lockwood D. E., Richardson S. H. and Wilkins T. D. (1982) Biological activities of toxins A and B of *Clostridium difficile*. *Infect. Immun.* **35**, 1147.

104 Lyerly D. M., Sullivan N. M. and Wilkins T. D. (1983) Enzyme-linked immunosorbert assay for *Clostridium difficile* toxin A. *J. Clin. Microbiol.* **17**, 72.

105 Sullivan N. M., Pellet S. and Wilkins T. D. (1982) Purification and characterization of toxins A and B of *Clostridium difficile*. *Infect. Immun.* **35**, 1032.

17 Carcinoma of the colon and gut bacteria

S. P. Borriello

Introduction   347
Epidemiology   348
Diet   348
Case control studies   350
International studies   352
Bile acids as potential carcinogens and co-carcinogens   353
  Lithocholic acid   354
  Deoxycholic acid   355
Other potential carcinogens and co-carcinogens   355
  Cholesterol   355
  Tryptophan   356
  Methionine   357
  Tyrosine   357
N-nitrosamine production   357
  Retoxification of hepatic metabolites of environmental polycyclic aromatic
    hydrocarbons   358
Potential microbial carcinogens of unknown origin   359
Conclusion   359
References   360

INTRODUCTION

Carcinoma of the large bowel is the second most common cause of cancer-mediated death in both Great Britain and the United States accounting for up to 17 000 and 47 000 deaths per annum respectively.

A number of workers have suggested that more than 90% of human cancers are due to environmental factors and, as such, are preventable. Higginson[41] by reference to cancer registry data, investigated the incidence of cancer in a number of countries and compared the highest and lowest incidences of cancer by site. He selected the lowest incidence in any country for a given site as the minimum inevitable level for that cancer and proposed that incidences greater than this level were due to environmental factors and therefore preventable. On this basis, it could be argued that if the causative agent(s) is identified, at least 80% of all colonic cancer could be prevented. Many investigators have devoted their energies to identifying these agents. Much useful information has been generated from epidemiological studies, and a number of resultant observations have prompted various workers to postulate a microbial role in the aetiology of this disease.

347

EPIDEMIOLOGY

The relative incidence of large bowel cancer has been determined for many countries.[22] In general, large bowel cancer is much more common in developed countries with a high standard of living than in countries with a lower standard of living; the disease is much more common in northwest Europe and North America than in Africa, Asia and South America.[22] Studies of migrants to the USA have shown that these differences in cancer incidence cannot be explained merely on a racial basis.

Japanese migrants to the United States acquire an incidence of colon cancer similar to that of the host nation, which is much higher than the incidence for Japanese living in Japan; this change can occur within the lifetime of the first generation migrant.[13] The longer Japanese migrants live in the United States, the closer their incidence of colon cancer approaches that of Americans.[39]

Studies have also been made of migrants to the USA from 12 other countries — England and Wales, Canada, Australia, Czechoslovakia, Germany, Ireland, Italy, Mexico, Norway, Poland, Sweden and the USSR.[37,81] Among these migrants the standard mortality rates differed little from each other and from that of native-born Americans, with the conclusion that the risk of colon cancer had become modified to attain the level of risk of the country of domicile. Interestingly, the Seventh Day Adventists in the United States who consume a vegetarian diet, have an incidence of colorectal cancer which is lower than the national average.[67]

In addition to these international and migrant studies colon cancer incidence within a country has also been investigated. In some low incidence countries such as Hong Kong,[20] Japan,[87] and Colombia[18] there is an excess risk for people in the higher income groups compared to the population as a whole. In these countries, the high income groups tend to consume a more 'westernized' diet when compared with the lower income groups.

Studies of racial groups within a country show that for countries where the various racial groups form part of a fairly homogeneous total with respect to cultural characteristics such as diet, then they will demonstrate similar incidence rates of large bowel cancer.[23] In contrast the four racial groups in South Africa — white, coloured, Bantu and Indian — have greatly different incidences of colon cancer;[22] these groups also have different cultural characteristics.

Any proposed aetiology for this disease must be able to take into account the above observations. The environmental factor that satisfies this criterion, and has therefore received most attention, is diet.

DIET

Several epidemiological studies have indicated a possible relationship between colorectal cancer and diet and it is widely accepted that diet may be a major aetiological factor. Dietary components that have been shown to be associated include beef,[38] animal protein,[26,36] unrefined carbohydrate,[14] fibre,[15,57] and dietary fat.[4,26,88] Most individual dietary components fit neatly into the two main schools of thought, the 'dietary fibre' theory, and the 'dietary fat' theory. The fibre theory asserts that the incidence of colon cancer is inversely related to the amount of dietary fibre.[15] Some of the data in support of this theory have been critically questioned[47] and the problems of defining dietary fibre are discussed by Huang *et al.*[48] who also state 'It cannot be denied that the fibre theory is simple, attractive and appears to be firmly based on common sense. When subjected to research studies, however, the situation appears much more complex than expected. Although some progress is being made, the data are often contradictory and confusing'. In contrast the many observations of a positive correlation between dietary fat and animal protein with colorectal cancer are well substantiated. When free and bound fat are considered separately the best correlation with this cancer was found to be with bound fat.[26] Bound fat — mostly derived from meat — and animal protein such as beef, are highly intercorrelated and these observations which support the relation of colorectal cancer to beef and animal protein are consistent with a relation to dietary fat.

Because dietary studies have failed to reveal any correlation between colorectal cancer and direct-acting dietary carcinogens or co-carcinogens, Aries *et al.*[2] postulated that a carcinogen or co-carcinogen is produced *in situ* probably by the action of bacteria on some benign substrate, the level of which is determined by the diet. This postulate is not without precedent. If cycasin (methylazoxy-methanol-β-1-glucoside) is fed to normal rats, tumours are produced in the gut, liver and kidney. In contrast, when fed to germ-free rats the cycasin is excreted unchanged in the faeces and the animal suffers no toxic effects. In addition parenterally administered cycasin is nontoxic. It is presumed that in normal rats the potent carcinogen methylazoxymethanol is released from its harmless glucoside cycasin by bacterial β-glucosidase activity, with resultant hepato-toxicity and subsequent intestinal carcinogenesis. The germ-free animals however lack this microbial enzymatic activity and the host intestinal mucosal β-glucosidase has a narrow substrate range which is inactive on cycasin. These observations have been well reviewed by Laqueur and Spatz.[56] This is a good example of an administered dietary component being metabolized to a carcinogen by the enzymatic activity of the gastrointestinal flora.

The obvious question raised by the postulate of Aries *et al.*[2] is the nature of the benign substrate in humans. In order to explain the relationship between dietary fat and colorectal cancer incidence it has been proposed that the benign substrate is a component of the bile-acid pool which is determined in part by dietary fat intake, and that the bile acids are metabolised in the gut by bacterial activity to yield carcinogens or co-carcinogens.[2,46] Evidence from international,[46] intra-national[20] and case control studies[47] has shown an association between high levels of faecal steroids and colorectal cancer, and in particular an association with the mean faecal concentration of dihydroxycholanic acid.

There is a structural similarity between steroids and the polycyclic aromatic carcinogens,[49] and it has been suggested that full aromatization of the bile acid nucleus can yield a carcinogen metabolite based on cyclopentaphenanthrene.[17] A theoretical pathway for the production of a polycyclic aromatic steroid has been proposed.[46] All of the steps required to metabolise conjugated primary bile acids to free 3-keto derivatives such as 3-oxo-5β-chol-24-oic acid, which can act as a substrate for the introduction of stable double bonds, have been described *in vitro* for a great number of gastrointestinal microorganisms which are common to the gastrointestinal tract of subjects from different parts of the world.[25] However, the introduction of a double bond into ring A of this steroid nucleus and other un-saturation processes such as the introduction of double bonds into ring B have only been described for certain members of the genus *Clostridium*.[3,34,35] These clostridia were termed nuclear dehydrogenating (NDH) clostridia. If the association between faecal steroids and large bowel cancer is related to the ability of the gastrointestinal flora to metabolise these steroids to unsaturated derivatives, then the bacteria of interest are those which can perform a unique step in this metabolic pathway. Such bacteria are the nuclear dehydrogenating clostridia. The postulate would therefore require that persons at high risk for the development of colorectal cancer, whether due to country of domicile or pre-disposing gastrointestinal disease, should harbour more NDH clostridia, both in terms of numbers and frequency, than low risk subjects. A number of studies have been performed to investigate this relationship.

CASE CONTROL STUDIES

An association between large bowel cancer and clostridia with the ability to de-hydrogenate the steroid nucleus at the $\Delta 4$ position and introduce a double bond, was first shown in a case control study by Hill *et al.* in 1975.[47] This study compared the faecal carriage of NDH clostridia in cancer patients with that of subjects with upper-alimentary-tract disease, nonmalignant large bowel disease, and nongastrointestinal disease. They found that 82% of large bowel cancer patients harboured NDH clostridia in their stools compared with a carriage rate of only 43% in the comparison groups. Analysis of their data shows that 36% of patients with nongastrointestinal disease harboured these clostridia. Since this study there have been three other case control studies[6,8,31] which have included data on carriage of NDH clostridia (Table 17.1).

Table 17.1   Percentage carriage of nuclear dehydrogenating clostridia

Controls*	Colon cancer	Postoperative colon cancer	Adenomatous polyps	Familial† polyposis	Reference number
34 (62)‡	70 (33)	39 (33)	41 (17)	72 (50)	8
40 (10)	—	25 (8)	—	30 (20)	6
24 (25)	—	—	40 (25)	—	31
41 (87)	82 (44)	—	—	—	47
Total					
36 (184)	74 (77)	37 (41)	40 (42)	60 (70)	

* Includes patients with large bowel disorders of no malignant potential, patients without large bowel diseases, and healthy adults. † Includes 'postoperative familial polyposis subjects'. ‡ Number of subjects studied.

In one study it was shown that numbers of faecal NDH clostridia discriminate well between patients with colorectal cancer and control subjects with no large bowel disorders;[8] with carriage rates of 70% and 30% respectively. Postoperatively the colorectal cancer group (POC) carried NDH much less frequently than the preoperative group (39% compared to 70%). The POC patients that did carry, tended to do so in high concentrations. In case control studies, patient groups with gastrointestinal disorders carried NDH clostridia more frequently than the control group, but less frequently than the subjects with colorectal cancer (Table 17.1). Familial polyposis subjects segregated as a high risk group from the point of view of carriage of NDH clostridia.[6,8]

Analysis of the data of Bone *et al.*[6] reveals that NDH clostridia were found in the stools of 55% of the group composed of those with familial polyposis and the asymptomatic polyposis siblings. Despite the fact that the familial polyposis subjects segregated into a high risk group from the point of view of clostridial carriage, the NDH/bile acid theory for colorectal cancer also requires the presence of high faecal levels of secondary bile acids. Bone *et al.*[6] have shown that the average rectal bile acid (RBA) concentration in these patients is low and that in addition the primary bile acids made up the bulk of the RBA detected. So, although familial polyposis patients represent a high risk group for the development of colorectal cancer both from a clinical and NDH clostridia point of view, they fail to do so with respect to type and concentrations of RBA.

Of the polyps of no known genetic determination, the colorectal adenoma is accepted by the majority of gastroenterologists to be the most important precursor lesion for large bowel cancer, with strong clinical, histopathological, epidemiological, and experimental evidence to support its premalignant nature.[60] The risk of malignant change varies considerably and is related to both the size and histological nature of the adenoma.[5,28,59]

In the study by Borriello[8] 41% of this group harboured detectable numbers of faecal NDH clostridia which is comparable to the carriage rate in the control group. However, of this 41%, the majority tended to carry relatively high numbers of these clostridia which also constituted a significant component of their total clostridial flora, unlike the situation in the control subjects. From an overall quantitative point of view the carriage of NDH clostridia in this group was not dissimilar to that of the control group. This overall pattern was also found by Finegold *et al.*[31] However, it has been shown that adenomatous polyp patients have elevated levels of faecal bile acids (FBAs) compared with patients with other gastrointestinal disease,[74] and that patients with benign gastrointestinal polyps have FBA levels not dissimilar to those of subjects without gastrointestinal disorders.[47] A combination of high FBA levels and carriage of NDH clostridia has proved to be a superior discriminatory factor than either of these parameters alone when trying to differentiate colorectal cancer patients from controls.[47] One must accept, therefore, that consideration of FBA levels in combination with carriage may differentiate better the adenomatous polyp group from the control groups. FBA levels may also improve the discriminatory factor generated by NDH clostridia analysis alone, in the other groups in these studies. The overriding questions are whether or not the large numbers of NDH clostridia noted in cancer patients and high risk groups indicate an aetiological role for this organism or whether they are simply due to the possibility that the diseased colon provides an environment conducive to the growth of these clostridia. In short, are they causative or consequential factors of the disease? Even if adenomas and other known predisposing gastrointestinal diseases produce an environment favourable to colonization by NDH clostridia, it is possible that the established clostridia then play an important aetiological role in the transformation of the benign polyp to a malignant state. The only way to establish whether the association is causal or consequential is by prospective studies. One such study is in progress and early results are indicative of a causal nature (M. J. Hill personal communication).

INTERNATIONAL STUDIES

The faecal carriage of NDH clostridia in different countries (Table 17.2) has been studied in an intranational comparison of subjects of differing socioeconomic status in Hong Kong,[20] an international study comparing Denmark and Finland,[50] a study by Drasar *et al.*[24] of the faecal clostridia of subjects from England, Wales, Scotland, USA, Japan, Hong Kong and Uganda, and a study by Borriello *et al.*[9] of English and Nigerians. In the Hong Kong study there was overall a low carriage rate of NDH clostridia, but no relationship was found between risk of development of colorectal cancer, as determined by socioeconomic status, and NDH clostridia carriage.[20] It was not clear what proportion of the subjects harboured NDH clostridia, nor what numbers of NDH clostridia were present in these subjects, but apparently only four of 92 strains of the lecithinase-negative clostridia were able to produce 3-oxo-5β steroid Δ 4 dehydrogenase, indicating that 6% of the population studied harboured these micro-organisms.[20] A study by the International Agency for Research on Cancer Intestinal Microecology Group[50] showed a carriage rate for NDH clostridia of 40% in Denmark, and 38% in Finland. However, actual numbers of NDH clostridia in the stools of these two populations were not given. Although Denmark, a high incidence country, has a four-fold greater incidence of colorectal cancer than Finland, a low incidence country, this difference was not reflected in differences in the rate of NDH clostridia carriage.

Table 17.2 Carriage of NDH clostridia in different populations

Country	No. of subjects studied	Relative colorectal cancer risk	% carriage of NDH clostridia	Reference number
Denmark	57	High	40	50
England	53	High	32	9
Finland	53	Low	38	50
Hong Kong	64	Low	6	20
Nigeria	17	Low	0	9

The study of Drasar *et al.*[24] is more difficult to evaluate. In this study importance was attached to the relative carriage rates of *C. paraputrificum*, which is the clostridium that most frequently possesses 3-oxo-5β steroid Δ 4 dehydrogenase activity.[33] *C. paraputrificum* was found more frequently in the stools of the high incidence countries — USA and United Kingdom — than in those of low incidence countries, Uganda, Japan and Hong Kong. However, not all strains of *C. paraputrificum* possess 3-oxo-5β steroid Δ 4 dehydrogenase, and clostridia other than *C. paraputrificum* can possess this enzymic capability.[33] It is therefore unfortunate that this study did not state the actual recovery rate and concentrations of clostridia with demonstrable Δ 4 dehydrogenase activity. NDH clostridia could not be found in the faeces of Nigerians,[9] which contrasts with the fairly high carriage rate of a relatively high number of NDH clostridia in subjects from the UK (Table 17.2). This low NDH clostridia carriage rate in low colorectal cancer incidence populations was shown by Crowther *et al.*[20] and indirectly confirmed by the study of Drasar *et al.*[24]

BILE ACIDS AS POTENTIAL CARCINOGENS AND CO-CARCINOGENS

Although the possible production of polycyclic aromatic hydrocarbons from steroids is an attractive hypothesis, it will remain just that until the existence of these compounds in human stool is demonstrated. However, investigations have demonstrated a number of previously unsuspected associations for high and low risk populations in both international and case control studies.

A number of the products of the microbial metabolism of primary bile acids have been shown to be co-carcinogenic or mutagenic (Table 17.3), and have been found in above-average concentrations in the stools of subjects at high risk for the development of colorectal cancer and colorectal cancer subjects. Of these secondary bile acids, lithocholic and deoxycholic acid have received the most attention.

Table 17.3 Bile acids and metabolites as carcinogens

Bile acid	Activity	Model	Ref. no.
Deoxycholic	Co-carcinogenic	Mouse rectum	63
	Mutagenic	Drosophila	21
	Mutagenic	Neurospora	51
Lithocholic	Co-carcinogenic	Mouse rectum	63
	Enhancement of	Bacteria	
	mutagenicity	(Ames test)	53,80
	Transformation	Hamster embryo cells	55
Cholic	Co-carcinogenic	Rat	72
Chenodeoxycholic	Co-carcinogenic	Rat	72
Bile	Co-carcinogenic	Rat	16,64

Lithocholic acid

Lithocholic acid is formed in the distal intestine by the activity of bacterial 7α-dehydroxylase on the primary bile acid chenodeoxycholic acid. This major faecal bile acid, of known pyrogenic and hepatoxic activity, is present in above-average concentrations in the stools of subjects from populations at high risk for the development of colonic cancer.[74] Lithocholic acid has also been shown to enhance chemically induced tumorigenesis in the intestine[63] and liver[40] of rats, to enhance the mutagenicity of suboptimal amounts of 2-amino-anthracene[80] and benzo(a) pyrene[53] in the Ames mutagenicity test, and to transform Syrian hamster embryo cells.[54] Lithocholic acid is conjugated in the liver to taurine or glycine (about 40%)[19] and also exists as the water soluble 3α-sulphate, which can account for up to 80% of the biliary lithocholic acid at any given time.[65] Sulphation occurs in the liver and is a detoxifying process that also apparently facilitates excretion, because the sulphate is poorly absorbed by the intestinal mucosa. Both lithocholic acid and lithocholic acid-3α-sulphate can escape the small bowel enterohepatic cycle and seep into the large bowel where they are available for metabolism by the gastrointestinal flora. Little is known about the further metabolism of this bile acid in the large bowel. However, recent work has shown that lithocholic acid (LA) and its 3α-sulphate can be metabolised by gut bacteria *in vitro* to yield 3-keto lithocholic acid, iso-lithocholic acid, 5β-cholanic acid and $\Delta 2$ and $\Delta 3$ cholenate[8,90] and that the group of organisms most active in this respect are the clostridia.

The metabolism of the 3α-sulphate of lithocholic acid probably represents a retoxifying process and it is possible that some of these metabolites may be potential carcinogens. Recent studies suggest that LA derivatives should not necessarily be considered as innocuous endogenous compounds as LA enhances the mutagenicity of carcinogens of different chemical classes and transforms mammalian cells. In addition, this bile acid has been shown to be present in higher concentrations in the faeces of patients at high risk of contracting colon cancer. It has been suggested that the more unsubstituted and degraded bile acids are more potent pharmacological agents than di- and trihydroxy compounds,[66] and the cholenates produced resemble the unsaturated ring-A bile acids postulated as potential carcinogens by Hill in 1971.[42] There is some evidence that the faecal flora of patients at high risk of contracting colon cancer more readily convert lithocholic acid 3α-sulphate to unsubstituted unsaturated metabolites such as $\Delta 2/\Delta 3$-cholenates.[54] It has also been shown that one genus, the clostridia, has a primary role in this metabolism, and that known individual strains can produce isolithocholic acid, 5β cholanic acid and the cholenates. Most significantly the clostridia that are thought to be important in the introduction of a double bond at the $\Delta 4$ position of ring A of bile acids — NDH clostridia — and that have an association with colon cancer (see above) are also those that are most active in metabolising lithocholic acid 3α-sulphate to the unsaturated cholenates.[8,90] If further evidence is forthcoming of an assciation between high faecal levels of $\Delta 2$- or $\Delta 3$- cholenate and colon cancer risk, then there is obviously a good case to be made for a primary aetiological role for clostridia.

Deoxycholic acid

This secondary bile acid is the product of microbial 7α-dehydroxylation of the primary bile acid cholic acid. It has been shown to enhance chemically induced tumorigenesis in the rat intestine, and has also been shown to be mutagenic to drosophila and neurospora (Table 17.3). In view of the known co-carcinogenicity and mutagenicity of this compound it is of interest that there is a good correlation between the faecal concentrations of this bile acid and colorectal cancer incidence in nine populations.[46] This association has also been shown in a case control study; in every one of 14 colorectal cancer patients the concentration of faecal deoxycholic acid was above an arbitrary cut-off point of 1.65 mg/g dry wt, compared with 8 of 41 control subjects.[43] In addition in this study 13 of 14 colorectal cancer patients had a combination of high levels of faecal deoxycholic acid and nuclear dehydrogenating clostridia which occurred in only 6 of 41 control subjects. A study of the faecal constituents of patients with colon cancer and adenomatous polyps showed an increased faecal concentration of deoxycholic acid in these patient groups compared with normal controls.[74]

Japanese in Hawaii, who are at high risk for the development of colorectal cancer, have higher concentrations of faecal deoxycholic acid than subjects in Akita, Japan, who are at low risk.[62] However, no difference in faecal deoxycholic acid concentrations could be demonstrated between subjects from areas of Denmark and Finland who have a four-fold difference in colon-cancer incidence.[50]

Other observations that are consistent with an association between secondary bile acids and microbial activity are those of Mastromarino *et al.*[58] They reported that the activity of faecal bacterial 7α-dehydroxylase, which converts the primary bile acids cholic and chenodeoxycholic acids into the secondary bile acids deoxycholic and lithocholic acids respectively, was higher in colon cancer or polyp patients than in control subjects. These data support the concept that in colon cancer and polyp patients there is a greater conversion of primary bile acids to their respective secondary metabolites than in lower-risk control subjects.

OTHER POTENTIAL CARCINOGENS AND CO-CARCINOGENS

The primary bile acids are not the only endogenous substances that can be metabolised by gut bacteria to potential carcinogens or co-carcinogens. They are not even the only sterols so metabolised. A number of other substances that could act as substrates for the microbial production of carcinogens/co-carcinogens are outlined in Table 17.4 and will be discussed below.

Cholesterol

Cholesterol is metabolised in the gut to yield three major metabolites coprostanol, coprostanone and cholestenone, and a number of minor metabolites.

Table 17.4 Microbial production of potential gut carcinogens/promoters

Substrate	Products	Type of activity
Bile acids	See Table 17.3	See Table 17.3
Cholesterol	Cholesterol epoxide (?)	Carcinogenic
Tyrosine	Volatile phenolics	Promoting
Tryptophan	Indolics	Promoting and mutagenic
Methionine	Ethionine	Carcinogenic
Various basic amino acids	N-nitroso compounds	Carcinogenic
Lecithin	N-nitroso compounds	Carcinogenic
Host conjugates and metabolites of Benzo [a]-pyrene	Retoxified Benzo [a]-pyrene	Carcinogenic

These neutral sterols have been shown to exist in above average concentrations in the stools of patients with ulcerative colitis and adenomatous polyps,[69,74] who are high risk groups with respect to the development of colorectal cancer. A correlation between high concentrations of faecal neutral sterols and colon cancer has been found in various populations.[46] Americans who consume a mixed western diet and are a high risk population, excrete high levels of cholesterol metabolites compared with Chinese, Japanese, and American Seventh-Day Adventists, who are at low risk.[71,73] Patients with colon cancer have elevated levels of faecal neutral sterols.[47] In contrast to these results Moskovitz *et al.* in 1979 reported lower levels of faecal coprostanol and coprostanone in colon cancer patients compared to control subjects;[61] and no significant differences in faecal neutral sterol concentrations could be demonstrated between subjects in Finland compared with subjects in Denmark and America, both of which have a higher incidence of colorectal cancer.[50,68] It would appear that a causal relationship between microbial metabolites of cholesterol and colorectal cancer is unlikely. However, the triol cholesterol metabolite (5α-cholestan -3β, 5α, 6β-triol) has been demonstrated in faeces.[70] A likely precursor of this metabolite is cholesterol epoxide, a known carcinogen.[30] Although epoxidation could be by mucosal mixed-function oxidases, gut bacteria are involved in producing the substrate for this reaction. Analysis of stools from various patients and population groups for the triol metabolite may yield some interesting correlations.

Tryptophan

Tryptophan is metabolised to a wide range of urinary excreted metabolites.[76] Many of these metabolites have been shown to be mutagenic and carcinogenic or co-carcinogenic, and have been implicated in bladder cancer.[12] Of this wide range of tryptophan metabolites, indole, 8-hydroxyquinaldic acid and quinaldic acid are produced only by bacterial activity and not by mammalian enzyme systems. In addition, all of the pathways for the production of hepatic metabolites of tryptophan have been demonstrated in bacteria, and it is not unlikely that the gastrointestinal flora is also involved in the production of these metabolites, and contributes to the total amounts excreted. It is possible that some of these metabolites are involved in the aetiology of colorectal cancer. Bone has shown that the faecal concentration of tryptophan is much higher in patients with large bowel cancer than in controls, and that in a study of six populations there was a relation between the incidence of large bowel cancer and faecal tryptophan concentrations (Bone quoted by Hill[44]).

Methionine

A number of bacteria can convert methionine to its S-ethyl analogue, ethionine *in vitro*.[32] The ethionine produced was not incorporated into protein, and so if produced *in vivo* it would be available for interaction with host tissue. Ethionine has been shown to be carcinogenic,[29] but to date there has been no report of the faecal concentrations of ethionine in various disease states and healthy controls.

Tyrosine

Tyrosine is metabolised by gut bacteria to yield phenolic metabolites. The major phenols produced are phenol, *p*-cresol and *p*-ethylphenol and a range of phenolic acids. These metabolites are absorbed from the gut and excreted in the urine. A number of these phenols, including phenol and *p*-cresol, have been shown to be promoters of chemically induced carcinogenesis in the mouse skin.[86] The amounts of volatile phenols in the urine of six patients with newly diagnosed large bowel cancer were no different from those in healthy controls;[7] faecal levels were not reported. A pilot study by head-space gas-liquid chromatography of faecal levels of phenol and *p*-cresol indicated that colon cancer patients had elevated levels of faecal *p*-cresol compared to controls, although no significant differences in phenol concentrations were apparent (Borriello, unpublished).

N-NITROSAMINE PRODUCTION

N-nitroso compounds are an extremely potent group of carcinogens which can be formed by the action of nitrite on a suitable nitrogen compound at neutral pH in the presence of bacteria. Consequently wherever nitrite, bacteria and nitrosatable amines coexist there is the potential for nitrosamine formation.

Bacterially-produced amines arise mainly from the decarboxylation of amino acids resulting in the formation of the corresponding amine with the liberation of carbon dioxide. In addition ethylamine, trimethylamine and dimethylamine can be formed by N-dealkylation of choline which is a product of the metabolism of lecithin. Therefore two of the components required for the formation of nitros-amines (bacteria and nitrosatable amines) are present in the colon; and the bacteria present that can form these amine metabolites are present in higher numbers in the faeces of colon cancer patients compared to controls.[52] It is more difficult to assess if the third component, nitrite (or nitrate which is readily reduced to nitrite by microbial nitro-reductase), is present in the large bowel and available for nitrosamine formation. It is thought that in humans most dietary nitrate is rapidly absorbed and excreted in the urine, so that little would be expected to reach the large bowel.[25] In addition if any nitrate or nitrite reached the large bowel it would probably be quickly degraded by microbial nitrate and nitrite reductase. However, it is the opinion of this author that some nitrate or nitrite could be available in the large bowel for nitrosamine formation, and that the most likely source would be from colonic secretions, as nitrate has been shown to be present in other body secretions that have been investigated, such as stomach and saliva. However, although a possible N-nitroso mutagen has been demonstrated in human faeces[84] more exacting methods that are free of artifactual synthesis of nitrosamines indicate that none are to be found in stool.[89]

Because organotrophic N-nitroso compounds are precarcinogens that require activation to yield the ultimate carcinogen, N-nitroso compounds formed at other sites in the body may reach the large bowel where they are subsequently activated. However, there is no good epidemiological or animal model evidence to link dietary nitrate levels or nitrosamines with colon carcinogenesis, and nitrosamines have been shown to be remarkably stable in faecal emulsions *in vitro*.[89] The situation in patients with ureterosigmoid anastamosis is rather unique and pertinent to the nitrosamine-colorectal cancer story. The diversion of urine, which is rich in both nitrate and nitrosatable amine, into the colon of these patients presents a situation where relatively large amounts of nitrate, nitro-satable amine and nitrite forming bacteria coexist. This would appear to be a situation ideally suited to the *in vivo* production of N-nitroso compounds. There is evidence that these patients are at an increased risk of developing colonic adenocarcinoma,[83] and that their 'faeces' are a rich source of mutagens.[45]

However, mutagens and co-carcinogens other than the N-nitroso class could also be produced in these patients.

Retoxification of hepatic metabolites of environmental polycyclic aromatic hydrocarbons

Polycyclic aromatic hydrocarbons (PAH) such as benzo(a)-pyrene, arise mainly from the combustion of organic matter, and they are widely distributed in nature. Many of these PAH are known to undergo entero-hepatic circulation and are detoxified in the liver to appear in bile, principally as glucuronide or sulphate conjugates. These would be deconjugated in the large bowel by microbial β-glucuronidase and sulphatase activity to release hydroxy-PAHs, which are themselves noncarcinogenic. However, after deconjugation some bacteria are able to dehydroxylate the hydroxy-PAH product and release the parent car-cinogen. This has been demonstrated for rat and human faecal flora for bile metabolites of benzo(a)-pyrene and, it was also shown that the bacteria that released the greatest amounts of parent hydrocarbon were *C. paraputrificum*,[75] which are found more frequently in the faeces of colorectal cancer patients and subjects at high risk for the development of this disease.

POTENTIAL MICROBIAL CARCINOGENS OF UNKNOWN ORIGIN

Some of the most exciting work to have emerged recently is the description of a mutagen in human faeces[11,27] which is mutagenic for *Salmonella typhimurium* TA-100 without microsomal activation in the Ames mutagenicity assay.[1] Data on the prevalence of this mutagen in the faeces of high and low risk populations is a little confusing. In a case control study the proportion of individuals with measurable levels of faecal mutagen in 17 patients with colon cancer and 17 age-matched control patients with haemorrhoids, was the same in the two groups.[10] Analysis of faeces from high and low risk groups on an intranational basis has shown that more individuals in a population at high risk for colorectal cancer (white South Africans) excreted mutagen in their faeces than did individuals in a population at low risk (black South Africans[27]). Although a positive correlation between the presence of this mutagen and colorectal cancer has not yet been demonstrated, it remains an intriguing observation that may well prove to have some bearing on the aetiology of this disease.

Preliminary evidence indicates that gut bacteria play a role in the production of this mutagen.[85] However it has not proved possible to identify which organisms are involved, mainly as a result of trying to work with three unknowns — an unidentified mutagen, an unknown precursor and no indication of which group of organisms is involved. In the opinion of this author a fruitful line of research to unravel this problem would be to look at the effect of antibiotic administration on faecal levels of mutagen in known excretors. If a significant reduction of faecal mutagen concentration occurs then one would hope that its precursor(s) would be present in these faeces. Coincubation of these 'precursor laden faeces' with whole faecal flora or various individual genera of micro-organism should result in mutagen production and yield valuable information with respect to which organisms are involved.

CONCLUSION

It is quite obvious that components of the gastrointestinal flora can produce compounds with carcinogenic, co-carcinogenic and mutagenic activity, and that some of these compounds can be found in human faeces. To what extent these compounds are involved in the aetiology of colorectal cancer is still far from certain, although it is likely that one of these microbially produced products may play a role in the aetiology of this disease in some cases. Certainly, if gut bacteria are ever shown to be involved in the aetiology of adenomatous polyps or ulcerative colitis, both diseases carrying an increased risk for the development of colorectal cancer, then gut bacteria could be at least indirectly involved in the aetiology of colorectal cancer.

To date most of the work in this field has concentrated on the production of compounds involved in induction of the disease and little work has been done on the production of possible protective factors that may be absent in the faeces of colorectal cancer patients and high risk subjects. In this respect the recent description of lignans in man,[79,82] and the observation that they may be produced by human gut bacteria[78] is of interest, as plant lignans have been used, with some success, for the treatment of cancer.[77]

It is hoped that work in progress around the world will yield more information relating to a possible association between the gastrointestinal flora and the aetiology of colorectal cancer and thus indicate possible methods of prevention of the disease.

REFERENCES

1   Ames B. N., McCann J. and Yamasaki E. (1975) Method for detecting carcinogens and mutagens with the salmonella/mammalian microsome mutagenicity test. *Mutation Res.* **31**, 347.

2   Aries V. C., Crowther J. S., Drasar B. S., Hill M. J. and Williams R. E. O. (1969) Bacteria and the aetiology of cancer of the large bowel. *Gut* **10**, 334.

3   Aries V. C., Goddard P. and Hill M. J. (1971) Degradation of steroids by intestinal bacteria. III. 3-oxo-5β — steroid Δ^1 — dehydrogenase and 3-oxo-5β — steroid Δ^4 — dehydrogenase. *Biochim. Biophys. Acta* **248**, 482.

4   Armstrong B. and Doll R. (1975) Environmental factors and cancer incidence and mortality in different countries with special reference to dietary practices. *Int. J. Cancer* **15**, 617.

5   Bacon H. E. and Eisenberg S. W. (1971) Papillary adenoma of villous tumor of the rectum and colon. *Ann. Surg.* **174**, 1002.

6   Bone E., Drasar B. S. and Hill M. J. (1975) Gut bacteria and their metabolic activities in familial polyposis. *Lancet* i, 1117.

7   Bone E., Tamm A. and Hill M. (1976) The production of urinary phenols by gut bacteria and their possible role in the causation of large bowel cancer. *Am. J. Clin. Nutr.* **29**, 1448.

8   Borriello S. P. (1981) Clostridial flora of the gastrointestinal tract in health and disease, PhD Thesis, University of London.

9   Borriello S. P., Drasar B. S., Tomkins A. and Hill M. J. (1983) Relative carriage rates of nuclear dehydrogenating clostridia in two populations of different colorectal cancer risk. *J. Clin. Pathol.* **36**, 93

10 Bruce W. R. and Dion P. W. (1980) Studies relating to a fecal mutagen. *Am. J. Clin. Nutr.* **33**, 2511.

11 Bruce W. R., Vorghese A. J., Furrer R. and Land P. C. (1977) A mutagen in human feces. In: *Origins of human cancer*, p. 1641, Eds H. H. Hiatt, J. D. Watson and J. A. Winstein, Cold Spring Harbor, New York.

12 Bryan G. T. (1971) The role of urinary tryptophan metabolites in the aetiology of bladder cancer. *Am. J. Clin. Nutr.* **24**, 841.

13 Buell P. and Dunn J. E. (1965) Cancer mortality among Japanese issii and nisei of California. *Cancer* **18**, 656.

14 Burkitt D. P. (1971) Epidemiology of cancer of the colon and rectum. *Cancer* **28**, 3.

15 Burkitt D. P. (1974) An epidemiological approach to cancer of the large intestine. *Dis. Colon Rectum* **17**, 456.

16 Chomchai C., Bhadrachari N. and Nigro N. D. (1974) The effect of bile on the induction of experimental intestinal tumors in rats. *Dis. Colon Rectum* **17**, 310.

17 Coombs M. M., Bhatt T. S. and Crofts C. J. (1973) Correlation between carcinogenicity and chemical structure in cyclopentaphenanthrene. *Cancer Res.* **33**, 832.

18 Correa P., Duque E., Cuello C., *et al.* (1972) Polyps of the colon and rectum in Cali, Colombia. *Int. J. Cancer* **9**, 86.

19 Cowen A. E., Korman M. G., Hofmann A. F. and Cass O. W. (1975) Metabolism of Lithocholate in healthy man. I. Biotransformation and biliary excretion of intravenously administered lithocholate, lithocholylglycine, and their sulfates. *Gastroenterology* **69**, 59.

20 Crowther J. S., Drasar B. S., Hill M. J., MacLennan, R., Magnin D., Peach S. and Teoh-Chan C. H. (1976) Faecal steroids and bacteria and large bowel cancer in Hong-Kong by socio-economic groups. *Br. J. Cancer* **34**, 191.

21 Demerec M. (1948) Mutations induced by carcinogens. *Br. J. Cancer* **2**, 114.

22 Doll R. (1969) The geographical distribution of cancer. *Br. J. Cancer* **23**, 1.

23 Doll R., Muir C. S. and Waterhouse J. (1970) *Cancer in Five Continents*, vol. 2, Springer-Verlag, Berlin.

24 Drasar B. S., Goddard P., Heaton S., Peach S. and West B (1976) Clostridia isolated from faeces. *J. Med. Microbiol* **9**, 63.

25 Drasar B. S. and Hill M. J. (1974) *Human Intestinal Flora*, Academic Press, London.

26 Drasar B. S. and Irving D. (1973) Environmental factors and cancer of the colon and breast. *Br. J. Cancer* **27**, 167.

27 Ehrich M., Aswell J. E., Van Tassell R. L., Walker A. R. P., Richardson N. J. and Wilkins T. D. (1979) Mutagens in the feces of 3 South-African populations at different levels of risk for colon cancer. *Mutation Res.* **64**, 231.

28 Enterline H. T. (1974) Pathology of colonic polyps as it relates to surgical management. *Ann. Clin. Lab. Sci.* **4**, 145.

29 Farber E. (1963) Ethionine carcinogenesis. *Adv. Cancer Res.* **7**, 383.

30 Fieser L. F. (1954) Some aspects of the chemistry and biochemistry of cholesterol. *Science* **119**, 710.

31 Finegold S. M., Flora D. J., Attebury H. R. and Sutter V. L. (1975) Fecal bacteriology of colonic polyp patients and control patients. *Cancer Res.* **35**, 3407.

32 Fisher J. F. and Mallette M. F. (1961) The natural occurrence of ethionine in bacteria. *J. Gen. Physiol.* **45**, 1.

33 Goddard P., Fernandez F., West B., Hill M. J. and Barnes P. (1975) The nuclear dehydrogenation of steroids by intestinal bacteria. *J. Med. Microbiol.* **8**, 429.

34 Goddard P. and Hill M. J. (1972) Degradation of steroids by intestinal bacteria IV. The aromatisation of ring A. *Biochim. Biophys. Acta* **280**, 336.

35 Goddard P. and Hill M. J. (1973) The dehydrogenation of the steroid nucleus by human-gut bacteria. *Biochem. Soc. Trans.* **1**, 1113.

36 Gregor O., Toman R. and Prusova F. (1969) Gastrointestinal cancer and nutrition. *Gut* **10**, 1031.

37 Haenszel W. (1961) Cancer mortality among the foreign born in the US. *J. Natl Cancer Inst.* **26**, 37.

38 Haenszeal W., Berg J. W., Segal M., Kurihara M. and Locke F. B. (1973) Large bowel cancer in Hawaiian Japanese. *J. Natl Cancer Inst.* **51**, 1765.

39 Haenszel W. and Kurihara M. (1968) Mortality from cancer and other diseases among Japanese in the United States. *J. Natl Cancer Inst.* **40**, 43.

40 Hiasa Y., Konishi Y., Kamamoto Y., Watanabe T. and Ito N. (1971) Effect of lithocholic acid on DL-ethionine carcinogenesis in rat liver. *Gann* **62**, 239.

41 Higginson J. (1968) The theoretical possibilities of cancer prevention in man. *Proc. R. Soc. Med.* **61**, 723.

42 Hill M. J. (1971) Gut bacteria, steroids and cancer of the large bowel. In: *Some Implications of Steroid Hormones in Cancer*, p. 94, Eds D. C Williams and M. H. Briggs, Heinemann, London.

43 Hill M. J. (1975) The etiology of colon cancer. *CRC Critical Reviews in Toxicology*, p. 31.

44 Hill M. J. (1979) Intestinal bacteria and cancer. *Ann. Ist. Super. Sanita.* **15**, 43.

45 Hill M. J. (1980) Bacterial metabolism and human carcinogenesis. *Br. Med. Bull.* **36**, 89.

46 Hill M. J., Drasar B. S., Aries V. C., Crowther J. S., Hawksworth G. B. and Williams R. E. O. (1971) Bacteria and aetiology of cancer of the large bowel. *Lancet* **i**, 95.

47 Hill M. J., Drasar B. S., Williams R. E. O., Meade T. W., Cox A. G., Simpson J. E. P. and Morson B. C. (1975) Faecal bile-acids and clostridia in patients with cancer of the large bowel. *Lancet* **i**, 535.

48 Huang C. T. L., Gopalakrishna G. S. and Nichols B. L. (1978) Fiber, intestinal sterols, and colon cancer. *Am. J. Clin. Nutr.* **31**, 516.

49 Inhoffen H. H. C. (1953) The relationship of natural steroids to carcinogenic aromatic compounds. *Prog. Org. Chem.* **2**, 131.

50 International Agency for Research on Cancer Intestinal Microecology Group (1977) Dietary fibre, transit-time, faecal bacteria, steroids and colon cancer in two Scandinavian populations. *Lancet* **i**, 207.

51 Jensen K. A., Kirk I., Kolmarg G. *et al.* (1951) Chemically induced mutations in neurospora. *Cold Spring Harbor Symp. Quant. Biol.* **16**, 245.

52 Johnson K. A. (1977) The production of secondary amines by the human gut bacteria and its possible relevance to carcinogenesis. *Med. Lab. Sci.* **34**, 131.

53 Kawalek J. C. and Andrews A. W. (1977) The effect of bile acids on the metabolism of benzo (a) pyrene and 2-aminoanthracene to mutagenic products. *Fed. Proc. Fed. Am. Socs Exp. Biol.* **36**, 844.

54 Kelsey M. I., Molina J. E. and Hwang K. K. (1979) A comparison of lithocholic acid metabolism by intestinal microflora in subjects of high − and low − risk colon cancer populations. *Front. Gastrointest. Res.* **4**, 38.

55 Kelsey M. I. and Pienta R. J. (1979) Transformation of hamster embryo cells by cholesterol-α-epoxide and lithocholic acid. *Cancer Lett.* **6**, 143.

56 Laqueur G. L. and Spatz M. (1968) Toxicology of cycasin. *Cancer. Res.* **28**, 2262.

57 Malhotra S. L. (1967) Geographical distribution of gastrointestinal cancers in India with special reference to causation. *Gut* **8**, 361.

58 Mastromarino A., Reddy B. S. and Wynder E. L. (1976) Metabolic epidemiology of colon cancer; enzymic activity of fecal flora. *Am. J. Clin. Nutr.* **29**, 1455.

59 Morson B. (1974) The polyp-cancer sequence in the large bowel. *Proc. R. Soc. Med.* **67**, 451.

60 Morson B. (1978) *The Pathogenesis of Colorectal Cancer*, W. M. Saunders, Philadelphia.

61 Moskovitz M., White C., Barnett R. N. *et al.* (1979) Diet, fecal bile acids, and neutral sterols in carcinoma of the colon. *Dig. Dis. Sci.* **24**, 746.

62 Mower H. F., Ray R. M. and Shoff R. *et al.* (1979) Fecal bile acids in two Japanese populations with different colon cancer risks. *Cancer Res.* **39**, 328.

63 Narisawa T., Magadia N. E., Weisburger J. H. and Wynder E. L. (1974) Promoting effects of bile acids on colon carcinogenesis after intrarectal instillation of N-methyl-N-nitro-N-nitrosoguanidine in rats. *J. Natl Cancer Inst.* **53**, 1093.

64 Nigro N. D., Bhadrachari N. and Chomchai C. (1973) A rat model for studying colonic cancer: effect of cholestyramine on induced tumors. *Dis. Colon Rectum.* **16**, 438.

65 Palmer R. H. (1972) Metabolism of lithocholate in humans. In: *Bile Ducts in Human Disease* (Back and Gerok), p. 65, Shattauer, Stuttgart.

66 Palmer R. H. (1972) Bile acids, liver injury and liver disease. *Archs. Intern. Med.* **130**, 606.

67 Phillips R. L. (1974) Cancer and Adventists. *Science* **183**, 471.

68 Reddy B. S., Hedges A., Laakso K. and Wynder E. L. (1978) Fecal constituents of a high-risk north American and a low-risk Finnish population for the development of large bowel cancer. *Cancer Lett.* **4**, 217.

69 Reddy B. S., Martin C. W. and Wynder E. L. (1977) Fecal bile acids and cholesterol metabolites of patients with ulcerative colitis, a high risk group for the development of colon cancer. *Cancer Res.* **37**, 1697.

70 Reddy B. S., Narisawa T., Maronpot R., Weisburger J. H. and Wynder E. L. (1975) Animal models for the study of dietary factors and cancer of the large bowel. *Cancer Res.* **35**, 3421.

71 Reddy B. S., Weisburger J. H., and Wynder E. L. (1975) Effects of high risk and low risk diets for colon carcinogenesis on fecal microflora and steroids in man. *J. Nutr.* **105**, 878.

72 Reddy B. S., Weisburger J. H. and Wynder E. L. (1978) Colon Cancer: Bile Salts as Tumor Promoters: In: *Carcinogenesis Vol. 2. Mechanisms of Tumor Promotion and Cocarcinogenesis*, Eds T. J. Slaga, A. Sivak and R. K. Boutwell, Raven Press, New York.

73 Reddy B. S. and Wynder E. L. (1973) Large bowel carcinogenesis: Fecal constituents of populations with diverse incidence rates of colon cancer. *J. Natl Cancer Inst.* **50**, 1437.

74 Reddy B. S. and Wynder E. L. (1977) Metabolic epidemiology of colon cancer. Fecal bile acids and neutral sterols in colon cancer patients and patients with adenomatous polyps. *Cancer* **39**, 2533.

75 Renwick A. G. and Drasar B. S. (1976) Environmental carcinogens and large bowel cancer. *Nature* **263**, 234.

76 Rose D. P. (1967) The influence of sex, age and breast cancer on tryptophan metabolism. *Clin. Chim. Acta.* **18**, 221.

77 Savel H. (1964) Clinical experience with intravenous podophyllotoxin. *Proc. Am. Ass. Cancer Res.* **5**, 56.

78 Setchell K. D. R., Lawson A. M., Borriello S. P. *et al.* (1981) Lignan formation in man — microbial involvement and possible roles in relation to cancer. *Lancet* **ii**, 4.

79 Setchell K. D. R., Lawson A. M., Mitchell F. L., Adlercreutz H., Kirk D. N. and Axelson M. (1980) Lignans in man and animal species. *Nature* **287**, 741.

80 Silverman S. J. and Andrews A. W. (1977) Bile acids: co-mutagenic activity using the Salmonella/mammalian-microsome mutagenicity test. *J. Natl Cancer Inst.* **59**, 1557.

81 Staszewski J. and Haenszel W. (1965) Cancer mortality among the Polish born in the US. *J. Natl Cancer Inst.* **35**, 291.

82 Stitch S. R., Toumba J. K., Groen M. B., Funke C. W., Leemhuis J., Vink J. and Woods G. F. (1980) Excretion isolation and structure of a new phenolic constituent of female urine. *Nature* **287**, 738.

83 Urdaneta L. F., Duffel D., Creevy C. D. and Aust J. B. (1966) Late development of primary carcinoma of the colon following ureterosigmoidostomy: report of three cases and literature review. *Ann. Surg.* **164**, 503.

84 Wang T., Kakizoe T., Dion P., Furrer R., Varghese A. J. and Bruce W. R. (1978) Volatile nitrosamines in normal human faeces. *Nature* **276**, 280.

85 Wilkins T. D., Lederman M., Van Tassell R. L., Kingston D. G. I. and Henion J. (1980) Characterization of a mutagenic bacterial product in human feces. *Am. J. Clin. Nutr.* **33**, 2513.

86 Wynder E. L. and Hoffman D. (1968) Experimental tobacco carcinogenesis. *Science* **162**, 862.

87 Wynder E. L., Kajutani T., Ishikawa S., Dodo H. and Takano A. (1969) Environmental factors of cancer of the colon and rectum. II Japanese epidemiological data. *Cancer* **23**, 1210.

88 Wynder E. L. and Shigematsu T. (1967) Environmental factors of cancer of the colon and rectum. *Cancer* **20**, 1520.

89 Lee L. J., Archer M. C. and Bruce W. R. (1981) Absence of volatile nitrosamines in human faeces. *Cancer Res.* **41**, 3992.

90 Borriello S. P. and Owen R. W. (1982) The metabolism of lithocholic acid and lithocholic acid-3-α-sulfate by human fecal bacteria. *Lipids* **17**, 477.

Index

Abscesses
  animal model 310
  antimicrobial ineffectiveness 318
Adenoviruses and diarrhoea **170** *et seq.*
  children 171
  structure 171
Adenylate cyclase and
  B. cereus 155
  C. perfringens 153
  E. coli 86, 93
  Salmonella 52
  Shigella 65
  V. cholerae 107
'Adhesins' 265
Adhesiveness
  E. coli 87, 329
  K88 87, 88, 329
  K99 88, 93
  987P 88, 93
  sIgA 10
  V. cholerae 107
Aeromonas **117** *et seq.*
  adults 118
  antibiotics 118
  children 117
  clinical features of disease 117, 118
  enterotoxin 197
  epidemiology 117, 118 122
  extra-intestinal 118
  hydrophila 117
  laboratory diagnosis 119
  oxidase test 119
  pathogenesis 118
  protection by cholera toxoid
    immunization 204
  punctata 117
  toxins 118
  water 118
'Aggressins' 265
Alkalescens-Dispar group 69
Ammonia metabolism 295
Amoebic dysentery **212** *et seq.* (and see
    Entamoeba histolytica)
  clincial features 214
  control 216
  epidemiology 213
  laboratory diagnosis 215
  pathogenesis 214

serology 215
  treatment 215
Anaerobic bacteria
  in healthy gut 290
  overgrowth syndromes 310, 303
  surgical sepsis **308** *et seq.*, 319 *et seq.*
Ancylostoma duodenale 225 et seq.
Angiostrongylus costaricensis 220
Anisakis species 220
Anthelmintics 222
Antibiotics to prevent gut sepsis 316, 320,
    321
Antitoxin assay
  E. coli LT 89
  E. coli ST 90
  V. cholerae toxin 89
Appendicectomy and sepsis 320 (and see
    Sepsis of gut and bacteria)
Ascaris lumbricoides 209, 219, **224** *et seq.*
Astroviruses and diarrhoea 172
  animals 173
  children 172
  structure 172
Australian Aborigines and diarrhoea 189
  Campylobacter 190
  carrier rates 199
  infants 189
  Salmonella 271
  water contamination 199

Bacillus cereus gastroenteritis 149, **154** *et
    seq.*
  causative organism 154
  clinical features 155
  control 156
  enterotoxins 155
  epidemiology 154
  laboratory diagnosis 155
  milk 278
  rice 154, 278
Bacitracin and PMC 333
Bacterial overgrowth syndromes
  aetiological factors 286
  breath tests 299
  direct tests 300
  indirect tests 299
  malabsorption 298 *et seq.* (and see
    Malabsorption)

sample collection   310
sample processing   303
treatment   302
tropical sprue   287
urinary indican   300
Bacteroides fragilis in
  healthy colon   293
  sepsis of gut   308 *et seq.*
  virulence factor   310
Baird-Parker medium
  in staphylococcal gastroenteritis   152
Balantidium coli   212
Bephenium hydroxynaphthoate for
  nematodes   220, 222
Bicozamycin for traveller's diarrhoea   284
Bifidobacterium in
  neonate   2
  adult   293
Bifidus factor   8
Biken test   89
Bile acids and colon cancer   349 et seq.,
    353 *et seq.* (see also Colon cancer and
    bacteria)
Bile salts (see also Colon cancer and
    bacteria)
  breath tests for malabsorption   299
  colon cancer   349 *et seq.*
  deconjugation   294
  steatorrhoea   194
  urinary indican test for
    malabsorption   300
'Bili-vaccination' for typhoid   256
Bismuth subsalicylate for
  E. coli diarrhoea   93
  traveller's diarrhoea   284
Bismuth—sulphite medium   54, 136
'Blind-loop' syndrome   290, 297 (and see
    Bacterial overgrowth syndromes)
Borborygimi   296
Borrelia sp.   293

Caliciviruses and diarrhoea   173
  animals   173
  serotypes   173
  structure   173
Campylobacter **55** *et seq.*
  animals   57, 58, 190
  antibiotics   59
  biotypes   56, 57
  bubulus   56
  carriers   190
  catalase test   56, 60
  clinical features   58
  coli   56
  colonies   58

dogs   190
enterotoxins   58
epidemiology   56
fetus   55
food-borne   57
identification   55
incidence   56
jejuni   56, 57
laboratory investigations   59
meat contamination   278
media   59
milk   57
mucolsalis   56
naladixic acid resistant   59
outbreak   271
pathogenesis   57
poultry   57, 248
Sereny test   58
serotyping   60
Skirrow's medium   59
sputorum   55
thermophilic   56, 59
treatment
venerealis   56
Cancer of colon (see Colon cancer and
    bacteria)
Capillaria philippenensis   220
Carcinoma of colon (see Colon cancer and
    bacteria)
Cary-Blair medium   109
Cercariae of *S. mansoni*   229
Cestodes **234** *et seq.*
  D. latum   234
  D. caninum   235
  H. diminuta   235
  H. nana   235
  T. saginata   234
  T. solium   236
Childhood gastroenteritis **187** *et seq.*
  Aborigines in Australia   189
  Campylobacter   190
  deaths   188
  enterotoxigenic bacteria   191 *et seq.*
  extent   188
  gastrointestinal mucosa   197
  lactose intolerance   198
  malnutrition   187, 198, 192, 197, 201
  monosaccharide absorption   195
  parasites   192
  prevention   201
  steatorrhoea   194
  upper intestine contamination   193 *et
    seq.*
  viruses **160** *et seq.*,   191
  water contamination, relation to   199

Chinese hamster ovary (CHO) cells and
    E. coli 89
    Salmonella 52
Cholera **104** *et seq.*, 258
    antibiotics 111, 254
    carriers 105, 110
    clinical features 104
    chlorpromazine 111
    control 111
    El Tor cholera 104
    epidemics 104, 105, 108
    food-borne 108
    immunization 111
    laboratory diagnosis 109
    lactating women 112
    oral-rehydration therapy 110
    outbreak control 111
    pathogenesis **105**, 190, 259
    public health measures 111
    serological diagnosis 110
    toxins 106
    toxoid 112
    treatment 110
    vaccine 108, 111
    Vibrio cholerae (see *Vibrio cholerae*)
    water-borne 108
Cholera-red colour 105
    cholera toxin (choleragen) 89, 195, 106,
        107
Cholesterol and colon cancer 355
CLED medium and vibrios 115
Clonorchis sineses 230
Clostridium beijerinkii and PMC 336
Clostridium botulinum and
    food 277
    infant botulism **13** *et seq.*
Clostridium butyricum in necrotizing
        enterocolitis 17
Clostridium difficile **327** *et seq.* (see also
        Pseudomembranous colitis)
    age 330
    alteration of gut flora 335
    bacitracin 333
    β-glucosidase 336
    clinical features 328
    cross-infection 294
    counterimmune electrophoresis 340
    cytotoxin 328 *et seq.*, 338, 339, **341**
    detection 339
    diarrhoea 330
    enterotoxin 338
    enzyme immunoassay 341
    hamster 329, 333, 335
    healthy gut 331
    identification 339

infant gut 294, 328
inhibition by faecal bacteria 336
ion-binding resins 334
isolation from faeces 339
Lactobacillus acidophilus 336
metronidazole 333
necrotizing enterocolitis 17
p-cresol 336, 339
pathogenesis of disease 328
prevention of colonization 337
second toxin 338
tetracycline 334
toxins, comparison 338
treatment 331 *et seq.*
vancomycin 332
Clostridium paraputrificum and colon
        cancer 353, 358
Clostridium perfringens
    clinical features of gastroenteritis 153
    enterotoxins 152
    incubation of gastroenteritis 149, 150
    laboratory diagnosis of
        gastroenteritis 153
    meat, and 278
    necrotizing enterocolitis 16
    outbreaks of gastroenteritis 152
    pathogenesis of gastroenteritis 153
    prevention of gastroenteritis 153
    serotyping 153
    water 275
Colicine-typing of *S. sonnei* 72
Coliform counts in water 272, **274** *et seq.*
    outbreak of *Campylobacter* 272
Colon bacteria in health 290, 292 (see also
        Sepsis of gut and bacteria and Colon
        cancer and bacteria)
Colon cancer and bacteria 295, **347** *et seq.*
    adenomas 350
    animals 349, 353, 357, 358
    bile acids 349 *et seq.*, 351, 353
    carcinogens 349 *et seq.*, 355 *et seq.*
    cholesterol 355
    C. paraputrificum 353
    co-carcinogens 349 *et seq.*, 355 *et seq.*
    cycasin 349
    deaths per annum 346
    deoxycholic acid 355
    diet 348 *et seq.*
    entero-hepatic circulation 358
    epidemiology 348
    ethionine 357
    faecal bile acids 351
    faecal steriods 349 *et seq.*
    fat in diet 349
    fibre in diet 349

international studies 352
lignans 360
lithocholic acid 353, **354** *et seq.*
methionine 357
mutagen 359
NDH clostridia 350 *et seq.* 354
nitrate and nitrite 358
N-nitrosamine 357
p-cresol 357
polycyclic aromatic hydrocarbons 358
polyps 350, 355 *et seq.*
racial groups 348, 352, 356, 359
tryptophan 356
tyrosine 357
Colonization factor antigens
  I 88
  II 88
  E. coli 88
Colostrum, cells in 11
Contaminated small bowel syndrome 194
  et seq.
Coronaviruses and diarrhoea 172
  healthy people 172
  piglets 172
Cyclic AMP and
  B. cereus 155
  E. coli 86, 93
  Salmonella 52
  V. cholerae 107
Cyclic GMP and
  E. coli 87
Cysticercus of
  T. saginata 234
  T. solium 237

Deoxycholate citrate medium
  Salmonella 54
  Shigella 67
  S. typhi 136
Deoxycholic acid and colon cancer 353,
  355
Dicrocoelium denditicum 230
Diphyllobothrium latum 235
Dipylidium caninum 235
Duodenal bacteria (see Jejunum bacteria)
Dysentery (see *Campylobater* and *Shigella*)

Echinostoma ilocanum 230
Electron microscopy and
  Campylobacter 58
  virus visualization 174
El Tor cholera 104, 109 (see also *Vibrio
  cholerae*
Hong Kong outbreak 106, 109

Entamoeba histolytica 209, 212 *et seq.*
  (and see Amoebic dysentery)
  control 216
  epidemiology 213
  laboratory diagnosis 215
  life cycle 213
  morphology 213
  pathogenesis 290
  pathogenicity 212
  taxonomy 212
  treatment 215
  water borne 274
Entamoeba species 213
  hartmanni 213, 216
  histolytica (see *Entamoeba histolytica*)
  invadens 213
  moshkovskii 213
  poleki 213
Enteric fever (see Paratyphoid fever and
  Typhoid fever)
Enterobacteriaceae 54, 68, 69, 8?
Enterobius vermicularis **219** *et seq.*
Enterochelins 11
Enteroinvasive *E. coli* (EIEC)
  antibiotics 92
  biochemical reactions 91
  epidemiology 90
  laboratory investigation 91
  pathogenesis 91
  Sereny test 92
  Shigella likeness 91
  treatment 92
  vaccines 92
Enteropathogenic *E. coli* (EPEC) —
  infantile
  epidemiology 80
  heat-labile toxin (LT)
  heat-stable toxin (ST)
  hospitals 79, 81
  laboratory investigations 83
  outbreaks 83
  pathogenesis 82
  serogroups 80
  summer diarrhoea 80
  toxins 80, 82
  water borne 82
Enterotoxigenic bacteria 196, 197
  and see under individual bacteria
  Aeromonas 117 *et seq.*
  E. coli 86 *et seq.*
  V. cholerae 103 *et seq.*
Enterotoxigenic *E. coli* (ETEC)
  adhesive factors 87
  antisera 90

Biken test 89
CFA/I, CFA/II 88
developed countries 84
developing countries 85
epidemiology 83, 86
Gm-1 ganglioside 89
heat-labile enterotoxin (LT) 86, 89
heat-stable enterotoxin (ST) 87, 90
infantile enteritis 83
laboratory techniques 89
K88 87, 293
K99 88
pathogenesis 190
pili 87
plasmids 87
serogroups 84
traveller's diarrhoea 84
Eosin-methylene blue agar for isolation of
    Salmonella 54
    Shigella 67
Epidemiology of
    Aeromonas enteritis 118
    amoebic dysentery 213
    ascariasis 224
    B. cereus enteritis 154
    Campylobacter enteritis 56
    C. difficile gut disease 329
    childhood gastroenteritis 188
    cholera 108
    clostridial gastroenteritis 152
    colon cancer 348
    enteroinvasive *E. coli* 90
    enteropathogenic *E. coli* 81
    enterotoxigenic *E. coli* 83
    giardiasis 217
    hookworm 226
    nematodes 221
    non-cholera vibrios 114
    P. shigelloides 121
    salmonellosis 49
    S. japonicum 223
    S. mansoni 229
    Shigella dysentery 62
    staphylococcal gastroenteritis 150
    strongyloidiasis 228
    trichuriasis 223
    T. saginata 225
    T. solium 237
    tuberculosis of gut 248
    typhoid fever 130
    V. parahaemolyticus 115
    Yersinia 242
Escherichia coli **79** *et seq.* (see also
    Enteroinvasive *E. coli*,
    Enteropathogenic *E. coli* and

Enterotoxigenic *E. coli*)
Aberdeen alpha and beta 79
enteroinvasive 80, 90 (and see
    Enteroinvasive *E. coli*)
enteropathogenic 80 (and see
    Enteropathogenic *E. coli*)
enterotoxigenic 80, 83 (and see
    Enterotoxigenic *E. coli*)
enterotoxin 80
healthy gut 293
heat-labile toxin 80, 86, 89, 93
heat-stable toxin 80, 90, 93
inhibition of enterotoxin activity 93
K88 antigen 87, 293
K99 antigen 88
leukaemia and signs 313
serotyping 79, 80
water, in 275
Eubacterium aerofaciens 293

Fasciola species 230
Fasciolopsis 230
Flagellar (H) antigens
    E. coli 81
    phase — I of *Salmonella* 55
    phase — II of *Salmonella* 55
    Salmonella 55, 136
    S. typhi, relationship to vaccine 256
Food-borne disease
    breast milk and protection 277
    control 277
    G. lambhe 282
    meat 278
    outbreak investigation 281
Food-handlers
    examination 279
    gastroenteritis 279
    Salmonella 51
    Shigella 62
Fusobacterium prausnitzii 293

Gastrodiscoides hominis 230
Gastrointestinal mucosa
    ammonia metabolism by flora 295
    bacterial flora 293
    malnutrition 197
Giardia lamblia 209, **216** *et seq.*
    clinical features 218
    epidemiology 217
    food-borne 282
    laboratory diagnosis 218
    life cycle 216
    morphology 216
    outbreak 271
    pathogenesis 217

taxonomy
  treatment 218
  water-borne 271
Gm-l ganglioside and
  E. coli 86, 89
  V. cholerae 107
Gram Negative (GN) both for
  Shigella 67
Granulocytopaenia (see Leukemia and
  sepsis)
Guanylate cyclase and
  E. coli 87
Gut associated lymphoid tissue
  (GALT) 6, 27, **33** *et seq.*
  cell-mediated immunity 40
  development 36
  immune responses 37, 261
  immunoglobulins 28, 261
  interepithelial lymphoid tissue 33, 40
  J-chain 6, 28–29
  lamina propria 33
  mesenteric lymphnodes 35
  morphology 33
  Peyers patches 32, **34**, 38
  plasma cells 33
  T cells 34, 38–40
  theliolymphocytes 33

Halophilic vibrios 103, 113
  lactose-positive 115
  Vibrio parahaemolyticus 114
Healthy gut bacteria **290** *et seq.*
  different regions 292
  selection factors 291
Heat-labile enterotoxin (LT) of
  Aeromonas 118
  B. cereus 155
  Campylobacter 58
  detection 89
  E. coli **86**
  Salmonella 52
  V. cholerae 106
Heat-stable enterotoxin (ST) of
  Aeromonas 118
  B. cereus 155
  Campylobacter 58
  E. coli 90
  Salmonella 52
Heiberg vibrio groups 113
Hektoen enteric medium 54
Helminthic infections 209, **218** *et seq.*
  enterobiasis 219
  nematodes 219, *et seq.*
  trematodes 229 *et seq.*
Heterophyes heterophyes 230

Hexylresorcinol for nematodes 230
Hookworm infection 209, **225** *et seq.*
Hymenolepis diminuta 235
Hymenolepis nana 235

IgG (see Immunoglobulins of the intestine)
IgM (see Immunoglobulins of the intestine)
Ileal loop model to detect toxins of
  Aeromonas 118
  B. cereus 155
  C. perfringens 153
  E. coli 80, 82, 86, 90
  P. shigelloides 121
  Shigella 65
  V. cholerae 107
  V. parahaemolyticus 116
Ileum bacteria in health 290, 292 (see also
  Jejunum bacteria)
Immunoelectron microscopy for diarrhoea
  viruses **175** *et seq.*, 273
Immunoglobulins in
  milk 9
  serum 30
Immunoglobulins of the intestine **28** *et
  seq.*
  biliary route 32
  concentration 29
  IgA 6, 10, 28
  IgG 28
  IgM 28
  monomeric Igs 31
  polymeric Igs 32
  secretory IgA 28
  transport to the lumen 31
Inaba serotype of *V. cholerae* **105**, 258
Infant botulism **13** *et seq.*
  clinical features 14
  pathogenesis 13
  treatment 14
Infant gut flora, development of **1** *et seq.*
  breast milk 7
  diet 4
  factors controlling 3
  gastric barrier 4
  immunological factors 6
  maternal factors 7
  non-immunological factors 3
  secretions 5
Infantile enteritis and
  E. coli 79
  rotaviruses 168
Infant mouse test and
  Aeromonas 117, 118, 197
  E. coli 80, 90, 93
  Plesiomonas 121

Interepithelial lymphoid tissue 33
Intestinal lymphoid system (see Gut
    associated lymphoid tissue)
Intestinal microecology **192** *et seq.*
'Invasins' 265
Iodochlorhydroxyquine
    (entero-vioform) 284

J-chain of sIgA (see Gut associated
    lymphoid tissue)
Jejunum bacteria in
    health 290, 292
    processing of samples 303
    tropical sprue 298
    sample collection in malabsorption 301
John Snow and cholera 108, 201

Kanagawa phenomenon
    and *V. parahaemolyticus* 115–116
Katayama fever 233
Kauffmann—White scheme for
    Salmonella 55

Lactobacillus acidophilus and PMC 336
Lactoferrin 9
Lactoperoxidase 8
Lactose intolerance 198
Larvae of
    A. duodenale 226
    A. lumbricoides 224
    N. americanus 226
    S. stercoralis 227
    T. trichiura 223
Leukemia and sepsis 312
    antimicrobials **323** *et seq.*
    pathogens 312
    preventive antimicrobials 314, 325
    prophylaxis 314, 325
Levamisole for nematodes 222
Lignans and cancer 360
Lithocholic acid and colon cancer 353,
    354
LT (see Heat-labile enterotoxin)
Lymphocytes (see Gut associated lymphoid
    tissue)
Lysozyme 8

MacConkey medium for
    E. coli 83
    Shigella 67
Malabsorption 290 (and see Bacterial
    overgrowth syndromes)
    clinical presentations 298
    diagnosis 299
Malnutrition (see Childhood gastroenteritis)

Meat and
    food-borne disease 278
    inspection 278
Mebendazole for nematodes 220 *et seq.*
Mesenteric adenitis due to *Yersinia*
    species 245
Mesenteric lymph nodes 35
Metabolism of drugs by gut bacteria 295
Metagonimus yokogawi 230
Methionine and colon cancer 357
Methylene-blue reduction test of milk 277
Metronidazole for
    amoebic dysentery 216
    giardiasis 218
    overgrowth syndromes 302
    prevention of gut sepsis 316, 318, 320
    pseudomembranous colitis 333
Milk
    antibodies 10, 11
    bacteriological examination of 276
    bifidus factor 8
    breast milk 8, 277
    Campylobacter 57
    cells 11
    contamination 276
    lactoferrin 11
    lactoperoxidase 8
    lysozyme 8
    pasteurization 277
    Salmonella 276
    ultra-heat treated 277
    Yersinia in 241, 243
Miracidia 229
Monosaccharide absorption
    enteric organisms' effects 195
Mutant-hybrid (MH) vaccines for
    Shigella 263
Mycobacterium tuberculosis of gut 241,
    248 (and see Tuberculosis of gut)

Natural antibodies 36
Necator americanus 225 *et seq.*
Necrotizing enterocolitis 15 *et seq.*
    aminoglycosides 18
    cross-infection 18
    C. difficile 17
    C. perfringens 16
    diagnosis 18
    microbes associated 16
    prevention 18
    treatment 18
    Nematodes **219** *et seq.*
    A. costaricensis 220
    A. duodenale 225
    A. lumbricoides 224

Anisakis species   220
C. philippinensis   220
E. vermicularis   219
hookworms   225
N. americanus   225
S. stercoralis   227
Trichostrongylus species   220
T. trichiuris   223
Neutropaenia and sepsis (see Leukaemia and sepsis)
Niclosamide for cestodes   235, 236, 238
N-nitrosamine and colon cancer   357
Niridazole for nematodes   230, 233
Non-cholera vibrios   103, **113**
   clinical features   113
   epidemiology   114
   pathogenesis   114
   treatment   114
Non-halophilic vibrios   103
Normal gut bacteria (see Healthy gut bacteria)
Norwalk agent (virus) diarrhoea   165, **166** *et seq.*
   incubation   166
   oysters   166, 273
Nuclear dehydrogenating clostridia and colon cancer   350 *et seq.*

Ogawa serotype of *V. cholerae*   **105**, 258
Oncomelania snails   233
Operations and gut sepsis   308, 323 (and see also Sepsis of gut and bacteria)
   antimicrobials   321
   classification   317
   colo-rectal surgery   318
   prophylaxis   314 et seq.
   reduction of colonic flora   315
Opisthorchis species   230
Oral-rehydration therapy   **202**, and in cholera   110
   rationale   106
   virus diarrhoea   164
Outbreaks of gastroenteritis   280, **281** *et seq.*
Overgrowth by bacteria (see Bacterial overgrowth syndromes)
Oxaminquine for *S. mansoni*   232

Paratyphoid fever   **135** *et seq.* (and see Typhoid fever)
   carriers   135
   clinical features   135
   food-borne   135
   laboratory diagnosis   135
   S. paratyphi A   135

S. paratyphi B   135
S. paratyphi C   135
Parvoviruses and diarrhoea   174
   animals   174
   children   174
   structure   174
Pasteurization of milk   277
Pathogenesis of
   Aeromonas gastroenteritis   118
   amoebic dysentery   214
   ascariasis   224
   B. cereus gastroenteritis   155
   Camphylobacter enteritis   155
   C. difficile gut disease   328
   cholera   105
   clostridial gastroenteritis   153
   enteroinvasive *E. coli*   91
   enteropathogenic *E. coli*   82
   giardiasis   217
   hookworm   226
   infant botulism   13
   nematode infections   221
   non-cholera vibrios   114
   P. shigelloides enteritis   121
   salmonellosis   52
   S. japonicum infection   223
   S. mansoni infection   231
   Shigella dysentery   64
   staphylococcal gastroenteritis   151
   strongyloidiasis   228
   T. saginata   235
   T. solium   237
   traveller's diarrhoea   84
   trichuriasis   223
   typhoid fever   131
   viral diarrhoea   160
   V. parahaemolyticus   115
   Yersinia   243
Pathogenetic mechanisms of diarrhoea   190 (see also under individual diseases)
Peptostreptococcus productus   293
Peyers patches   **34**
   IgA   6, 32
   immunoglobulins   32, 34
   S. typhi   131
Phage typing
   Salmonella   55
   Shigella   72
Piperazine for nematodes   222
Plasmids
   E. coli   94
Plesiomonas shigelloides   119, **120** *et seq.*
   antibiotics   121
   chemical features   120

epidemics 120
epidemiology 121
laboratory diagnosis 121
pathogenesis 121
treatment 121
water 118
Polycyclic aromatic hydrocarbons and
    colon cancer 328
Polyps and colon cancer 350
Poultry
    Campylobacter 57, 278
    Salmonella 49
Proglottids of
    T. saginata 234
    T. solium 237
Prophylaxis of sepsis (and see Sepsis of gut
    and bacteria and Leukaemia and
    sepsis)
    in leukemia 314, 315
    in surgery of the gut 314 *et seq.*
Prostaglandins and
    Salmonella 52
    V. cholerae 107
Protozoal infections 212 *et seq.*
    B. coli 212
    C. mesnili 212
    D. fragilis 212
    E. coli 212
    E. hartmanni 212
    E. histolytica 212
    E. polecki 212
    Enteromonas 212
    G. lamblia 216
    I. butschlii 212
    Isopora sp. 212
    Trichomonas hominis 212
Pseudomembranous colitis **328** *et seq.* (see
    also *Clostridium difficile*)
    cholestyramine 334
    diagnosis 330
    faecal enemas 335
    hamster model 329
    laboratory diagnosis 339
    pathogenesis 328
    prevention 337
    steroids 337
    treatment 331 et seq.
Public health aspects of
    gastroenteritis **269** *et seq.*
    bacteriological examination of milk 276
    bacteriological examination of
        water 275
    Campylobacter 278
    C. pefringens 278
    control of enteric diseases 280

developing countries 270
drinks 283
food-borne disease 277
food-handlers 279
gut bacteria in water 270
outbreak investigation 281
outbreaks of water-borne
    gastroenteritis 271
prevention for travellers 282
Salmonella 278, 281
sanitation 274
sewage 272, 274, 282
S. aureus 279
swimming pool water 273
travellers and enteritis 282
viruses in water and sewage 272
water supplies in developing
    countries 274
Pyrantel for nematodes 222

Rappaport's medium 54
Rotaviruses
    animals 169, 177
    antibodies 179 et seq.
    disinfectants 169
    electron microscopy 174, 175, 177
    electropherotypes 183
    ELISA test 180, 182
    epidemiology 168
    immunity 169
    immunoelectron microscopy 177
    immunofluorescence 179
    laboratory isolation 169. 170
    'long' forms 183
    neutralizing antibodies 180
    RNA 182
    serological reactions 179
    serotypes 170, 182
    'short' forms 183
    structure 166
    tissue culture 177 et seq.
    transmission 168
    vaccine possibilities 169, 170

Sakazaki vibrio serotypes 113
Salmonella
    abortus-equi 49
    agona 50, 200
    animals 48, 49
    animal feeds 50
    biochemical reactions 48
    biphasic 55
    braenderup 55
    carriers 51, 198, 279
    children 50

cholerae-susis 47, 55
dublin 49
eastbourne 52
enteritidis 47, 50
enterotoxins 52
epidemiology 49
hadar 50
heidelberg 55, 200
hirschfeldii 129
host groups 49
humans 48
identification 54
isolation techniques 54
isolations in UK 49
isolations in USA 49, 52, 129
kiel 55
Kauffmann-White scheme 55
meat, in 278
oranienburg 199, 271
panama 280
paratyphi 49, 53, 55, 135, 195, 200 (and
  see Paratyphoid fever)
phage-types 50, 137
pullorum 49
ruki 55
schottmulleri 129
serotyping 54
typhi 47, 53, 55, 129, 268, 279 (and see
  Typhoid)
typhimurium 48, 50, 55
water, in 200
Salmonellosis **48** *et seq.* (and see
  Salmonella)
antibiotics in 53
clinical features 53
epidemiology 49
laboratory investigations 54
pathogenesis 52, 190
treatment 53
Sanitation requirements 274
Schistosoma intercalatum 230
Schistosoma japonicum 4229, **232** *et seq.*
Schistosoma mansoni 229 *et seq.*
Sea-water viruses 273
Secretory IgA 28
development of gut flora 6
Selenite F broth 54
  S. typhi 136
Sepsis of gut and bacteria **307** *et seq.*
animal model 310
antimicrobials **314** *et seq.*, 321
appendicectomy 320
bacteria 308 et seq.
biliary surgery 322
classification of operations 317

colo-rectal surgery 322
gastroduodenal surgery 322
host factors 311
operations requiring antimicrobial
  prophylaxis 316
pathogenesis 308
pathology 309
'prevention' 314 *et seq.*
'prophylaxis' 314, 319
timing of antimicrobials 317
virulence factors of bacteria 31
Sereny test
  Campylobacter 58
  Shigella 65
Selemonas sp. 293
Sewage
bacteriological monitoring 282
disposal 274
Sewer-swab 282
Shell-fish 280
Shiga's bacillus (*Shigella dysenteriae* 1) 60,
  64, 261
epidemics 64
Shigella 60 *et seq.*, 261 *et seq.*
ambigua 61
antibiotics 66
arabinotarda 61
biochemical reactions 67
biotypes 69
boydii 61, 64, 68
children, 62
clinical features 65
colicine typing of *sonnei* 72
dysenteriae 60, 61, 64, 68, 281
dysentery 60
epidemiology 62
enterotoxin 65, 262
etousae 61
extraintestinal 66
flexneri 61, 63, 65, 68, 70, 261
food-borne 62, 67
G-C content 69
incubation period of dysentery 65
infecting dose 65
isolations in UK 63
laboratory investigations 67
largei 61
Manchester biotype 69
metadysenteriae 69
MH vaccine
Newcastle biotype 69
pathogenesis 64, 190, 262
phage-typing 72
rabauleunsis 68
rio 61, 68

schmitzii 61
Sereny test 65
serogroups 61
serotypes 61, 69
Shigas bacillus, 60, 64, 261
shigas 61
sonnei 61, 63, 66, 68, 72, 261
S$_m$ D vaccine 62
species 61
treatment of dysentery 66
vaccines 66, **261** *et seq.*
water, and 67
Shigella-salmonella (SS) medium for
 Salmonella 54
 Shigella 67
 S. typhi 136
Skin permeability factor assay 52
Smollett, Tobias and London water 177, 200
Somatic (O) antigens
 E. coli **79** *et seq.*
 non-cholera vibrios 113
 Salmonella 55, 136
 Shigella 61
ST (see Heat-stable enterotoxin)
'Stagnant loop' syndrome 290 (and see Bacterial overgrowth syndromes)
Staphylococcus aureus gastroenteritis 149, **150** *et seq.*
 clinical features 151
 deoxyribonuclease 152
 enterotoxins 151
 epidemiology 150
 food-handlers 279
 laboratory diagnosis 151
 leukemia and sepsis 313
 outbreaks 279
 pathogenesis 151
 prevention 152
 sepsis in gut surgery 308
Steatorrhoea **194** *et seq.*, 298
 contaminated small bowel in children 194
 micelle formation impaired 198
Stomach
 acidity 290
 bacteria 280, 292
Streptomycin-dependent (SmD) mutants of
 Shigella 262
 S. typhi 257
Strongyloides stercoralis 209, 219, **227** *et seq.*
Suckling mouse test (see Infant mouse test)
Summer diarrhoea and *E. coli* 80

Taenia saginata 234 *et seq.*
Taenia solium 234 *et seq.*
TCBS medium (thiosulphate-citrate-bile salts-sucrose) for
 non-cholera vibrios 113
 V. cholerae 109
Tetracycline for
 overgrowth syndromes 302
 prevention of gut sepsis 316, 320
 pseudomembranous colitis 334
Theliolymphocytes (see Gut associated lymphoid tissue)
Thiabendazole for nematodes 222
Tissue culture for diarrhoea viruses **177** *et seq.*
Traveller's diarrhoea
 antimicrobials 94, 254, 284
 enterotoxigenic *E. coli* 84
 precautions to prevent 282
 treatment 283
Trematodes 229 *et seq.*
 C. sinensis 230
 D. dendriticum 230
 E. ilocanum 230
 Fascaiola sp. 230
 Fasciolopsis 230
 G. hominis 230
 H. heterophyes 230
 M. yokogawi 230
 Opisthorcis 230
 S. intercalatum 230
 S. japonicum 232
 S. mansoni 229
Trichostrongylus species 220
Trichuris trichiura 209, 219, **223** *et seq.*
Trimethoprim—sulphamethoxazole to prevent infection in leukemia 325
Trophozoites of
 E. histolytica 213, 215
 G. lamblia 217
Tropical sprue **287** *et seq.*
 clinical features 298
 diagnosis 299
 enterobacteria 290
Tryptophan and colon cancer 356
Tuberculosis of gut 241, **247** *et seq.*
 clinical features 247
 control 248
 epidemiology 248
 laboratory diagnosis 247
 treatment 248
Typhoid fever 130 *et seq.*, 254
 ampicillin
 amoxycillin

anaemia 138
antimicrobial therapy **141** *et seq.*
blood culture 136
bradycardia 132
carriers 140, 144, 257
children 133
chloramphenicol 141
clinical features 132
clot culture 136
complications 137
cotrimoxazole 143
counterimmunoelectrophoresis 137
epidemiology 130
fever 132
gal E vaccine 257
gelatin string capsule test
haemagglutination test 140
haemolytic uraemic syndrome 138
haemorrhage 138
'hepatitis' 132, 138
incubation period 132
laboratory diagnosis 135
leukopenia 132
mecillinam 143
meningitis 138
myocarditis 139
pathogenesis 131
perforation 132, 137, 141
phage types 144
pivmecillinan 144
plasmids 141
prevention 145
relapse 142
rose-spots 133
schistosomiasis 133
sickle-cell trait 133
serology 136, 140
SmD vaccine 257
splenomegaly 132
strontium selenite broth 136
S. typhi resistant strains 130
trimethoprim 143
Ty 21a vaccine 257
urinary carriers 140
vaccines 145, **254**
vaccinated subjects and serology 136
Vi antibodies 140
Vi antigen 137
Tyrosine and colon cancer 357

Upper gut bacterial colonization
  296 *et seq.*
  children 193 *et seq.*

Vaccines for gut infections **253** *et seq.*
  E. coli 92

future possibilities 264
gal E of *S. typhi* 257
MH of *Shigella* 263
rotaviruses 169
Shigella 66, **261** *et seq.*
SmD 257, 262
S. typhi 145, **254** *et seq.*
V. cholerae 112, **258** *et seq.*
viruses 265
Vancomycin and PMC 332
'Vero' toxin in *E. coli* 82
Vibrio alginolyticus 103, 114
Vibrio cholerae 103, **105**, 268
adherence 107
agglutination 110
antibiotics 111
antitoxin assay 89
bacteriophages 105
carriers 15, 108, 110
choleragen 15, 106, 107
control 111
El Tor biotype 104, 105, 108, 271 (see
  also El Tor cholera)
epidemiology 108
environmental 110
Gm-1 ganglioside
haemagglutination 105, 106
haemolysin 106, 108
laboratory isolation 109
LPS 261
O-antigen 110
resistant strains 109, 111
serotypes, Inaba, Ogawa, Hikojima 105
toxins 89, 106
transport media 109
treatment 110
vaccine 109, 111
Vibrio fetus 55, 103
Vibrio parahaemolyticus 103, **114** *et seq.*
epidemiology 115
haemolysis 116
laboratory diagnosis 116
Kanagawa-test 115 *et seq.*
pathogenesis 115
salt-colistin broth 116
treatment 116
Vibriostatic compound 129
and *Aeromonas* 119
Viruses and diarrhoea **159** *et seq.* (see also
  Norwalk agent, Adenoviruses,
  Coronaviruses, Rotaviruses and
  Caliciviruses)
animal infections 161, 165
clinical features 160
detection of viruses 165, **175** *et seq.*
dose effect 161

electronmicroscopy 174
immunoelectron microscopy 175 *et seq.*
pathogenesis 160
recovery 165
R forms 175
S forms 175
tissue culture 177
treatment 162
villus cells 161, 162
water, in 272
Vitamin B$_{12}$ deficiency
absorption defect 194
Vitamin K synthesis 294
Viprynium for *Enterobius* 222

Water
bacterial contamination of 199, 200, 270
chlorine-resistant virus in, 272
coliform counts 272, **274**
developing countries **274** *et seq.*, 283
drinking 283
Entamoeba histolytica 274
Giardia lamblia 274
outbreaks of enteritis in USA 271
piping of 274, 276
purity standards 276
Salmonella in 199, 200
sea water 273
Schistosoma mansoni 274
Salmonella typhi, protection from 256
swimming water 273
viruses 272
Widal test in enteric fever 136–137

Wilson-Blair medium 54, 136
Winter vomiting and Norwalk agent 166

Xylose lysine deoxycholate medium 54
S. typhi 136

Yersinia enterocolitica **241** *et seq.* (and see *Yersinia* infections)
biochemical features 242
clinical features
epidemiology 242
isolation from the gut 282
laboratory diagnosis 245
milk 242, 277
serogroups 242
Yersinia frederiksenii 242
Yersinia infections 241 *et seq.*
clinical features 244
control 246
epidemiology 242
laboratory diagnosis 245
milk 241, 277
pathogenesis 243
treatment 246
Yersinia intermedia 242
Yersinia kristensenii 242
Yersinia pseudotuberculosis **241** *et seq.*
biochemical features 242
clinical features 244
serogroups 242
Y1 cells to detect toxins of
Aeromonas 118
E. coli 89
V. cholerae 108